Praise for
Denny and Susan Waxman

"Denny has been changing the world of conventional thinking regarding health for the past 40 years and has had the courage to stand tall against the powerful forces of industry and government . . . my kind of character!"

—Craig Borten, Academy Award nominee,
Best Original Screenplay, *Dallas Buyers Club*

"Our bodies are amazing machines that require an intricate balance for good health. Denny Waxman has deciphered this amazing riddle and knows how to bring us back to homeostasis through a combination of ancient and modern dietary applications. He is a gifted healer and I have had the pleasure of seeing him transform and heal many people—including myself."

—Stewart Raffill, Hollywood writer/director

"This book is a treasure! It is a great handbook, packed with information and instructions, that if followed, will result in the enhancement of one's Health of Mind, Body, and Spirit."

—Martha Clayton Cottrell, M.D.

"Denny Waxman's practice and teaching on macrobiotics carry in them the essence of Buddhist teachings on interbeing, happiness, and compassion. Through his message and conviction that personal health is the basis for planetary health, I see in him a truly engaged Buddhist."

—Anh-Huong Nguyen, meditation teacher and
author of *Walking Meditation*

"After graduating from the University of Chicago Medical School, I worked as a research physician for a large multinational pharmaceutical company. I was steeped in the scientific method and the value of clinical trials. I thought that for every disease, there must be a medication that could help the condition. However, after having the good fortune of marrying a woman who was macrobiotic and had studied with Denny Waxman for many years, I have come to appreciate the power that lifestyle and food have over one's health. I now realize that a macrobiotic diet offers the possibility for a deeper level of health than is available with the dietary recommendations of conventional medicine. I am grateful to Denny for his depth of knowledge and his great experience in applying macrobiotic principles to human health. His teachings have allowed me to enjoy a happier and more vigorous life."

—Jeffrey Dubb, M.D., Philadelphia

"Anyone who reads this book and follows Denny Waxman's advice will experience better health, greater happiness, and deeper insight into the meaning of life."

—Tom Monte, author of
The Complete Guide to Natural Healing

"Denny Waxman's system of teaching is flexible, unique, and refreshing. A really cool book."

—Jessica Porter, author of *The Hip Chick's Guide to Macrobiotics:
A Philosophy for Achieving a Radiant Mind and a Fabulous Body*

"*The Ultimate Guide to Eating for Longevity* could well be the most powerful and practical book you will ever own. It shows you *why* food choices have such power to improve your health, then shows you *how* to put that power to work in easy, sensible steps. I highly recommend it!"

—Neal D. Barnard, M.D., FACC, Adjunct Associate
Professor of Medicine, George Washington University
School of Medicine, and President, Physicians Committee
for Responsible Medicine

"Denny and Susan are surely two of the most qualified people in the world to guide Americans to greater levels of health and happiness and to extend that "great life" to great longevity. Delicious food, a philosophy of life based on gratitude and joy—there is nothing but goodness in this book. The incredible power of macrobiotics is one of the best kept secrets in the world. Here are the keys to discover its benefits in your life."

—Martin Halsey, founder and director of La Sana Gola,
Italy's largest natural foods cooking school;
www.lasanagola.com

"As a spiritual teacher I am profoundly grateful to Denny and Susan for making the necessary connection between us and the food we eat, the environments we live in, and all the expanding and contracting energies of the cosmos which sustain our lives and determine its quality. Their newest book, *The Ultimate Guide to Eating for Longevity*, is as much a healthful approach to living as a holistic spiritual practice."

—Rowena Mae MacGregor, M.Div., Episcopal priest
and macrobiotic health coach

"Mr. Denny Waxman was one of my early students and is outstanding in his knowledge and dedication to macrobiotics. I am proud to have him as one of my associates and regard him one of the leading educators and outstanding teachers of the macrobiotic lifestyle."

—Michio Kushi, leader of the international
macrobiotics community

The Ultimate Guide to Eating for Longevity

The macrobiotic way to live a long, healthy, and happy life

DENNY WAXMAN
and SUSAN WAXMAN

FOREWORD BY T. COLIN CAMPBELL

PEGASUS BOOKS
NEW YORK LONDON

THE ULTIMATE GUIDE TO EATING FOR LONGEVITY

Pegasus Books Ltd.
148 W. 37th Street, 13th Floor
New York, NY 10018

Copyright © 2019 by Denny Waxman and Susan Waxman

First Pegasus Books edition August 2019

Photography by Kateri Likoudis

Interior design by Maria Fernandez

Library of Congress Cataloging-in-Publication Data is available.

ISBN: 978-1-64313-068-2

10 9 8 7 6 5 4 3 2 1

Printed in the United States of America
Distributed by W. W. Norton & Company

This book is dedicated to all people past, present, and yet to come who share our dream of personal, social, and planetary health and abundance for all.

Disclaimer

The information contained in this book is intended solely to provide guidance and to increase the reader's awareness about the dietary and lifestyle practices that can create lasting health. If you suspect that you have a medical problem, we urge you to seek competent medical help and be aware that a second medical opinion is often the best course to achieve the best outcome for any particular condition.

Contents

Food Section

Recipes and Meal Plans

Testimonials

"No disease that can be treated by diet should be treated with any other means."

—Maimonides

"He who has health has hope, and he who has hope has everything."

—Arabic Proverb

FACTS AND LESSONS LEARNED FROM GUIDING DR. ANTHONY SATTILARO TO HEALTH FROM TERMINAL PROSTATE CANCER.

Dr. Anthony Sattilaro was the president of Methodist Hospital in Philadelphia. In May 1978, he was diagnosed with terminal prostate cancer that had spread to his whole body. In August 1979, the cancer was gone. After further medical tests in 1981, his doctors declared him to be in complete remission.

My first client, Mona Schwartz, was at my house when Dr. Sattilaro came for a consultation with me. He had found out about me by accident after picking up some hitchhikers who were cooks at my summer camp. When he left, Mona urged me to look after Dr. Sattilaro the same way that I had looked after her. I invited Dr. Sattilaro to eat at my house every day and guided him with food recommendations: more of this, less of that, focus here, etc. I helped him to develop the skill to make decisions that support health.

He attended lectures and seminars about macrobiotic eating and never missed a cooking class. The macrobiotic community in Philadelphia at the time also fully supported and encouraged him throughout the recovery process. I introduced him to Michio Kushi, who also became a part of his recovery.

Dr. Sattilaro documented his recovery at every step. His story was published first by the *Saturday Evening Post* and *Life* magazines and later in his book *Recalled by Life*, which became an international best seller. The articles are available to read on my website.

I learned many lessons about what it meant to me to be a counselor through guiding Dr. Sattilaro. I gained a deep confidence in my own ability to help people create lasting health, especially when I had the ability to guide them closely. Terminal illness means modern medicine does not have the understanding or the technology to help or reverse it. I have personally observed hundreds of people reverse terminal illness. My life's work has evolved into doing what medicine can't. Hippocrates, the father of Western medicine, recommended diet and lifestyle practices as the best medicine.

Macrobiotics is about the cultivation of spiritual, mental, and physical health. Even in sickness, the emphasis is still on the cultivation of health. As we increase health, sickness naturally diminishes in our life. "Recovery" in macrobiotics is a spiritual revolution in which we learn how to guide and create our own health and life.

Active participants in their own recovery always do better. They take the time to find out what to do and get involved with creating their own health. The journey toward health is an energizing adventure, and education is a very important part of the process.

Proper support is vital for any recovery; support is more than approval, it is a collaboration. Real support means "let's do this together" and moves us toward our goal of health.

In my experience, there are three common points that lead to recovery. The first is finding good guidance. The second is education through books and seminars. The third is putting together a good support team. People who make recovery their number one priority are the ones who recover.

The following testimonials are from some of my clients. People accomplished seemingly miraculous transformations after accurately and vigorously applying the principles in this book. Some people have chosen to combine these principles with traditional medical treatments while others have used them alone. In either case, please consult with your medical professional before making these dietary and lifestyle modifications. It is also important to find a medical professional who will support you in your healing journey. I am sure you will be inspired from these experiences. Our bodies have amazing healing abilities when we treat them with love, care, and respect.

"Each patient carries his own doctor inside him."
—Norman Cousins

THE STORY OF JOHN AND TOINI WILLIAMS, SENIOR MAINTENANCE REPAIR

Four days after our wedding, I was diagnosed with testicular cancer. In support of my desire to try a natural healing approach, my wife Toini got some books on macrobiotics. We discovered Denny Waxman through *Recalled by Life* by Dr. Anthony Sattilaro. We went to see Denny and began a journey that transformed our lives and how we view health.

I strictly followed Denny's dietary recommendations for two years. The tumor shrank, and the pain went away. I felt so good, I went off the diet and the cancer spread fast and suddenly. Cat scans and other tests revealed that I had stage 3 testicular seminoma. To my great fortune, two doctors on staff at Methodist Hospital in Philadelphia (where Dr. Sattilaro worked) were macrobiotic themselves and were a great encouragement to me as I underwent the chemo and radiation that was to follow. Once the chemo and radiation halted the cancer, I was told that any more chemo would kill me. After surgery, I decided to seriously return to the diet to heal. One huge side effect of all the treatment was that I would not be able to father children.

When we told Denny about it, he assured us that within two years of following his dietary and lifestyle recommendations, I could eliminate all the toxins and reverse the effect of the chemo and radiation. In just a little over two years' time, our first son was born on Christmas morning. Another son and two daughters were to follow, our youngest born to us when we were forty-four years old.

At a newborn-baby checkup with our third child, the doctor asked about my medical history. When I told him about my bout with stage 3 testicular cancer and the treatments, he looked confused. He thought I had undergone treatment AFTER my wife was pregnant, and when he found out he was amazed. He stated that men who go through the treatments for this cancer cannot father children.

Although healing from cancer and fathering children when I was told I wouldn't be able to are dramatic aspects to this story, the everyday benefits are what make up a life of transformation.

Denny's intuition and recommendations, even over the phone, are invaluable for health crises. It is uncanny how he can recommend a drink or dish that will eliminate physical problems. Our seventeen-year-old daughter recently said she feels confident she can deal with most everyday illnesses herself using her knowledge of the diet. I feel truly blessed to know Denny Waxman, and grateful that he dedicated his life to the study of macrobiotics and strengthening health.

THE STORY OF NANCY WOLFSON-MOCHE, NOURISHMENT EDUCATOR, COUNSELOR, AND BLOGGER

Prior to getting married, I sought help from Denny for a few different conditions that were completely resolved after following his recommendations. When I got married at forty-two, I began trying to conceive. After several months, and after learning I was not eligible for any high-tech fertility treatments due to my elevated FSH level, I went to see Denny. I worked closely with him, and over the course of a year my FSH dropped by 25 points. Soon after that, I became pregnant at age forty-four. Denny guided me through a healthy pregnancy and I worked closely with him during the first few years of my daughter's life. He was always responsive, open, and highly professional. Over the following five years we worked closely to tweak and fine-tune my diet and lifestyle. With Denny's guidance and support, I was able to have a second baby at the age of fifty-one.

Denny is a brilliant, generous, patient, and wise counselor, teacher, and thinker.

"The doctor of the future will no longer treat the human frame with drugs, but rather will cure and prevent disease with nutrition."

—Thomas Edison

THE STORY OF SIGRID GEERLINGS, SENIOR ASSOCIATE FOR NEW THEME, INC.

I think I might be the medical version of an X-File, which rather thrills me. I'm referring of course to the TV show about FBI cases concerning unexplained phenomena, filed away and forgotten. Similarly, my carcinomas' disappearance thanks to macrobiotics will not be included in any medical statistics or even written up in my personal medical file as such; it was deemed unexplainable by my surgeon. Yet the truth about the way the body can heal itself is out there.

About two years ago, I had really bad migraines. My husband had been macrobiotic twenty years earlier and told me to call Denny Waxman. When I called Denny to make an appointment I mentioned that my son, who was four at the time, had speech delay and a number of other vague global delay symptoms that were deemed either extremely serious or totally transient, depending on which professional gave what opinion. My son and I both went to see Denny, and in both our cases we were helped enormously by making just the basic changes. My son improved overnight!

Shortly after that, a mammogram and a needle biopsy showed that I had DCIS, or Ductal Carcinoma In Situ, which is a stage 0 cancer, with III grade cell necrosis. My medical treatment options ranged from a full mastectomy of both breasts, and medication for life—since I was "lucky" enough to have the right kind of cancer—to a lumpectomy with radiation. When I told one of my doctors that I wanted to try macrobiotics for six months, he allowed that for that period of time, my condition probably wouldn't become life-threatening, so I felt quite safe to delay and hopefully avoid medical intervention. The very next day, I received a call that they had looked at the biopsy slides again and found a suspicious-looking spot that might be interpreted as an inflammatory cancer. They urged me at least to get a lumpectomy right away. I thought they tried to scare me into going the medical route. At my most cynical, I thought they wanted me on board because I would make a pretty good candidate for their HER2 clinical study, being fairly young and healthy. Instead, I went back to Denny.

I took the Strengthening Health Intensive, which changed my whole being. From that weekend on, I cooked gorgeous and delicious food, took walks, rubbed my skin, tried to meditate, and received amazing Shiatsu massages.

About four months after I took the Strengthening Health Intensive, my breast started to hurt. Denny and I suspected that the metal marker left at the site of the biopsy was causing the pain. I needed surgery to have it removed. The tissue my surgeon took out was completely clear of DCIS.

Before the surgery, my surgeon said: "Hey, if it's gone, we'll say macrobiotics cured it." After the results came back, she said: "I can't say macrobiotics cured it. Maybe the needle biopsy removed it all, maybe it went away by itself." She Scullied me, and I'm sure the word "macrobiotics" never made it into my medical file; it's an unexplained disappearance of cancer. I believe . . .

THE STORY OF STEVE GITTELMAN, WOODWORKER, AND SUSAN HEINEMAN, FINANCIAL EDUCATION & T'AI CHI INSTRUCTOR

My partner Steve was diagnosed with Alzheimer's at age fifty-seven. After the diagnosis, he agreed to change his diet. We decided to explore the macrobiotic path and began counseling with Denny Waxman. Steve followed the recommendations and hoped the food would help him.

Denny Waxman's counseling during those years was crucial for both Steve and me. I credit Denny's guidance and the diet for bringing stability and a sense of confidence and well-being into Steve's life. Denny gave us purpose, direction, clarity, and hope.

As a result of working with Denny Waxman, the following changes took place for Steve:

- Chronic dandruff gone
- Lowered and normalized cholesterol
- Gradual, effortless 50-pound weight loss, balancing to his ideal 160
- Stabilized blood sugar levels
- Improvement in mood, attitude, clarity of thinking, freedom of movement, overall well-being

THE STORY OF JACK SCHULTZ, CEO/PRESIDENT JERSEY SHORE STEEL: GREEN STEEL MANUFACTURER

Five years ago, I underwent a total knee replacement. My wife, Carole, is very careful concerning her diet and she suggested that I exercise the same discipline concerning mine. Under the direction of Denny Waxman, and with the help of his wife, Susan, and Carole, a healing diet was recommended.

I remained in Philadelphia for six weeks, doing my exercises and watching my diet. After the initial six weeks, my surgeon and his staff were so pleased with my progress that they felt it was unnecessary for me to return to Philadelphia for the normal twelve-week post-op checkup. When I returned to Williamsport to continue my therapy, the therapist inquired where I had had the operation since she had never seen anyone recover as quickly as I had. I attribute my quick recovery, my loss of forty pounds, and the fact that I was able to get off the pain medication so quickly, to the discipline I followed concerning my diet.

Foreword

by T. Colin Campbell

I am honored to be invited to write a foreword to Denny and Susan Waxman's book on macrobiotics for health, longevity, and lifestyle. Denny has followed and taught this macrobiotic lifestyle since the 1970s and now has produced this second edition of his groundbreaking book.

The macrobiotic lifestyle was brought to this country from Japan by Michio and Aveline Kushi after World War II. The Kushi's, who were students of George Ohsawa, followed a dietary lifestyle with origins in the Zen tradition.

In 1999, Michio Kushi invited me to present a lecture at the Smithsonian Institution's National Museum of American History in Washington, D.C., when his contribution and many of his papers were enshrined in a collection honoring his work. Kushi, with his wife Aveline, had been for many years vigorously promoting this dietary lifestyle in lectures throughout the world. I was awed and inspired by Kushi's motivation to embrace macrobiotics after his profound experience living at ground zero in the aftermath of the detonation of the Nagasaki atomic bomb. This intense experience, Kushi said, made him determined to dedicate his life to the promotion of food as a means to create a more peaceful world, and a life of health, peace, and longevity for all members of the human race. Denny Waxman, as a student and disciple of Kushi, embraced this same commitment to counsel and teach macrobiotics as a lifestyle and to heal ailments of the human body.

My personal interest in diet and health began in the 1950s at Cornell University, and was derived from my own experimental research significantly funded by the National Cancer Institute of the National Institutes of Health (NIH). My findings led me to develop, in the 1980s, a similar dietary lifestyle approach based upon whole plant food—like macrobiotics, similarly focused on the broad health improvement value of a diet composed of vegetables, whole grains, and fruits. I was then invited to present to the Kushi Institute in Becket, Massachusetts, and reciprocated by inviting Michio Kushi to present to my class on plant-based nutrition at Cornell University. Since then, I lectured to the Kushi program in Amsterdam, Holland, and for the last seven years to the Holistic Holiday at Sea cruise in the Caribbean. As chair of a national committee on public nutrition information established by my professional research society, the American Institute of Nutrition, I learned of the efficacy of the macrobiotic diet from an unpublished collection of data assembled by Kushi health practitioners showing a rather remarkable benefit of this diet on cancer patients. Unfortunately, this information was never published, thus was mostly ignored by the traditional cancer research community. Ironic, in light of the clear historical record of ancient and developed cultures embracing natural foods as medicine and the healing potentialities of organic whole plant-based foods.

Now, thankfully, Denny Waxman, who is also the founder of the Strengthening Health Institute (SHI), is carrying on this incredible nutritional and lifestyle legacy by publishing this book with his wife Susan, who serves as the codirector of SHI. After many years of promoting, teaching, and documenting the health benefits that may be achieved, Denny and Susan have updated and incorporated new material in this magnificent book and the best material from their previous best seller, *The Complete Macrobiotic Diet*. In my opinion, Denny and Susan now carry the torches of Ohsawa and Kushi into the new millennium as the leaders of the macrobiotic movement.

I highly recommend this book both for its practical usefulness, historical significance, and reference by future generations, and for its continuing contribution to the science, lifestyle, and benefits of the macrobiotic movement.

The Waxmans' new book deserves a high place on the book shelves of all who work in this amazing field of plant-based nutrition and those who choose to live or seek a healthy lifestyle and whose goal is to strengthen their health.

—T. Colin Campbell, PhD,
Jacob Gould Schurman Professor Emeritus of
Nutritional Biochemistry at Cornell University,
coauthor of the best-selling books
The China Diet (2005) and *Whole* (2013)

Introduction

"Just because you're not sick doesn't mean you're healthy."
—Author Unknown

In 1992, I was sitting on the beach in Portugal. Watching the waves come in and back out. My mind was occupied. Over the years, I've observed thousands of people practice macrobiotics—some with great success and some with none at all. I sat there trying to pinpoint what the difference was between a successful practice and a failed one. I thought about the clients who felt macrobiotics was too much, too restrictive, or too difficult. Those phrases repeated in my mind. I gazed at the water moving back and forth.

I started thinking about my past and my own journey into macrobiotics. It all started when I found a book by George Ohsawa on my bed. I am not really sure how it ended it up there, but I read the book cover to cover. The book opened up a new path and direction for me. The next day, I went out and bought brown rice, sea salt, and mu tea (Eastern herbal drink). I rushed home to cook my first meal. The taste was interesting—not good, not bad—but I felt wonderful and inspired. And so it was the start of my first ten-day rice fast as described by Ohsawa in his book.

The second day went the same as the first. The rice was—not good, not bad. I felt great. However, on that third day of my new regimen the cravings kicked in. I found myself in the supermarket, buying a half-gallon of Breyers Vanilla Fudge ice cream, a box of graham crackers, and a quart of orange juice. By the time I reached the checkout counter, I'd eaten almost everything in the cart. I was completely lost, confused, and disappointed. I knew in my heart that macrobiotics was the way of life that I had been looking for but I didn't know how to stick to it. I realized I needed help.

As luck would have it, while having lunch at a health food store, I spotted a man with a very intense look. For some reason, I thought he might be macrobiotic and I was right. That was the day I met Stanley. As it turned out, Stanley was opening a macrobiotic restaurant. We became partners and leased space in an underground mall called Sansom Village. A few days after we signed the lease, we found out the space was not zoned for a restaurant. So instead we opened Essene Market & Café, a food market with a lunch counter.

In my partnership with Stanley, he introduced me to Rod and Peggy. We became friends and they gave me the macrobiotic diet guidelines. They suggested I eat vegetables with my brown rice. It became the advice I needed. I found myself satisfied, more energized, and the food delicious. I couldn't believe the difference.

And even more amazing, I saw the same changes in the people coming to our store. I noticed regulars who returned every day to eat at our lunch counter looked better. Their skin was more vibrant, their eyes brighter, and their appearance quickly changed. All from just that one meal several days a week.

Splash! I came back to reality. The water moved back and forth from the beach. I sat there and it dawned on me. If one meal is that powerful then any change in your diet makes an impact. Macrobiotics needs to be more flexible and open. Teaching macrobiotics by constantly talking about what you should not do only leads to people craving their bad habits. If you have an idea in mind that health is restricting and all-or-nothing then you feel the pressure to be perfect. Perfection is not possible. The demand of perfection makes you feel hopeless and give up. Instead, it should be about adding healthy habits and meals. Lifestyle changes are hard. It is important to have flexibility and understand that changing your habits and practices happens gradually.

It has been more than twenty years since being at the beach in Portugal. But the discovery that day changed the way I have seen and taught macrobiotics. It has improved my ability to work with clients and led to me the discovery of the Strengthening Health Approach to Macrobiotics or SHI Macrobiotics as it is now known. I saw students more likely to stay with it as soon as I made it clear it was okay to start with one healthy practice and build from there. For clients, it took the pressure off of giving up everything and changing everything at once. Instead, clients would find one meal to have such dramatic results—that when they were ready, they would come back to me asking for the next step. This SHI macrobiotics method continues to grow and evolve as people and society change.

WHAT THIS BOOK IS ABOUT

The concept of health is in vogue and getting more people interested in health again. However, current ideas about health lack clear direction, consensus, or guidelines about how to achieve it. If you wish to be healthy, there is still the struggle to understand the inconsistent information about diet, lifestyle, and exercise. Leaving you feeling negative, depressed, and lost. This problem became my inspiration. In this handbook are practical guidelines based on practices and patterns observed from the world's long-standing civilizations that still exist untouched by modern diseases. And recommendations from my experience as a macrobiotic counselor, as I have adapted these guidelines to modern life. I hope to share that health is within your reach when you build easy yet powerful practices into your life and have the knowledge of what creates lasting health.

For this handbook, I wanted to identify the biggest health challenges and address each of them. These are the three major problems:

1) The Struggle to Cut Through the Confusion and Contradictory Advice

Modern diets have created confusion about health and food, and have spread misinformation about plant-based diets and macrobiotic life-style. That is why I wanted to dedicate the first part of this handbook to resolving food myths. The food myth section wil give you a strong understanding of food and nutrition, so you no longer have to second guess yourself and eating choices.

2) How to Start and Learn What to Do

Modern diets focus on short-term goals which lead to an all-or-nothing way of thinking. You have to cut all bad habits at once—if not you have failed. I have found that this process of restricting only leads to negativity and eventually giving up. Instead, the approach in this handbook is to build healthy habits in 7 steps at your own pace.

3) Find Food to Prepare, Take Home, Enjoy It

To help you start cooking at home, our last section has meal plans by Susan, an expert in macrobiotic cooking. She also provides you with handy tips, food lists, and recipes.

Keep in mind while reading this handbook that these guidelines are based in common sense and have certainly passed the ultimate test of time.

WHY HABITS AND PRACTICES FROM LONG-STANDING CIVILIZATIONS?

Japan has one of the highest degrees of health and life expectancy in the world.

What it really comes down to is traditional foods and simple practices that Japan continues to follow. Japan consumes three kinds of foods for longevity: a wide variety of unique fermented foods, sea vegetables, and soy products. These foods together with their lifestyle practices of making time for their meals, eating on small plates, and eating together make all the difference.

Keep in mind, Japanese Americans tend to have high rate of chronic disease but people who eat traditional Japanese food are the ones who live the healthiest and longest.

The same goes for Mediterranean civilization. People who eat a traditional mediterranean diet of grains and beans (rice, beans, lentils), vegetables, nuts, and fruits show low chronic disease. And again the Mediterranean life is focused on spending time together and taking time for meals.

All of this shows that modern diets are clearly missing foods, habits, and practices that create longevity.

HEALTH IS A CHOICE AND IS ACCESSIBLE TO ALL

"Happiness depends upon ourselves."

—Aristotle

We have the ability and capacity to create either sickness or health in our own lives. This is the first thing I learned from my first macrobiotic book that stopped me in my tracks and convinced me to pursue this way life. This thought that we have the capacity create our own health and happiness still echos in my mind after more than fifty years.

What if I shared with you the reality that it is in fact you, whatever your circumstance—that health is within your reach because health comes from within?

There is no thing that is going to make you healthy. It is a step-by-step reorientation and reeducation that connects you back to yourself and the entire world that you are a part of. As long as you believe that some (perhaps magical) thing is going to make you healthy, you are most likely moving in the wrong direction. We have the ability to grow our health throughout our life. At the same time, health is a journey. Each step in a healthy direction has value, no matter how small. It may even have a value that you can not even imagine. This approach is open and can grow endlessly at your own pace, if you use the principle of adding before taking away.

On the other hand, stopping harmful foods and lifestyle practices does provide benefits in the short term. But for the most part, they do not contribute to lasting health. Stopping things that we have built habits of to support ourselves can leave us feeling unsupported, unfulfilled, and even defeated if we end up going back to them. In other words, a negative can not lead to lasting health. Only a positive can do that.

ADDING VS TAKING AWAY

"The journey of a thousand miles begins with a single step."

—Lao Tzu

Everyone seems to be increasingly busier these days, but it is always possible to improve our health—if we know which steps to take. This handbook has been designed to clarify those steps. As you add these practices and understanding, you will see the transformation occur and experience the benefits. This will inspire you to invigorate your practice and keep creating more health around you.

The goal is to change the percentage of unhealthy to healthy in your diet and lifestyle practices. The more you increase healthy things, you automatically decrease unhealthy. This needs to be the guiding principle for short- and long-term health. Taking away leads to restriction, dissatisfaction, and eventually rebellion. It can also lead to nutritional deficiencies because restrictions do not nourish or encourage our appetite for making healthy choices. Overall, we do not learn anything positive or gain from restriction.

The premise for much of these recommendations comes from the experience and understanding that anything you can do is better than nothing and that small, incremental steps over time provide the longest lasting benefit. If you add one new thing each week, you will be surprised at how your life can transform from one year to the next. If it is one new thing each week, you will have experienced fifty-two health-supporting practices over the course of the year. How many of those will become a habit or practice for you in your everyday life?

Health craves health. One healthy thing automatically leads to another. Healthy foods encourage healthy activity. And healthy activity in turn encourages healthy foods. Adding opens up our appetite and curiosity and healthy lifestyle practices. It also automatically provides more balanced and complete nutrition. The bright side is, there is no limit to adding: it is a lifelong process of discovering foods, cooking styles, cuisines, and meals.

The goal is not perfection, but to have a sufficient amount of health-supporting practices to continue in your journey toward health. It Is Not What You Don't Do—It Is What You Do Do.

Incorporate as many things as you can comfortably without feeling stressed. If you start to feel overwhelmed, scale down, or back off a little bit. (The journey of 1,000 miles must begin with a single step.) Zero to one is everything. One to one hundred is easy.

Remember, the body is a self-healing organism that has evolved and adapted over millions of years. Anyone can take steps through their diet and lifestyle to improve their health. This cannot be reiterated enough. It is in what you do, not what you don't that creates lasting health. How we regain or achieve health, and by extension, our own happiness, well-being, and peace is in our own power.

HEALTH IS A MOUNTAIN STREAM

Anything that aids good nutrition, good digestion, and good circulation helps our health.

Health is like a mountain spring, the right amount of water moving at a natural speed. Water in a natural mountain stream constantly cleans, renews, and renourishes itself. If the source is pure, great. But even if the source is not pure, if it has the right kind of activity, it is still sparkling. It can purify and renew itself. If water becomes deficient it slows down. It starts to putrefy if there isn't enough water or power for active movement. If there is too much force behind it or if there is too much water, it becomes destructive.

Our bodies are the same. If we can have a comfortable amount of nourishing foods and proper movement our body can constantly renew itself like a healthy mountain stream. The source doesn't need to be pure for a mountain stream to be healthy, and our nourishment doesn't need to be perfect. We do need to have the ability to digest and circulate. Food is the source of nourishment and energy. Activity is the pump, the circulator for our bodies.

Good macrobiotic practice means good digestion, from beginning to end of the process; good circulation; and good nourishment, both quality and quantity. Good health is the sum total of our nourishment, activity, and circulation.

From my observation, practicing strengthening health macrobiotics can help improve practically any health condition you can imagine, from diabetes to heart disease to high blood pressure to cancer. Proper activity and circulation along with nourishment contribute to lasting health.

HEALTH IS AN ADVENTURE

> "The purpose of life, after all, is to live it, to taste experience to the utmost, to reach out eagerly and without fear for newer and richer experience."
>
> —Eleanor Roosevelt

Remember health is an adventure. Everything changes; we are never standing still. Each day, we are either moving toward health or sickness. Modern life currently moves us toward sickness. This is why so many people are convinced that sickness is natural, or at the very least, inevitable.

What we forget is that in many communities around the world people live long and full lives because they share many diet and lifestyle practices in common. We see a pattern of human life where people lead active, productive lives, enjoy the greatest longevity on the planet, and die not from sickness, but when they have had enough of life. The commonalities with these communities are not only a grain, bean, and vegetable-based diet but also an orderly and active lifestyle.

This handbook identifies and shares the common and adaptable habits and lifestyles from the wisdom of these communities, and how it can be applied to common lifestyles in modern life. The guidelines have been adapted and customized to confront challenging aspects of healthy, mindful living in modern society. I wanted these recommendations to be achievable even by those with a busy lifestyle, who may find it hard to incorporate healthy dietary or lifestyle practices into their routines.

On a daily basis, we can find adventure, excitement, and self discovery. Over time, we can identify and appreciate our own uniqueness and our connection to all of life.

EMOTIONS AND OUR HEALTH

> "Health and cheerfulness naturally beget each other."
>
> —Joseph Addison

Emotions are inseparable from our health. There are natural and healthy emotions, like a mountain stream in equilibrium. We associate streams with tranquility, curiosity, joy. This is our natural emotional state. Our natural emotions, when consistent, encourage a healthy flow in our body and mind together. In an unnatural state, there is disruption. I am saying that emotions are not positive or negative, but that the state of our emotions is either natural and healthy, or disrupted. In disrupted, unhealthy states, our liquid is either stagnant or surging. Stagnancy, or lack of movement, can be expressed as desensitization, depression, or numbness. And surges, which seem like "boiling over," can be expressed as anger, aggression, or hysteria.

Emotions specifically depend on liquids. Without liquid, we would have no emotion. We can express this culturally in a series of questions: When are we more emotional? When do we visit bodies of water, and for what reasons? How does our language express the observation of emotions in others? What kinds of liquids do we use, and for purposes of expressing which emotions? These are all interesting questions to ask; I'll follow up with some answers, as quickly as I can.

People tend to be more emotional during the full moon. People will contemplate beside a lake, follow the path of a stream to explore, bring a loved one or a friend to the bank of a river to watch it flow, or to intake the power of the ocean. When we talk about emotions, we can refer to an overly sentimental person as sappy or wishy-washy, and at the other extreme barren or dry. It is interesting that we drink beer at sporting events, wine for intimate evenings, tea or water to relax, calm down, or meditate. The character of each of these liquids brings about different emotional states.

Water itself permeates every aspect of life, and the human body and the planet itself is composed mostly of water. Water is associated with the unconscious and is included in all types of ritual, whether something as simple as a celebration at a sporting event or a spiritual ceremony. There are ponds and lakes—places where water gathers. And there are streams, rivers, and oceans, which are places where water moves. This brings me back to the vision, or image, of health and the mountain stream's emotional complement: healthy flow.

Emotions also depend upon temperature. Emotion expresses itself when liquid comes to the surface of the body and evaporates. This partially explains how people living in or visiting hotter climates express emotions more readily than in colder climates where we may need to be "warmed up" first. The use of fire in cooking raises our temperature. Outdoor cooking, such as barbecue, brings out a lot of emotion. Using spices, stimulants, and alcohol also raises our temperature. The opposite, cold, interferes with our ability to express emotions smoothly. Cold affects our bodies through ice, out-of-climate foods, and chemicals (especially artificial sweeteners). Extremes of both hot and cold have disruptive effects on our emotions and in turn, our physical and mental health.

It follows then that the state of our emotional health has the capacity to affect the course of our overall health, either in a more natural and healthy flow or into a more disrupted and unhealthy flow. Because health craves health, a flowing and joyous emotional state helps us flow with healthy habits. This season is a perfect time while in the company of family or friends to return to our natural state of tranquility, curiosity, and joy.

HOW TO USE THIS HANDBOOK

"Twenty years from now you will be more disappointed by the things that you didn't do than by the ones you did do."
—Mark Twain

We have designed this handbook for you to start where you feel most comfortable. There are tips and information on diet, lifestyle practices, and eating habits. If you are not ready to change your diet, you can still create healthy change through your eating habits and/or lifestyle practices. The key is to go at your own pace and add more when you are ready. Even one step forward makes a difference and builds over time. We want you to feel encouraged by your progress with each step rather than feel disappointed or like a failure for not doing everything or as much as you wanted to. Any effort benefits your health. For example: making it a priority to sit down and eat with no distractions during lunch improves your metabolism, energizes you, and stimulates awareness of when you are full. Eating more slowly makes you more conscious about what you are eating and aids digestion and appreciation of food.

In-Depth Look at Your Health, Food, and Emotions: Introduction to Food Myths (p. 29)
Eating Habits: Steps 1–3 (p. 53)
Lifestyle Practices: Steps 4–7 (p. 119)
Diet: Food Section (p. 181)

Remember, how you eat and lifestyle practices are just as important as what you eat.

Connecting with the
Spirit of Health

"We are one and inseparable from Nature and the environment."
—a rough translation of *Shindo Fuji*,
which George Ohsawa used to formulate the
macrobiotic philosophy and lifestyle

GIVING THANKS FOR OUR FOOD

"The noblest question in the world is What Good may I do in it?"
—Benjamin Franklin

The orderly cycles of Nature guide this book and my macrobiotic practice. Through aligning with these orderly cycles, we reconnect with all aspects of Nature. For life on this planet, we observe this orderliness through days, seasons, years, and growth cycles. Food is our connection to Nature. When eating plants directly from Nature, we create a direct connection, which fosters a care and love of self and planet. When we eat plants that have already been processed by animals, we create an indirect connection. All food has three types of nourishment: physical, energetic, and spiritual.

Physical nourishment is the basic constituent of food, the raw material that we digest and process. Physical nourishment gives us energy and becomes our blood, tissues, and organs. The principal categories of physical nourishment are minerals, proteins, carbohydrates, fats, vitamins, and enzymes.

Energetic nourishment is the nourishment we derive from the food as a result of its life cycle—from growth to our plates. For plants, energetic nourishment begins with the quality of both the seed and the soil within which they grow. The process continues and includes the harvest, how the plants grow, how we process, store, distribute, and finally prepare them for consumption. Energetic nourishment is the food quality.

Modern agriculture has lost touch with the common sense of our ancestral agriculture. We have a worldwide history of small, local farms producing nourishing food on a community basis. There is a clear connection between healthy soil, healthy plants, and healthy people. How can we expect to have healthy people without healthy food?

Spiritual nourishment is the nourishment derived from the health and intention of the person or people preparing the food. Our care and love transforms the physical and energetic properties of the food into the most nourishing food. This type of food gives us the most satisfaction and inspires in us a profound sense of gratitude. Everyone knows how wonderful holiday meals are and the way they can stand out in our memory.

Food is our life. Without food, there is no life. When we start with food that is naturally grown and processed and prepared with care and love, we have something that is unfortunately rare in today's society. Food prepared with care and love, even without using the highest quality ingredients, is still satisfying and nourishing. Most people will agree that the spiritual aspect of nourishment is the most satisfying, followed by the energetic. The energetic aspect is enhanced when the food grows naturally and originates close to where we live. Food from your garden always tastes the best.

> "When eating fruit, remember who planted the tree; when drinking water, remember who dug the well."
> —Vietnamese Proverb

Giving thanks before and after a meal literally wakes up the goodness in the food. We become aware by appreciating and acknowledging the entire process of our food. We give thanks for the whole network that connects us to that food, which in turn allows us to be nourished and satisfied at a much deeper level. Our gratitude for food opens us to health, to life, and all of its possibilities.

HEALTH CRAVES HEALTH

"Preserve and treat your food as you would your body, remembering that in time food will be your body."
—B. W. Richardson

Everything is interconnected, interrelated, and interdependent. After we make the decision to be healthy, we need to consider all aspects of our life, including our daily habits, activities, environment, and relationships.

Health is our natural state and inheritance as humans and creatures of this planet. Health is physical, emotional, mental, and spiritual. Your body is always trying to maintain and move toward health. It really comes down to the basics of learning about and experiencing good food, healthy eating habits, natural activity, and having or cultivating a good attitude. As we continue with these practices and habits, we build stronger and stronger confidence in our innate ability to regain and maintain our health.

We know this because if we develop a serious health problem, it takes far less time to return to health than it did to become sick in the first place. It often takes many years to spoil our health, yet most people could turn their health around in six months to a year. If we allow it, our body is always trying to maintain or return to health. Most people think that being healthy seems to require a lot of discipline. The focus is on taking away rather than adding.

My experience is the opposite. Adding is more important than taking away. Giving things up does not lead to lasting health. When I started to add healthful foods to my diet, I realized that I had started to crave more foods that supported my health all of the time. It became apparent that it wasn't only food. My desires started to extend to other areas of life. At the same time, I started to lose interest in things and even people that weren't supportive of my health and life. I believe this pattern is common for everyone. The opposite is also true. Once we start to eat unhealthful foods, we surround ourselves with more destructive food, habits, and tendencies. This is why fast foods and junk foods have been able to take over so strongly.

Health is simple. I find it interesting that many people think that health is not attainable for two main reasons.

One, people think that becoming healthy requires too much effort.

The second main reason is they think that genetic and/or environmental factors undermine our daily efforts. It is easy to assume that sickness is inevitable no matter what we do. It has recently been discovered that there are factors that have more influence than genetics alone. Epigenetics offers scientific support that daily choices are responsible for the activation and expression of genes that regulate the disease process, including cancer genes. Diet and lifestyle factors have the ability to turn gene markers on or off. In my experience, daily things, not special things, create health. Good food, natural activity, and a healthy attitude are the most important factors to create lasting health.

Lasting health is our ability to grow and nourish our health on all levels throughout our life. There is no limit to our vitality, memory, sense of joy, or appreciation of life. The keynote of spiritual health is gratitude and appreciation, which leads to mental and emotional health, which in turn produces physical health. It does not work in the opposite direction. At base, health is a spiritual condition, secondly mental and emotional, and lastly physical. Health is a spiritual condition, that is a sort of reawakening.

Gratitude and appreciation open us to life and all of its possibilities. Even if we are not raised with a deep sense of appreciation and gratitude, we still have the ability to achieve this spiritual quality. Life's challenges offer us the opportunity to develop this appreciation. Often enough, people with a deep sense of appreciation have the greatest ability to overcome life's challenges.

As the world changes, we must learn to adapt to faster paces, greater demands, and what seems like less time to smell the roses. It becomes important to learn about what leads to lasting health and how to incorporate healthy diet and lifestyle habits at your own pace.

As busy as we may be, we all have to eat. Within our individual framework, we can learn to make the healthiest choices possible, given our options, circumstances, and goals. There is an endless ability to be creative and flexible when moving in the direction of health.

Health craves health. We start with good eating habits. Then we add healthful foods and cooking styles into our way of eating. We further the process with natural activities and try to create a healthy home environment. These things work together to move us in the direction of health. This process becomes self-sustaining: that is, it does not require discipline.

> "What we are doing to the forests of the world is but a mirror reflection of what we are doing to ourselves and to one another."
>
> —Mahatma Gandhi

Personal health and planetary health are the same. Healthy people want to live in a healthy home environment, and the desire extends to a healthy natural environment. As we take better care of our own health, all of our choices begin to support our community and environment. As we become more calm, more peaceful, and more positive, we begin to spread these things around us. When we eat naturally grown and processed foods, we don't spoil the environment. When we eat grains and beans directly, as opposed to feeding them to animals, we make enough food available for everyone. We are also, in turn, naturally much kinder to animals. We also no longer need to clear-cut forests to raise animals. The desire to seek health is an open-ended cycle.

Health is contagious. Healthy people naturally want community-supported agriculture organizations (CSAs), farmers' markets, and other practices that promote a healthier environment; it is not a matter of discipline, but desire. The proliferation of CSAs, farmers' markets, seed exchanges, and artisanal food products reflects the growing number of people who are experiencing the life-changing effects of craving health.

One Thing Leads to Another—Health Is an Open-Ended Process
Going for a walk stimulates your appetite for healthy foods. Having plants in your home cleans the air. Choosing products that don't outgas

electrical or air pollution can lead to finding products that you enjoy having. Healthy foods stimulate your desire for healthy activity.

LASTING HEALTH, A SPIRITUAL QUALITY

Illness surrounds us; heart disease, cancer, dementia, and diabetes have reached epidemic levels. From this, it is natural to assume that we are likely to die from at least one degenerative illness. However, there are cultures and communities around the world whose older members are just as vital and bright as those much younger. Take Okinawa, where they have the highest life expectancy. Their diet and lifestyle practices produce more centenarians than anywhere else in the world. Many people there have been able to delay, or even avoid, the "diseases of aging."

"The belly rules the mind."

—Spanish Proverb

George Ohsawa, the founding father of modern-day macrobiotics, created a unique definition of health. Michio Kushi further refined, adapted, and developed his definition. They divided health into three main areas: physical, mental/emotional, and spiritual health. Conditions of physical health are a strong physical and mental vitality, a good appetite for healthy food, and deep and refreshing sleep. You can achieve five points for each condition. Ideal physical health amounts to fifteen points. Mental/emotional conditions of health include good memory, being calm and patient, and being joyous and alert. Mental/emotional conditions of health receive ten points and amount to thirty in total. The condition of spiritual health is the endless appreciation for all of life, and the spiritual total is fifty-five points. You need this condition to be a healthy person, as it accounts for more than half of all the points. This definition is unique because it shows that we have the ability to grow and create our health throughout our life. This point system allows us to check our health on a regular basis, but it is most important on a seasonal or yearly basis.

Macrobiotics is a lifestyle through which we can grow spiritually and also develop our mental, emotional, and physical health, which allows us to lead the most exciting and fulfilling life. Lasting health is our ability to grow and nourish our health on all levels throughout our life. There is no limit to our vitality, memory, sense of joy, or appreciation of life.

Gratitude and appreciation open us to life and all of its possibilities. Even if we are not raised with a deep sense of appreciation and gratitude, we still have the ability to achieve this spiritual quality. Life's challenges offer us the opportunity to develop this appreciation. It is my long observation that people with a deep appreciation have the greatest ability to overcome life's challenges. Many of my clients have attributed their recovery to their sense of appreciation of life.

INDIGENOUS AND LOCAL FOODS

Indigenous Food: The Soil Principle

Indigenous foods are foods that are native to a growing region; they have evolved and adapted over long periods of time to particular, unique climates and ecosystems. Food grows in perfect balance with local conditions, in accordance with soil and water quality, temperature, humidity, patterns of sunlight, etc. To eat indigenous food is to eat foods that have adapted to the locality. Where a food was originally cultivated in relation to our own regions matters far more than whether or not the food is local.

When we eat food that is native or climatically similar to our own region, it is easier to digest, absorb its nutrition, and eliminate excess. Indigenous foods align us to our locality so we can connect more easily to what we eat and the natural conditions where we live. When we eat foods that are native to our climatic region, the food harmonizes our metabolism to that region. The pace of life is more active in the temperate climatic regions than in the tropics and subtropics.

When we eat food from the tropics and subtropics in a temperate zone, the food regulates our metabolism to the tropics and we disconnect from the natural pace of our own environment. From my experience, many foods from subtropical and tropical climates introduced to a temperate-climatic diet cause the blood to become more acidic than any other plant-based foods.

We lose minerals and other nutrients trying to neutralize the acidity. When we have acidic conditions, we become more susceptible to infectious, inflammatory, and degenerative illnesses. When our blood is more acidic, the hemoglobin loses its ability to bind with and transport oxygen throughout our body. Our ability to absorb nutrients also becomes compromised. Two types of foods that evolved in the tropics and subtropics are the thick-skinned tropical fruits and the nightshades.

I find it very interesting that five tropical foods have become so deeply ingrained in our diet, even though they all negatively affect our health: potatoes, tomatoes, sugar, bananas, and, more recently, coconuts. Out of these, cooked or sundried tomatoes that are ripe, are the least harmful and actually have beneficial qualities for people who have consumed a lot of animal foods in the past. They are all tropical and highly acidifying to our blood. We know that nightshades have a strongly acidifying effect. Those with arthritis are usually affected by eating these foods. The perception of these foods as healthful in a temperate region does not consider the role that local and indigenous foods play with our health.

From my observation, people with a healthy metabolism never have to think about their weight. Many of my clients who come for a variety of health problems naturally lose weight as they improve their health in other areas. When the body begins to function naturally again, it actively releases toxins and other forms of excess. Could it be that all these tropical foods are interfering with our ability to eliminate excess, as well as exacerbating the obesity epidemic?

An indigenous food can be considered indigenous along a line of latitude, not longitude. Which means we can choose foods east and west of where we live around the world. For example, cherry blossoms are enjoyed in both Washington, D.C., and Kyoto, Japan. For those in the temperate climatic regions, there is not as much flexibility in choosing foods north and south as the climate changes dramatically. It is best to choose foods within the temperate zones rather than the subtropics or tropics.

The problem, though, is not the banana or the coconut, it is the proportions of consumption of tropical fruits and nightshades in relation to the indigenous foods we eat. It is best to use these foods with care and discretion. If you are unsure about which foods are indigenous to temperate climatic zones, you can consult the food list in the back of this book.

Since food is our direct connection to the entire network of life, indigenous and local foods in combination are the foods that are most healthful for us, as they are best adapted to where we live.

Local Food: The Water Principle

The local food movement gains momentum day to day, week to week, farmers' market to farmers' market, season to season. Getting our food and exchanging with local growers increases our awareness of the life cycles of our food. It also gives us the opportunity to experience the changing seasons and connect with what grows in our area. We look forward to the first strawberry of mid-spring and for the first peach of the summer. We somehow understand that foods grown locally make more sense for the overall planet and ourselves, but apart from reducing our dependence on fossil fuels, local foods also help us to align with the rhythms of Nature.

Food becomes unique to a locality. The food grown in a specific area experiences the changes and patterns according to the conditions and quality of the weather, the water, the soil, and many other factors. Food local to our area has essentially had a similar experience to ours, except that food metabolizes the environment directly. We can feel this connection through our experience with spring fever. In plants, energy rises, sap begins to run, buds form, and we become excited to be out and experience the warmth and witness Nature coming back to life. When we eat local foods, we connect to the experience of the season and can receive better nourishment. Food absorbs minerals directly from the soil, and local foods allow us to absorb these minerals more efficiently.

Water is the most important thing to have locally, as it quickly loses its freshness. Since we use so much water for cooking and drinking, the quality of water is important. We recommend a water purification system such as Berkey (there may be other brands) over bottled water, reverse osmosis, or distilled water. Berkey removes contaminants, pathogens, fluoride, and arsenic. We have found this the most natural tasting water compared to natural spring water at the source.

Water from a spring does not taste the same, once we take it home, as it does while at the spring! Most leafy vegetables have a high water content; the higher the water content in a vegetable, the more important it becomes for the vegetable to be from a local source. Vegetables with high water content lose their nutritive value and freshness faster than vegetables that can be stored for a longer period of time. However, vegetables grown locally on good soil also store water better than others. If we get the vegetables locally, we maximize the nutritional benefit from the growth and harvest process as well as take in the available water in the plant.

The most important source of water is in food. We use water in food more efficiently than by just drinking alone. If we contrast this with the modern diet, we can see that almost all of the foods in the modern diet are dry foods, such as meat, poultry, cheese, eggs, and baked goods. These foods create an imbalance of thirst. People have perpetual thirst, but don't seem satisfied, whereas eating food that has a high moisture content satisfies our need for liquids more deeply.

All cooked grains, beans, pastas, vegetables, and soups have high water content. The taste of these foods becomes sweeter and more thirst-quenching as we chew them. These healthful foods allow us to become more satisfied with drinks and beverages that we choose to enjoy. The water in food refreshes us, and we cherish foods that are considered refreshing (e.g., lettuce, cucumbers, and of course watermelon). Refreshing is a vital nutrient.

Locality is less important to consider for vegetables that can be stored. Storing vegetables (cabbages, onions, carrots, sweet potatoes, hard fruits, etc.) used to carry people through barren winters. Harder vegetables have more adaptability, that is, they can store in a variety of environments without rapidly decaying. Fruits that can be stored, such as apples and pears, become more nutritious and better tasting during cold storage as the flavors and nutrients settle down and concentrate.

Grains, beans, dried vegetables, and seaweeds store for much longer than other foods. Therefore, these foods can come from farther away, even anywhere in the country, or from the same hemisphere. Foods from opposite sides of the equator have an opposite magnetic charge and should be avoided. These foods interfere with our body's functions as well as our connection to our locality. Finally, we cook our food using local, filtered water, which completes the cycle.

You can start to make a more local transition by using water content as the guide. Visit farmers' markets first to get leafy vegetables and local, seasonal fruits, and follow this with more substantial vegetables. Enjoy your way through the seasons as they change.

> "Here is your country. Cherish these natural wonders, cherish the natural resources, cherish the history and the romance as a sacred heritage, for your children and your children's children. Do not let selfish men or greedy interests skin your country of its beauty, its riches or its romance."
>
> —Theodore Roosevelt

As we start to choose more indigenous and local foods, we start to make a deeper and more satisfying connection to where we live. This enhances our ability to make healthful choices for our own lives. We start to create a balance through indigenous and local foods that also helps us to become more deeply satisfied from the foods we do eat. This balance continues to perpetuate itself. The reality is that the most healthful food is the most enjoyable food.

Acid & Alkaline
and Overeating

ACID AND ALKALINE

I found it necessary to reinterpret acid and alkaline to make it more effective and easier to understand. I am not a scientist, but this interpretation is based on my understanding of macrobiotics. This understanding has passed the test of time, as I've used it with clients over the years to create healthy alkaline conditions. People have said that grains and beans are acidifying, but that has not been my experience. I think you'll find when grains and beans are cooked in water with a little sea salt or kombu, and digested properly, they create alkaline conditions. If this wasn't so, macrobiotics would not have such a large number of recoveries from serious illnesses, which is what it is so well known for. My observation throughout the years is that macrobiotic children have been stronger and healthier than their peers not raised in this way. Healthy digestion, which starts with thorough chewing, is essential for creating a mildly alkaline condition.

When digested properly, complex carbohydrates, such as grains and beans, and temperate land and sea vegetables create a mildly alkaline condition in the blood. On the other hand, simple sugars, refined carbohydrates, and alcohol quickly become absorbed into the bloodstream, creating an acidic condition. Animal and dairy foods, tropical fruits, and nightshades also acidify the blood. We lose minerals, especially calcium, to neutralize the acidity. This loss of minerals weakens not only our bones, but our muscles, organs, and nervous system. It also weakens our digestive and thinking abilities.

For food to become alkalized, three important things must happen. First, we need to sit down to eat without doing other things. Second, food must be chewed well. Third, complex carbohydrates must slowly break down in the digestive process, alkalize in the duodenum, and finally be absorbed in the small intestine. A combination of complex carbohydrates creates the most healthy alkaline condition. In essence, the importance is to differentiate between good quality and poor quality carbohydrates, because the complex carbohydrates are the ones that break down slowly and pass through the duodenum.

Create alkalinity with food by eating a variety of complex carbohydrates that are digested slowly, and are absorbed in the small intestine. In life, anything that promotes good digestion and circulation promotes alkalinity: chewing our food, laughter, a nice walk outside, a great conversation, green plants, natural materials and activity, etc. Alkaline conditions allow hemoglobin to bind with more oxygen and transport it through our body. Indicators of an alkaline condition include a sense of inner peace and joy, having a positive attitude, feeling strong and energetic, good muscle tone, healthy skin, and youthful appearance.

Acidic conditions are caused by stagnation. Overeating is one of the most common causes of stagnation and acidity in our body. Contrast the freshness of a walk outside with one in a shopping mall or sitting in front of a computer all day. Common symptoms of acidity are fatigue, negativity, irritability, weak bones and muscles, and a weak resistance to illness.

You can get a pretty decent indicator of your overall condition by observing how you wake up and feel every day.

OVEREATING

Overeating is one of the most harmful and common habits that many people experience today. Eating while standing or doing other things sets the stage. The most common practices that break our connection with food are reading, watching TV, or listening to engaging radio broadcasts while trying to eat. These practices interfere with our digestion and feelings of satisfaction. Another cause for overeating is having a diet that is too simple and repetitive, whereby we try to get satisfaction by eating more and more food. Eating unhealthful foods causes a biological frustration and imbalance that causes us to overeat. One unhealthful food makes you crave another.

My analogy is this: if you have a comfortable number of people in a room, people tend to be thoughtful and accommodating to everyone else. However, if you double the number of people in the room, beyond the capacity of the room, the same caring people often become irritable and negative instead. The same goes for the food we eat. Once we eat beyond our capacity, we start to bring out the negative aspects of the food.

There is a physical limitation as to how much our digestive system can process and eliminate. Overeating can cause food to putrefy in our digestive system and create the buildup of toxins. This also produces a more acidic condition, as the food cannot move naturally and efficiently through our digestive system.

Another analogy is the mountain stream. As long as the stream can move and flow naturally, it continually cleans and purifies itself. However, if a boulder falls and breaks the natural movement of the stream, stagnation builds up around the boulder. Overeating creates stagnation which interferes with the natural movement of the digestive system. Overeating healthful food is harmful enough, and overeating unhealthful foods brings out the worst aspects of the worst foods.

Almost everyone overeats these days, and it may be difficult for you to tell if you are overeating. A good rule of thumb that they use in Okinawa is to "only eat to 80 percent capacity." If you're not sure what that feels like, try reducing the overall volume of food by 5 to 10 percent at each meal. Then try it again until you get down to a comfortable amount. Once you get used to this, you'll feel more energetic and clear-headed.

Food Myths

"Americans love to hear good things about their bad habits."

—T. Colin Campbell

The most pervasive myth is that healthier eating is based on restriction and giving up things that we may feel are very important for our well-being—emotional or otherwise. You achieve health by avoiding animal foods, avoiding soy, avoiding dairy foods, avoiding sugar, avoiding coffee, avoiding carbohydrates, avoiding gluten, avoiding this, avoiding that, avoid perhaps pretty much anything enjoyable. Stranger still, what is replacing all of this taking away?

The idea of restriction and avoiding things is so absolutely pervasive and detrimental that it is hard to escape. There is no model in nature or in life where restriction leads to flexibility, openness, healthy old age, or long-lasting health. We can however consistently be making decisions and actions that support our own health. And as it turns out, we have the ability to reconnect to a natural sense of health.

Restrictions and taking away can lead to imbalances and deficiencies, whereas adding healthy foods cannot. One thing that is common is that science and medicine constantly change their nutritional recommendations to the opposite. The end result is often: Are carbohydrates, proteins, fats, etc. beneficial or not?

UNDERSTANDING NUTRITION

When we began breaking food down into nutrients, we began to lose touch with food itself. Food has to replace nutrition. Activity has to replace exercise. Trying to move toward health has to replace simply avoiding sickness. This book is not against sickness; it is for health. Creating conditions for health naturally diminishes the prevalence of sickness. It is that simple.

The reality is we never really need to think about nutrients. If we eat a variety of plant-based foods according to some orderly guidelines throughout the year, we receive abundant nourishment in all areas.

Our body has the ability to choose what it needs when it needs it, in the exact quantities. This leads to complete and balanced nutrition. Here is a useful analogy: if you like to cook, then you keep a well-stocked pantry and refrigerator. Then when you decide on your meal, you pick whatever you need in the right amounts to create that meal.

When you eat a variety of plant-based foods from different categories, our bodies do exactly the same. What we eat today enters our blood plasma by tomorrow. Plasma is the liquid portion of our blood that carries nutrients and transports waste to be eliminated. It makes up about 55 percent of our blood, and renews itself every ten days. So choosing a variety of plant-based foods over a ten-day period creates the best quality blood. Essentially then, the more variety you include in your diet over a one- to two-week period, the more you will benefit.

With the modern approach in nutritional theory, each nutrient needs another nutrient to be utilized properly. It is impossible to calculate the amounts we need and the types of individual nutrients we need. When using this approach, we may even develop imbalances and deficiencies. The key to good nourishment, from a purely nutritional perspective, is to take the steps to create good eating habits that support digestion, and learn the orderly planning of meals.

We break food down from solid to liquid and then into energy. Food nourishes us on many levels: physically, emotionally, mentally, and even spiritually. It is much more helpful to use the perspective: "How can I nourish and satisfy myself in these different areas?" In this way, we can relearn how to nourish ourselves in the best possible way, guided by our body's intuition.

Essentially, we need a different approach to nutrition, or at the very least to move away from the belief that good nutrition is based on ingredients. Protein is probably the one nutrient of greatest concern and importance for most people. It is interesting to observe that our thinking has been clouded by superstition, by the myth that animal and dairy proteins are superior nutrients. The fact of the matter is that plant-based proteins provide the highest quality protein that does not tend to move us toward degenerative illness.

Whereas animal foods are combinations of second-hand nutrients and toxins from the animal eating plants, dairy foods for human consumption are third-hand nutrients and provide even more toxins from the animal. Each form of dairy is unique to a species, and is the perfect transitional food until the young are able to take plant-based foods. Therefore, these proteins tend to be highly acidifying and over time, contribute heavily to degenerative illness. The one nutrient that may need to be supplemented in those with plant-based diets is the micronutrient B-12.

The main source of B-12 worldwide is dirt, and is especially concentrated in manure, where it is a by-product of digestive fermentation. When food used to be produced by small farms with animals, the transformed manure returned to the soil. In turn, B-12 is found in the crevices of vegetables growing in the soil. We do not need much B-12 in our diet, so in many cases, eating completely organically grown vegetables provides us abundantly with B-12. B-12 deficiency is extremely rare in people following these guidelines. Some people are also more comfortable taking a B-12 supplement. The only sure way to know if you are getting adequate B-12 is with a blood test.

SOURCE OF ALL MAJOR NUTRIENTS

Dairy and Calcium

As far as calcium is concerned, another superstition is that the best calcium comes from dairy. The more animal and dairy foods in the diet, the greater the risks for developing osteoporosis. Excess animal and dairy foods tend to create acidifying conditions that tend to leach calcium from our bones, muscles, and nervous system. The most absorbable and usable calcium is in leafy greens, vegetables, and beans. Seeds and nuts (especially sesame seeds) further aid in building and maintaining strong bones, muscles, and nervous system. Greens and beans have been in human diets for many thousands of years. Traditional people largely did not have osteoporosis; it is a truly modern disease.

The Good and The Bad: Carbs

All of the world's long-standing civilizations were grain based. In addition, all people identify with, and are inseparable from their traditional grains. Common examples include rice in Asia, bread in Europe, corn in the Americas. This idea that grains were the most important food on the planet has been around for thousands of years, up until 1956 when the United States Department of Agriculture created "The Basic Four."

The Basic Four—meat and animal proteins, milk and dairy, vegetable and fruits, and starches—conquered the world. Cereal grains dramatically shifted from a place of honor and respect to almost taboo. To make matters worse, cereal grains became confused with breakfast cereals composed mostly of refined grains and added sugars. The traditional un-yeasted sourdough breads made from organic stone ground flours gave way to refined and enriched baked flour products. Both unrefined and refined grains became grouped together as "carbs" and were thought to be simply "fillers" or calories devoid of nutrients.

Contrary to popular belief, protein is not our principal nutrient. Glucose is our main nutrient and nourishes every cell in the body. Healthy glucose comes from grains, beans, and starchy vegetables, which are complex carbohydrates (or polysaccharides). These complex carbohydrates slowly break down into glucose, a monosaccharide. The fiber in these foods guides them through the entire digestive process, allowing them to be absorbed in the intestines in a healthy way.

On the other hand, simple sugars and refined carbohydrates are absorbed directly into the blood without going through the entire digestive process. This immediate absorption creates an acidic condition in the blood, whereby we lose minerals (especially calcium) and vitamins in attempts to neutralize the acidity.

We recommend reintroducing healthy, complex carbohydrates in the form of grains, whole grain products, beans, and starchy vegetables, as opposed to trying to avoid refined or processed grain products. Some examples of healthy carbohydrates are brown rice, barley, millet, oatmeal, bulgur, polenta, durum wheat semolina pasta, and un-yeasted sourdough bread. When we begin to incorporate whole grains, we naturally begin to develop a taste for beans and starchy vegetables.

Complex carbohydrates are the most satisfying and filling foods. They also provide the strongest energy, vitality, and flexibility for physical and mental activities. More and more professional athletes are discovering the power and importance of these foods.

Oil

Oil has a long tradition in cooking; both olive and sesame oil have been in use for thousands of years. Both olive and sesame oil can be pressed naturally without added heat or solvents. Even though oil is not a whole food, it has the ability to transform our foods. The use of oil in food preparation has recently come under question because it is not a whole food and is very calorie-dense. Because it has been in use for thousands of years, it leads me to think that the proper use of high-quality oil has important value.

Oil provides different benefits. Oil changes the taste and satisfaction of the food as well as the physical, mental, and emotional energy of the food. It can also create a heating or cooling effect, and increases our ability to absorb minerals and fat-soluble vitamins (A, D, E, and K) at the deepest levels of our organs, bones, and nervous system. If you use oil at the beginning of cooking, it has a more deeply nourishing and energizing effect and provides warmth. Whereas if you add oil at the end of cooking, there is a more dispersing effect, which tends to be more relaxing and cooling. When oil is used properly, it enhances the taste and texture of the food and does not taste oily because the oil has been integrated into the dish.

Try to find the highest quality, mechanically-pressed and unrefined sesame and olive oils for use as your primary oils. You can tell much about the quality by the taste and smell—similar to water. Think about the water in different cities, or at different times of the year. Sesame oil is drier than other types of oil; it has a lighter, more refined quality and encourages the intellect and practicality. Olive oil is richer and more moisturizing, and nourishes the emotions more. Imagine the differences in Japanese and Italian cuisine. You may want to experiment on your own, trying periods with or without oil in your food preparation. Always mind the quality and quantity of the oil.

Oil should never burn. When using oil at the beginning of cooking, slowly and gently add water before the first sign of sizzling to disperse and cool the oil. Do not wait until the oil is too hot or sizzles loudly. This method allows us to use less oil and combines the oil with the food more thoroughly. You may also add oil near the end after steaming or boiling to add a light, refreshing effect to a dish. These suggestions and insights have come from my experience with how we use oil at home, at seminars, and in my counseling practice.

Protein

One of the common misconceptions about vegan diets is that they are deficient in protein due to the lack of animal and dairy foods. However, all foods in their natural state contain protein; it is nearly impossible to have a protein deficiency. Eating a variety of grains, beans, vegetables, fruits, and naturally pickled and fermented foods provides the most complete and high-quality protein available.

The research of T. Colin Campbell brings to light epigenetics, and how our food choices regulate how our genes express themselves. It seems the combination of animal and dairy foods moves us closer to the potential to develop cancer. His research demonstrates that consuming casein (dairy protein) has a stronger potential to cause cancer than red meat. At first, I was surprised about these findings, but upon thinking, it makes perfect sense.

When we eat a whole-foods, plant-based diet, we are getting protein directly from nature. On the other hand, when we eat meat, we receive second-hand protein as well as the toxic waste produced by the animal through processing the protein. When we eat dairy foods, we receive third-hand protein, as the food went through another stage of processing in the animal. What we are told about the source of superior protein is actually much more inferior. Not only that, but the commercial conditions in which most animals are raised increases the amount of toxicity we receive from these animal products.

What we eat today enters our blood plasma by tomorrow. Plasma is the liquid portion of our blood that carries nutrients and transports waste to be eliminated. It makes up about 55 percent of our blood, and renews itself every ten days. So choosing a variety of plant-based foods over a ten-day period creates the best quality blood.

My long-term observation has been that people naturally lose their taste for animal and dairy foods once they base their diet on grains, beans, and vegetables. I find it interesting that most macrobiotic children are in the top 50 percent of their class for height and weight. They are generally raised on what is considered a low-protein diet. Macrobiotic children raised eating a variety of healthy foods are never thinking about individual nutrients. Food is a source of physical, emotional, mental, and spiritual nourishment.

Many of these children often have little taste for many protein-rich foods other than tofu and broccoli. Shifting our thinking away from food as a set of composite nutrients is one of the keys for adopting a healthy and satisfying way of eating. Nature provides for us abundantly, and choosing plant-based foods that nourish us directly gives us the additional satisfaction of feeling a deeper connection with nature.

Soy and Miso

Throughout its history Japan consumed little animal food, and almost no dairy. Breast and prostate cancer rates are very low. Could it be that the use of traditional soy products made that possible?

What Is Healthy Soy?

Soy has been called both a superfood and a danger to the thyroid, hormone, and nervous systems; it has been suggested that it may cause cancer. It is no wonder eating healthy feels impossible. What you need to know is that the quality of soy matters. To get the all these benefits from soy, buy organic, non-GMO. Instead of soy isolates used to make fake meat and dairy products, use a variety of traditional soy products including miso, shoyu, tofu, tempeh, natto, and soy milk. Soy isolates, like textured vegetable protein (TVP or TSP) are harmful due to the high level of processing. TVP is not a natural process. Soy meat substitutes such as

Tofurkey should be avoided. They are not tofu. Reserve soy chicken and hotdogs for special occasions.

What is Miso?

Miso is a unique food. It is a fermented soybean paste often made with brown rice or barley. It can be used as a seasoning in various types of sauces, spreads, soups, and for pickling other foods such as vegetables, tofu, or fish. Certain preparations of miso provide the most benefit. In macrobiotics, we recommend using barley or brown rice miso that has been aged two to three years. Miso soup can be enjoyed often or daily, and even two to three times a week will start to improve your health.

Health Benefits

A recent article reported that miso may prevent a number of modern illnesses. It provides protection from radiation and other environmental toxins and can be eaten for digestive and cardiovascular health.

A great way to get the amazing benefits of miso is to make it into a soup with wakame seaweed and vegetables. The benefit of properly prepared miso soup is that it immediately strengthens digestive health, blood quality, and circulation. Miso helps clean the intestinal villi and creates healthy bacteria and enzymes in the digestive tract. Enjoying miso soup regularly strengthens our digestion and alkalizes our overall condition.

SALT, SUN, AND STRESS

It is so strange and unfortunate that three things absolutely essential for life have become villains in our society: the sun, salt, and stress. There is hardly any rationale or evidence that these nefarious claims are true. They only become a problem when they become too much.

Salt

Today's diets blame salt for chronic diseases, high blood pressure, and hypertension. They claim a major decrease in salt will cure these problems. However, salt is an essential nutrient that every living creature needs in order to survive. What we have discovered in macrobiotics is that not all salt is bad and too little salt is just as harmful as too much. Instead, salt should be evaluated on what type of salt is used—refined salt or unrefined white sea salt—and when salt is added to food. This will determine if the salt will be harmful or beneficial to the body.

What Is Refined Salt?
Refined salt or table salt is sodium chloride that has been stripped of all minerals and elements. It is brined in sulfuric acid or chlorine, added with anticaking chemicals, and bleached. This means refined salt has extra additives and harsh chemicals that are not natural. If the salt is unnatural then the body cannot use it to perform vital functions.

On top of it, refined salt is heavily added to processed foods. The overprocessed foods and refined salt increase toxins and acidity in the body. That acidity decreases your health by weakening the immune system, making you vulnerable to health issues such as high blood pressure and hypertension. That is why it is important to not get rid of all salt but decrease intake of refined salt by eating less processed foods.

What Is Unrefined Sea Salt?
Unlike refined salt, unrefined white sea salt is a whole product that can be utilized by the body. Sea salt is evaporated from sea water and washed. It is never exposed to harsh chemicals, therefore the natural minerals and elements stay intact. Unrefined sea salt is also stable and balanced. That balance from the sea salt is transferred to our bodies and helps our blood to have an alkaline condition instead of acidic. This improves our immune system and healing ability. A high-quality unrefined sea salt tastes sweet before tasting salty.

Cooking with Sea Salt
Not only does the quality of salt matter, but incorporating unrefined sea salt during cooking is essential. Adding the salt while cooking allows the sea salt to blend and bring out the natural flavors without increasing your blood pressure. Never add salt after cooking or while eating. The strongest application of salt is the catalyst for most natural fermentation processes.

Benefits of Sea Salt

The benefits of sea salt include balance of blood fluids, prevention of low blood pressure, prevention of dehydration, ability to transmit nerve impulses, allowing nutrients and oxygen to travel to their destinations, keeping bones strong, and improving the immune system. Salt brings out and preserves the nutrients in food; it is essential for the absorption and utilization of carbohydrates. The properties of salt help us to create and maintain an alkaline condition, which strengthens immunity and aids in healing ability. Salt is also the basis of physical and mental resistance and memory. The way salt is used is very important. Salt helps us be active and strengthens our determination.

SUN

There is no mistake that we get vitamin D from the sun. All of life depends on the sun, and sunlight is an essential ingredient for an overall healthy life. It is important to overcome our fear of the sun and the many myths surrounding sun exposure as an enemy to health. It's very clear that the sun is our friend and absolutely essential for good health: physically, mentally, emotionally, and spiritually. The sun cleans and renews our energy. It promotes good health and prevents cancer. The sun also releases stagnation and toxification physically, emotionally, and mentally.

To get the most benefit sit up, stand, or take a walk outside in the sun. A vertical position (active, standing, or sitting upright) activates our metabolism and allows us to use the energy of the sun in the most healthy and beneficial way. When we are in a horizontal position, as in sunbathing, we deactivate our metabolism. Falling asleep in the sun feels similar to having an overly rich meal. Too much sunbathing is like eating too much rich food. It can also weaken immunity, causing the skin to dry out and age prematurely. Unhealthy skin and overexposure to the sun may result in the development of skin cancer. The sun is good until we become very slightly red. This is the sign that it is time to cover up or take cover.

STRESS

The great historian Arnold Toynbee interpreted history in terms of challenge and response. The development of civilizations is possible by their responses to neighboring people and the environment. It is stress. If the challenge is either too great or insufficient, a civilization is not able to develop. A lack of stress means we develop in a spoiled environment, and if the stress is too great, it can be crushing or stifling.

All three, salt, sun, and stress are great additions to our lives if we keep them balanced.

A MACROBIOTIC PERSPECTIVE ON GLUTEN ALLERGIES AND SENSITIVITY

Grains are currently under attack as a cause of many modern Western illnesses. The two most widely consumed grains in the world are rice and wheat. Attacks on rice are for arsenic contamination and phytic acid's role in mineral absorption. Attacks on wheat are for its gluten content and for being over-hybridized. This is not a scientific explanation about gluten sensitivity and allergies, as others have adequately explained gluten issues from a scientific perspective. Instead, I offer a macrobiotic perspective of the value and importance of these grains for our enjoyment and health. This is based on my understanding of diet and health and my experience with my students and clients over time. I have helped many people overcome their gluten sensitivities completely.

The common grains containing gluten are wheat, barley, and rye. These grains are among the most ancient grains, and wheat in particular has been cultivated as early as 16,000 B.C.E. in Egypt. All long-standing civilizations and their cuisines developed and evolved using grains as a primary source of nourishment. For more information about what a grain actually is, I provide an overview in Step 3.

Whole grains provide the ideal balance between minerals, proteins, and carbohydrates, making them the most complete source of nutrition of any food. Gluten is a combination of two proteins and is found in the endosperm (or starchy part) of certain cereal grains, and gives dough its texture. Grains essentially have encapsulated within them the entire life cycle from seed to fruit, so they are the vital food that provides and maintains the foundation of our nutrition.

There are three parts to the problem with the modern treatment of grains. First, it is true that many modern grains have become over-hybridized, sacrificing quality for yield. Second, modern milling practices (which use steel hammers and develop excessive heat) as opposed to the gentle quality of slow-grinding stone mills disturb the quality of the grain. Third, refining and enriching the grain disturbs the nutritional balance. This works like shattering a mirror and merely pasting it together and expecting it to look and function the same as before. Although enriched and refined grains have the same amount of nutrients as a whole grain, they are nutrients out of their original context and do not act the way the nutrients do in whole grains. It is likely that the combination of modern grain and our overall weakened health caused by imbalanced diet and lifestyle are the causes of gluten sensitivity, which is more like an allergic reaction. It's also important to differentiate between gluten allergy/sensitivity and celiac disease. These guidelines are not for people with celiac disease who should avoid gluten completely.

The science of epigenetics demonstrates that diet and lifestyle regulate the way genes express themselves, which means that autoimmune diseases may reverse themselves over time with healthy diet and lifestyle practices. Many people have reported recovery from degenerative illnesses through dietary and lifestyle changes. A healthy person has the capacity to enjoy nature and life at their fullest, which includes the complete enjoyment of the foods eaten for thousands of years by the world's long-standing civilizations. Food and environmental allergies have become rampant in our society. Allergies are results and indicators of imbalances, and are related to a weakened blood, lymph, and digestive quality, caused mostly by an overly rich or nutritionally imbalanced diet. Gluten sensitivity is an allergy of the digestive system. The base cause of digestive issues is the overconsumption of animal foods, especially red meat, poultry, eggs, cheese, and other dairy foods. Our digestive system is not designed primarily to digest and process animal foods efficiently.

Dairy foods confuse our immune system, and sugar paralyzes its ability to react appropriately. The immune system filters our blood and neutralizes acidity. Excessive consumption of dairy foods and poor quality fats clog and stagnate our immune system. They interfere with its ability to filter blood. In essence, the function of the immune system is to gather, localize, and neutralize toxins. The immune system does not fight—it harmonizes and balances. The highly expansive nature of simple sugars (such as white sugar and fructose) incapacitates our immune system's ability to gather and localize toxins when consumed above a certain level. Only the liver can metabolize fructose, whereas all of the cells in our body metabolize glucose. The combination of dairy foods and fructose especially affects the liver, the spleen, the pancreas, and the immune system in general. In Eastern medicine, the liver and gallbladder are nourished and balanced specifically from the grains containing gluten. In a diet too highly saturated with dairy foods and fructose (especially high fructose corn syrup and agave nectar), our liver and immune system functions are compromised and may react inappropriately to these grains.

Two things cause allergic symptoms: the cause of the problem and what relieves the problem. In other words, symptoms cannot tell us directly whether a problem is getting better or worse. My experience also shows that people produce symptoms when they are recovering their health, which makes the healing process seem scary to many. We've associated symptoms with illness itself, which is not the case.

There is a huge difference between boiled grains such as brown rice or bulgur wheat and baked or toasted grain products. Baked, toasted, fried, yeasted, refined, and enriched grains (such as doughnuts, cookies, pastries, and commercial breakfast cereals, to name a few) seem to cause the worst reactions. From my experience, many people who are gluten sensitive are not affected by wheat or barley cooked or boiled together with brown rice. If people react to wheat or barley cooked with brown rice, it is a sign that they may have a more serious issue that requires more time to recover from.

Our body is meant to run on complex carbohydrates, especially those found in whole grains, beans, vegetables, seaweeds, and other unrefined, plant-based foods. These foods go through the entire digestive process and are eventually absorbed by the small intestine. Simple carbohydrates (such as enriched and refined grain) become absorbed directly into the blood before they go through the duodenum where they would otherwise naturally go through an alkalizing process. Baking or toasting these refined grains using dry heat can convert complex carbohydrates into trisaccharides which also causes them to be absorbed by the blood more quickly and may spike the blood sugar.

Baking and toasting are important cooking methods and I am in no way suggesting that we stop enjoying them. However, their overuse with many refined foods and added sugars contributes to the imbalances in our health. Boiling grain aids in our ability to efficiently digest and absorb its nutrition.

For those with gluten sensitivity, there are methods to try to reintroduce grain. First, avoid the foods with gluten that you know cause you to experience a reaction. Then, slowly and systematically reintroduce barley, farro, or wheat cooked with brown rice. Then, one by one, reintroduce other boiled, unrefined grains. If they cause a reaction, wait at least ten days and then try again. Then when you're ready, try to introduce soup seasoned with naturally fermented miso. If you have difficulty or continue to experience reactions, you may want to consult with an experienced macrobiotic counselor.

There is a lot of confusion about soy products as well. My experience is that the traditional soy products, which include miso, natural soy sauce, tofu, and tempeh are all protective against estrogen-related illness. It's been found in China and Japan that traditional soy products are protective against breast cancer. In addition, these traditional soy products have a rich array of nutrition and are helpful in practicing a healthy vegan diet.

I hope you will not be dissuaded from eating foods that have been enjoyed by people for thousands of years that provide wonderful health benefits, taste delicious, and even give us emotional satisfaction and fulfillment.

THE
7 STEPS

SHI Macrobiotics proposes an orderly approach to eating and living. It is based on creating healthful eating habits, a balanced diet, and beneficial lifestyle practices. With this in mind, let's get started on the 7 Steps.

"Health, without which there is no happiness."

—Thomas Jefferson

EATING HABITS: FORMAT OF MEALS

1. Take time for your meals every day.
   - Sit down to eat your meals or snacks without reading, watching TV, or working.
   - Allow adequate time for your meals.
   - Eat slowly and chew well.
   - Stop eating three hours before bedtime.
   - Eat in an orderly manner.
   - Avoid mixing foods in the same mouthful.

2. Set your daily schedule.
   - Rise early and go to sleep before midnight.
   - Keep your mealtimes regular.

DIET: CONTENT AND QUALITY OF MEALS

3. Eat two or three complete and nutritionally balanced meals every day.
   - Plan every meal around cooked grains and grain products.
   - Complete and balance every meal with one or two vegetable dishes.
   - Have a serving of soup with one of your meals.
   - Buy the highest quality organically grown, unrefined, naturally processed, and non-GMO foods.

LIFESTYLE: APPROACH TO HEALTH

4. Make your daily life active.
   - Walk outside for at least thirty minutes every day.
   - Give yourself a daily body rub.
   - Life-related exercise provides the most benefit for lasting health.
   - Cultivate and take time for hobbies.

5. Create a more natural environment.
   - Surround yourself with green plants, especially in the bedroom, the kitchen, the bathrooms, and office or workspace.
   - Wear pure cotton clothing next to your skin.
   - Use natural materials such as wood, cotton, silk, and wool in your home.

6. Make your macrobiotic practice work.
   - Keeping to the format of meals improves your ability to make healthful food choices.
   - Keep a daily record of your meals to help you become more objective about your practice.

7. Cultivate the spirit of health.
   - Be open, curious, and endlessly appreciative of all of life.
   - Be flexible and adaptable in your practice.
   - Develop a strong will and the determination to create your own health.
   - Be accurate in your practice.
   - Create a good support network.
   - Learn to cook well.

"Ill-health, of body or of mind, is defeat. Health alone is victory. Let all men, if they can manage it, contrive to be healthy."

—Thomas Carlyle

THE ORIGIN OF THE 7 STEPS

Where do the 7 Steps come from? In other words, what is the model on which they are based? The answer is simple. They are based on my observation of Nature. If we observe Nature closely over time, two clear patterns emerge. The first is that Nature is orderly and consistent. As a result, its cycles are 100 percent predictable. For example, we know that the sun will rise and set every day. We know the exact time at which this will happen. We know the exact position the sun will occupy in the sky at any given moment. We can predict where it will be at any time in the future. We can project backward with the same certainty. The sun never takes a break, never takes a day off. If the sun fails to rise, either there is no more sun or our planet is out of orbit. Either way, our worries will be over! We also know that every month, without exception, the moon will move from new to full and back again, as surely as we know that every year, spring will follow winter and summer will follow spring. However, we can never be certain what any individual season, month, week, day, or hour will be like. Sometimes May is atypically rainy and cold while June can be as hot as August. From this observation we can conclude that Nature is orderly and consistent while at the same time it is endlessly variable and inconsistent. These are Nature's two patterns. Simple, yet it seems that in the practice of macrobiotics the two most difficult concepts to understand are those of balance and variety.

SHI MACROBIOTICS

SHI Macrobiotics is the next evolution of macrobiotic practice, and we have adopted and modernized it to make it more accessible and effective for people. There is much more emphasis on adding foods and lifestyle practices, going at your own pace, and using a wide variety of traditional cooking styles. This makes it a more relaxing and familiar approach to a healthy lifestyle.

> "Common sense and nature will do a lot to make the pilgrimage of life not too difficult."
>
> —W. Somerset Maugham

BALANCE

If, as I am proposing, our sense of balance comes directly from Nature, then the easiest way to achieve balance is to align with Nature's orderly cycles. To choose to align with endless variety, inconsistency, and change is obviously to choose failure. But we can easily align with the very orderly aspects of Nature—its cycles of sunrise, sunset, and seasons.

VARIETY

Let's take a look at the principle of variety as it applies to macrobiotics. In macrobiotics we believe that everything has its complementary opposite, some other aspect that completes it or brings it to wholeness or to oneness: day—night, man—woman, heat—cold, happiness—sadness, health—sickness, etc. This is true for Nature as well. Its orderly cycles are complemented and completed by its cycles of endless variety, change, and inconsistency. These are Nature's two aspects, or you might say Nature's front and back. The point is that the way we can best align with Nature's variety is through Nature's orderly cycles. This is key to our understanding.

APPETITE

With this in mind, I'd like to pose another basic question. Where does our appetite come from? What determines what our appetite is on any given day, month, or year? Many years ago, when there were a number of macrobiotic study houses in Philadelphia and the community was very closely knit, on any given day you could be sure that almost exactly the same meal was being served in all the different locations—dish for dish, sometimes ingredient for ingredient. Why? We could, I suppose, blame it on gossip. The macrobiotic grapevine is amazingly efficient! However, these different study houses were not sharing menu plans. There is a principle at work behind the similarity, and it is that the nature of each day calls for certain types of food, certain dishes. And so the people who were more aligned with Nature were all drawn to the same foods. In other words, their appetites were aligned with Nature and therefore with each other, so that when they planned their meals they chose nearly identical foods and cooking styles.

Our appetite, our taste, and sense of variety all come from Nature. Now let me take this a step further. Some people argue that having a set schedule is too rigid a way to live. But if we look at Nature, it's hard to say that Nature is rigid. Nature is full of change and inconsistency. Nature is asymmetrical and Nature has no lack of vitality. If you cut things down, they will grow again. Whatever we do to the earth, the earth has the ability to adjust, adapt, repair, and maintain itself. Based on this observation, we can say that Nature has great vitality.

> "After you have exhausted what there is in business, politics, conviviality, and so on—have found that none of these finally satisfy, or permanently wear—what remains? Nature remains."
>
> —Walt Whitman

VITALITY

Where does this vitality come from? I have an answer that satisfies me. You might agree with it, you might not. I believe Nature's vitality is the result of its orderliness. For example, if you grow up in an orderly family, one that has structure, routines, and traditions, one that values consistency so that you know what to expect, then automatically you have a kind of confidence and a vitality for life. Whereas if you grow up in a family where nothing is consistent and life is disorderly, you don't have that positive kind of vitality. Let's suppose, for the purpose of argument, that you have job security and that you know what's expected of you. In such a situation, you can work hard and efficiently without becoming exhausted. But if your job is in jeopardy from day to day and you're not sure what is expected of you, exhaustion sets in almost automatically. Am I right? You lose your energy. You lose your vitality. You lose your creativity. Can you see the influence order and structure exert over our lives and health? Order and structure are what give us vitality, adaptability and creativity, confidence, and a zest for life.

If you talk with very old people about their lives, you will discover that what most of them have in common is an orderly life. Set times for sleeping, waking, and meals, times that don't vary. These people are self-sufficient. They rarely, if ever, see doctors. They prefer to guide their own lives and to take care of all their needs themselves. Generally, they live simply. And, because over the years they have maintained this orderliness, they have been rewarded with good health, strong vitality, and long life.

STRUCTURE AND CREATIVITY

I read about an experiment that was done some time ago that is pertinent to what we're talking about. The researchers asked a certain number of people who had had no previous experience in the field of advertising to come up with slogans for various products. The subjects were offered no guidelines whatsoever. The same thing was asked of computers, but since computers can't function without being programmed, the computers were given very clear guidelines. The results didn't surprise me, although they may have surprised the researchers. The slogans the human subjects came up with were too boring and childish to attract any attention. The computers, on the other hand, produced highly creative material that was as good as any dreamt up by the world's most successful advertising agencies. The difference from the macrobiotic point of view was that the human subjects were given no guidelines, no structure, while the computers were given explicit instructions—this is what we want, this is what you may do, this is what you may not do. The point is that alignment with Nature's orderly cycles is the key to understanding variety. It is the key that unlocks freshness and creativity.

7 STEPS

Some of you may have seen the 7 Steps bookmark, all seven steps printed on a slender bookmark. When I lecture, I often say to people that now they know everything I know. People think I'm joking, but I'm not. I'm very serious. If you do these things and bring yourself into alignment with Nature, then you and I will be receiving life from the same source—including our appetite, food choices, ideas, and understanding. We all have the ability to align with Nature and its orderly cycles. All we need is the will and to be shown the way.

I hope that now you can appreciate why an explanation of Eating Habits: Format of Meals had to precede an exploration of the actual Diet: Content of Meals. Eating Habits are the controlling factor. The bottom line is that good eating habits create the ability to make healthful choices. Let's say I fill a table with the best quality and most delicious macrobiotic food and you eat nothing but food from that table. Will that be a guarantee of good health? I don't think so. You won't achieve good health until you learn how to choose the foods you need. We build our health one day at a time, one meal at a time. You must learn to choose appropriately.

The question is, of course, how do we do this? Again, the answer is by adhering to a structure, by incorporating the structure of the 7 Steps into our daily lives.

EATING HABITS: FORMAT OF MEALS

Take Time for Your Meals Every Day

Sit down to eat your meals or snacks without reading, watching TV, or working.

> "One of the very nicest things about life is the way we must regularly stop whatever it is we are doing and devote our attention to eating."
>
> —Luciano Pavarotti

This is the first step toward good health and will help you feel more satisfied. Sitting down to eat is an expression of our appreciation and respect for our food. Sitting down enables us to create order in our daily eating habits and it makes us more conscious of what we eat. The tendency is not to count the food we eat while standing. It just doesn't enter our consciousness. In fact, we usually stand when eating the foods we really don't want to eat or shouldn't be eating. If you tend to snack throughout the day, you will have trouble regulating your meals and perhaps have some difficulty with weight control. Generally, we don't realize how much food we ingest when we are eating constantly. Remember that many people eat not because they are hungry but out of a desire to soothe their nerves or lessen their frustration. For them, food acts as a tranquilizer. If this is true in your case, you will become more aware of it if you sit down whenever you snack. You may even decide you don't really want to eat at that time.

Chinese medicine says that food has both physical aspects and *chi* (or energetic) aspects. If you want to absorb the energetic aspects of your food, your stomach must be in the bent position it takes when you are seated, not in the elongated position it assumes when you stand. As I see it, different positions are for different activities. Standing is for being active and productive; reclining, which is a receptive position, is for sleep, sex, and rest; and sitting is a transitional position between the two postures. We eat during the day so that we have the energy to be active. We sleep at night so that the body, using the food consumed during the day, can repair and maintain itself.

SITTING, STANDING, AND LYING DOWN

Sitting is the link between standing and lying down. Think about how the seated position aligns with eating. The seated position is the one in which the change between the external and internal environments, between giving out and taking in, occurs. Sitting is the position for receiving nourishment, for strengthening the ability to absorb, digest, and assimilate food. It is also the position most congenial to the process of thinking. Try reading while standing up or lying down. Ideas are not as easily understood in these positions. Whether we are talking about absorbing, digesting, and assimilating food or ideas, sitting is unique.

If you eat while standing up, your stomach cannot accept the food properly. Standing interferes with the digestive process. When you sit down to eat, you will be more conscious of what you are eating and also how much you are eating. Since sitting is a more relaxed position than standing, you will probably eat less food because you will be digesting what you have eaten more thoroughly and will be satisfied with smaller amounts. When you are seated and you overeat, often you don't know it until you get up from the table. Then you think—oh-oh, I ate too much. In other words, what you are experiencing at that moment of awareness is a natural sensation of fullness. This gives you a gauge by which to measure how much is too much. On the other hand, if you eat standing up, you never know when you've had enough. You lose your natural sense of how much food it takes to satisfy you.

EASTERN AND WESTERN MEDICINE

In the early stages of medicine, during the era of Hippocrates, Eastern and Western medicine were very similar. Both were grounded in practical knowledge and common sense. Both taught the importance of diet and lifestyle in creating good health. In those days, health advice included instructions for properly handling all aspects of life. People were taught to sit up straight when eating and to chew their food thoroughly. These guidelines were considered rudimentary. Then as the East moved toward a more spiritual way of life and the West gravitated toward science and analysis, their commonly held ideas became increasingly divergent. However, certain of these ideas—like sitting down to eat and chewing properly—were passed on from one generation to the next in both the East and the West.

"Let food be thy medicine, and let medicine be thy food."
—Hippocrates

NOURISHMENT AND BALANCE

Ideally, a meal is a time for nourishing and balancing oneself. A meal is a time to be relaxed, open, and receptive to nourishment, and these attributes don't mix well with activity. Eating while doing other things such as reading, working, watching TV, talking on the phone, or driving interferes with your ability to receive nourishment. Light, quiet conversation is fine because it makes you more open and receptive. (Heavy, loud conversation tightens you up and closes you down.) My analogy is this: if we're talking and in the middle of our conversation I pick up a book, I close off to you. If you're eating, trying to receive nourishment from your food, and you do something else at the same time, you close off to your food. It's that simple. You aren't being fully nourished. Each of us takes different nourishment from the same food. Our ability to receive nourishment depends on how we eat and on our approach to eating.

Many of us don't like to sit down and eat without doing other things, especially when we are alone. When we eat alone, what happens? Thoughts and feelings come up, memories come up. Often we don't like what comes up, but if we learn to think of this as part of a cleansing process, of getting things out that don't belong inside us, it should be easier to eat without distractions. And if we can be patient and allow the unhappy thoughts and feelings to come up, they will be followed by happier ones. In the beginning, just try to let go of your thoughts as you would in meditation. Acknowledge each thought as it comes and then let it pass away.

Food is our strongest desire in life. Food also has the capacity to give us an incredibly deep sense of satisfaction. If we eat quietly and without distraction, we will feel deeply satisfied and fulfilled. However, many people don't allow this to happen. As soon as unhappy feelings come up, they automatically feel the need to do something, to jump up, to read something, to turn on the TV. It's very important to get past this. Let's say that when you begin to practice macrobiotics, you abruptly stop drinking coffee. A headache follows. You can either allow the headache to pass (and the pain might be very intense for a few days) or you can drink a cup of coffee and end it. You might not think so, but this situation is analogous to eating without doing other things. Eating while you distract yourself with something else is the same as taking the very thing (coffee) that was the cause of your problem (headache) in the first place. The cause is also the cure—albeit a very temporary one.

Of all my recommendations, I think sitting down to eat without doing other things is the most difficult one for my clients to practice. At the same time, it's the most important of all the steps. It's the one that sets our direction toward health or toward sickness.

Key Points:

- Sitting down to eat your meals and snacks without doing other things is the first step toward good health.
- When you eat without distraction, you absorb the most nutrition.
- You need to concentrate when you read a book or see a movie to get the most out of the experience. You need to participate fully in a conversation to be completely satisfied. This principle applies to your meals as well.
- Sitting down to eat without doing other things allows you to be more aware of what you are eating and to stop when you have had enough.
- You eat less and feel more satisfied.
- This is one of the most difficult steps. Try to always be conscious of it.

Allow Adequate Time for Your Meals.

The minimum time required to consume a meal is twenty minutes. Now, you might think that that's an arbitrary number, but it isn't. Let me explain. According to Eastern thinking, everything in the universe is energy, some of it materialized energy (us, for example) and some not (wind, for example). Energy is manifested in vibrations. And we know that vibrations have a natural tendency to align with each other—that's physics. I first realized this when I was in Switzerland, in a shop that sold cuckoo clocks. All the pendulums were exactly aligned. (I was so pleased with my discovery that I made the mistake of buying one of these clocks. It drove me crazy once I was home.) Or, take the example of women's menstruation. It's well known that after a short while women who share living quarters begin to menstruate at the same time. Therefore, it should not surprise you to learn that after twenty minutes in the same room, the rate of heartbeat, blood pressure, and breathing of those present tends to align. By the same token, if someone should enter the room whose rate of heartbeat, blood pressure, or breathing is very different from that of the group's—too different for alignment to occur—everyone will feel some discomfort, no one will be able to relax completely. Understandably, the person who entered the room will feel too uncomfortable to stay very long.

FIFTY CYCLES OF ENERGY EVERY DAY

Why does the process of alignment take roughly twenty minutes? Here is the reasoning: fifty cycles of energy (*ki*, the Japanese word for energy) flow through the body each day. This means that *ki* circulates through the entire body fifty times a day. One cycle takes just under thirty minutes. It takes 70 percent of the thirty-minute cycle, or about twenty minutes, for alignment to become significant. You can check on this yourself. When you go somewhere new, how long does it take until you really feel comfortable? How long does it take to settle into a serious conversation? It takes about twenty minutes. Still, many people sit down to eat a meal assuming that five to ten minutes is an adequate amount of time. It certainly isn't. If a friend says he has something really important to talk over with you and you say—great, I can give you five minutes—it's likely he or she will feel insulted.

You can't have a serious conversation in five minutes. You can introduce a subject, but you can't delve into it. In the same way, you can have an appetizer or a snack in five minutes but not an entire meal.

Breakfast is the most forgiving meal because we're active for a full day afterward. Dinner is the least forgiving. In other words, if you have a fifteen-minute breakfast, it's not the end of the world. But in a manner of speaking, a fifteen-minute dinner is. It doesn't count as a meal. I'm not talking about solid eating time. I'm talking about the time it takes to complete your meal—from the moment you sit down until the moment you get up from the table.

Let's say you're standing next to someone at a bar. Even if you don't say a word to that person, after twenty minutes your energy will be aligned. If you smile at that person, the alignment happens more quickly. If you talk together it happens more quickly still, and the alignment becomes stronger. I hope you can see now that quiet conversation during mealtimes, talking and eating together, fosters a strong and deep alignment. If you eat quietly without talking, you become more independent, but not as strongly connected to one another. Whether you eat alone or with others, the minimum time for a meal is twenty minutes.

Key Points:
- The minimum time for a meal is twenty minutes.
- Time yourself from the beginning to the end of the meal, not just while you are eating.
- Breakfast is the most forgiving meal in terms of time.
- It takes time for your body to adjust from being active to receiving nourishment, just as it takes time to settle into a good conversation.

Eat Slowly and Chew Well.

It's only common sense that in order to eat slowly you must be seated. You must also allow time in your mind for the meal. If you don't do this you won't be able to slow down. If, when you sit down, you are thinking that you're running late, that you don't have time for this meal, you won't be able to eat slowly. Once you pick up your fork, the pace is set and it's very hard to change it. In other words, eating slowly and chewing well require some preparation.

> "Chew your drink, and drink your food."
>
> —Mahatma Gandhi

CHEWING AND POSTURE

In order to chew well, we have to assume the correct posture. The posture for chewing and the posture for reading are exactly the same. If you have something to read that is important to you and requires deep understanding, then you had better sit up straight and tilt your head forward slightly. It is in this position that we can best absorb, comprehend, and retain. I think we can agree that if you sit up straight but tilt your chin up slightly, reading becomes more difficult. In order to chew, digest, and absorb information completely, we must sit up straight, head tilted slightly forward so the head spiral is pointing upward. The same holds true if our aim is to circulate, digest, and absorb what we eat.

In this position, sitting up straight with your head spiral facing upward, the food remains in your mouth as you chew—it doesn't slip down your throat—and you can circulate (chew) the food as many times as you wish—fifty times, a hundred times, five hundred times. In order to chew thoroughly and well, it's best to put down your utensils between each mouthful and place your hands in your lap. This increases your concentration and encourages thorough chewing.

Why do I place so much emphasis on chewing? Chewing strengthens digestion. If you chew your food well, you will develop your physical ability to digest and assimilate food.

CHEWING AND CIRCULATION

Chewing is a pump. It circulates all our body's energy and fluids, all blood, lymph, digestive, hormonal and cellular fluids. Each chew is like a pump circulating all our energy. Each chew is renewing our physical, emotional, mental, and spiritual health. To digest food properly, the minimum count is twenty-five. To quiet the mind and develop thinking, the minimum is fifty. To refine *ki* (energy), the minimum is one hundred.

In Eastern philosophy, the body is made up of different systems working together and complementing each other. The digestive system and the brain form one of these systems. The digestive system is designed to digest solid and liquid food, the brain to digest vibrational food—food that takes the form of thoughts and images.

CHEWING FOOD—CHEWING IDEAS

Once, while I was living in Japan, I was invited to a restaurant that specialized in *fugu*, a treasured Japanese delicacy. *Fugu* is very expensive. It has a delicious and delicate taste, but it is also highly poisonous. In fact, if it has not been properly prepared, it is usually fatal. Two days before I was scheduled to eat at this restaurant, a famous sumo wrestler died of *fugu* poisoning, a fact that only served to increase my nervousness. But it would have been a terrible loss of face to turn down such an honored invitation, so I went. I drank sake and ate *fugu* with my Japanese friends. None of them seemed unsettled by what had happened to the sumo wrestler, but I wondered if this was to be my last meal. I tried to behave naturally even though I was frightened, and eventually I managed to relax a bit. The *fugu* was delicious. To this day, I don't know whether it was the taste and texture or the danger it posed that made it so interesting to eat.

Later, I told this story to a well-known Japanese macrobiotic teacher, Herman Aihara. He had a good laugh and then said, "A macrobiotic person can't be poisoned. His body won't accept the poison. It will immediately be thrown out of his body. You didn't have to worry."

Maybe, maybe not. But what I do believe is that we can be poisoned by ideas as readily as (or perhaps more readily than) by food. If Eastern thinking is correct about the connection between the brain and the digestive system, then strengthening the digestive system is the easiest way to strengthen thinking ability. In other words, chewing your food and chewing your ideas amount to the same thing. If you chew your food well, you strengthen your ability to digest and assimilate ideas and thoughts. The action of chewing actually improves your thinking ability and your memory. A healthy mind can accept all ideas, chew them over, and either absorb or dispel them. I call this conscious chewing. The concept is applicable to all forms of nourishment, physical, mental, emotional, and spiritual.

CHEWING AND CONSCIOUSNESS

It's important to be conscious of how you eat. Most people eat automatically. They give little or no thought to eating mindfully. Being relaxed before sitting down to eat will help you take the time to chew properly. Doing some stretching, a few yoga postures, or even some deep slow breathing before you start may help you to unwind.

A five- to ten-minute break between cooking and eating can make a big difference in your ability to enjoy your meal and to concentrate on chewing well. Cooking tends to be tightening and that may contribute to overeating and under-chewing.

You've probably not thought much about chewing. The fact is that most people chew very little. Changing old habits is tough, so before you begin your new program of proper chewing, observe the way you and other people chew. You'll be surprised at what you see and, with a bit of reflection, you'll soon realize that your body deserves better treatment.

Solid food should be chewed until it turns to liquid. Aim to chew each mouthful of food fifty times. Start slowly. For the first two weeks chew each mouthful twenty-five times. Work your way gradually to fifty or, if you have the will and the patience, to a hundred. Once you become accustomed to well-chewed food, you will feel uncomfortable if you eat too quickly.

The more you chew, the more aware you become of your own needs. People today tend to be constantly on the run with little or no time to reflect on what is important to them in their lives. Chewing well will help you break that pattern. It leads naturally to a calmer and more orderly life. By thinking about what's appropriate for you to do next, you will begin to use your time more efficiently; and that, in turn, will help you accomplish more than you ever thought possible.

Everything in Nature occurs in an alternating pattern—movement followed by rest—action followed by inaction. Ideally our lives should reflect this process. We might think we are wasting time if we stop to take care of ourselves and chew our food but, in reality, valuing our quiet time will make our active time more productive.

If you can take at least one or two of your three daily meals alone, you will have the ideal opportunity to concentrate on chewing well. Even if you can chew well at only one meal, you will notice an improvement in how you feel and think. If you can form the habit of chewing well at every meal, your health and your outlook on life will improve dramatically. You can chew well even when dining with others. Take advantage of those times when your companion is talking to do your chewing.

CHEWING AND DIGESTION

Chewing well also releases the full power of saliva. Ideally, saliva has a pH factor of 7.2, which means it is slightly alkaline. Saliva digests complex carbohydrates by breaking them down from complex to simple sugars. (That's why grains, beans, and vegetables get sweeter the longer you chew them.) Chewing any food well prepares it to pass more smoothly and completely through the digestive system. Saliva can also neutralize imbalances in your food. Even if your diet is not well balanced, thorough chewing helps compensate for the imbalances.

When you chew well, your saliva mixes with the food and makes the food more alkaline, which means the food is better able to absorb the highly acidic secretions that are released in your stomach. If your blood is more alkaline, you will enjoy better health, stronger immunity, and a greater resistance to illness.

Simple carbohydrates and refined foods are absorbed quickly into the bloodstream, creating more acidic blood. Sugar and alcohol are simple carbohydrates. Many foods contain hidden sugar, and sugar can be disguised in various ways on food labels. Most cakes, pastries, cookies, and crackers contain sugar. Fruit is also a simple carbohydrate. Concentrated fruit juices are commonly used as sweeteners in many commercial and health food–related products. These are all absorbed quickly and they all create acidic blood. Fructose, or fruit sugar, which is found in fruit and honey, can also raise blood cholesterol.

Other foods that are absorbed quickly include white rice, white bread, white pasta, and potatoes. You can help neutralize their acidity by chewing thoroughly, but it's best to avoid these foods altogether once your cravings are minimized.

The problem with these foods is that by the time they reach the stomach, they will have been absorbed in the mucous membranes and therefore will not pass through the duodenum. Foods that are absorbed before passing through the duodenum create more acidic blood. The duodenum has strong alkaline secretions that increase the alkalinity of our food before it passes into the small intestine for final digestion and absorption.

Opposites attract. Chewing alkalizes food. Then the alkaline food attracts stomach acids and the protein content is digested. Food turns alkaline again as it passes through the duodenum where fats are broken down. Your food is then ready for the next stage—final digestion and absorption in the small intestine. Only food that is absorbed through the small intestine creates healthy, alkaline blood. The final stage is water absorption and bowel formation in the colon or large intestine, where the waste products are then excreted.

When your blood is acidic, valuable minerals, especially calcium, are lost from bones, teeth, or muscles. These stored minerals are needed to create the buffer action that breaks down strong acid and turns it into weak acid on its way to being converted to carbon dioxide and water. Mineral loss dilutes the blood and weakens resistance to illness. It weakens the bones as well.

Acid blood weakens the kidneys, heart, and lungs, all organs affected by excessive liquids. The kidneys must work harder to filter more blood and discharge more fluid, which leads to a loss of valuable nutrients (minerals, B vitamins, and vitamin C). The heart has to work harder to pump the increased blood volume. And the lungs must work harder also, in order to discharge the excess carbon dioxide and fluid. Think of the steam that emanates from our mouths when we exhale on a cold day. Think of how much more difficult it is to breathe easily when the weather is humid. Experiment. Try drinking a lot of fruit juice, beer, or soda before exercising. Check your heart and breathing rates and compare the readings with those taken when you drink fewer liquids.

As you can imagine, your health will be adversely affected by a loss of minerals. If you eat a steady diet of refined foods and white sugar, you will weaken your entire system and create a climate for the development of illness.

On the other hand, if you eat foods with healthful, nourishing complex carbohydrates and chew them well, you will enjoy the natural sweetness of good food that can be digested properly. Chewing regulates peristalsis, the automatic expansion and contraction of the muscles of the entire digestive system. Peristaltic movement is wavelike and forms a continuous pattern. Chewing stimulates peristalsis. The more you chew the more frequently the wavelike movement occurs and the more rapidly you move toward a state of balance.

The result is that elimination will return to normal and toxic conditions in the colon, conditions that could cause discomfort and disease, will be warded off. You will have reached the point at which the rhythm of your entire system flows in harmony with the rhythm of Nature and the universe.

Thorough chewing makes the salivary glands produce enzymes that stimulate the release of parotid hormones. These hormones help the thymus gland create T cells, which bolster the immune system.

As I said earlier, chewing also acts as a pump that circulates the body's fluids and energy. Chewing actually activates the blood and other fluid circulation in the body as well as regulating energy flow. If you are feeling physically or emotionally blocked, chewing will help to disperse the stagnation that is causing those conditions.

It activates the whole system and dispels negative energy.

BRIGHTEN UP YOUR DAY

After you have chewed thoroughly for a few days or longer, you will notice that you feel brighter and that you are thinking more clearly. This is also easy to test. Try chewing every mouthful of food, even soup and liquids, at least fifty times for four days. Notice the difference. Are you calmer? Is your thinking clearer? Is your energy brighter? If you feel adventurous, try another four days of chewing each mouthful of food at least a hundred times.

To make this a more useful test, it's best to count the number of chews per mouthful over the four-day period. Better chewing alone will strengthen your health but, as I said earlier, make sure that you are seated when you eat and not doing other things—not driving, watching TV, or reading.

RELIEVING STRESS

Most people think they are wasting time when they take time for their meals. The busier and more stressed they are, the more they think they're wasting time. Nothing could be further from the truth. Consider this: the more you rush your meal, the more stressed you become. It's really quite simple. Traditionally there were three times during the day when we stopped what we were doing in order to return to balance, to re-nourish ourselves and readjust our direction. They were called meals—not lunch or dinner breaks—three times a day when we could stop and think, what am I doing, where am I going, what do I want to be doing? If we don't take time for meals, we never develop the ability to ask or answer these questions, and the result is that we lose our direction in life, we lose control over our lives. This is what we see happening today. People are more confused and disoriented than ever before. They never take the time to stop and think about the important things. Meals are purposeful in that they give us the opportunity for this kind of self-reflection. Meals are great stress relievers, provided they are at least twenty minutes long. You will gain time, not lose it, when you take time for your meals.

Key Points:
- Start by chewing each mouthful twenty to thirty times and gradually increase to fifty.
- To improve your health and calm your mind more quickly, chew each mouthful of food at least fifty times.
- Thorough chewing also helps you eat less and feel more satisfied.
- Chewing circulates your body's energy and all its fluids (blood, lymph, hormones, digestive, etc.).
- Put your utensils down after each mouthful. This will help you chew more thoroughly.

Stop Eating Three Hours Before Bedtime.
"Dine with little, sup with less: Do better still; sleep supperless."
—Benjamin Franklin

Your body cleans and repairs itself while you sleep. Your stomach needs to be empty for this process to be efficient. It takes, on average, about three hours for food to leave the stomach. Therefore, it's best to refrain from eating for three hours before retiring. My analogy is this: it's impossible to clean a room packed with people. If you want to clean a room thoroughly and efficiently, you have to empty it of people. If you want to clean your body, you have to empty it of food.

During the day while we're up and about, we receive the benefits of the sun's energy. Just the opposite occurs at night when we are nourished by celestial energy from the moon, stars, constellations, and galaxy. Daytime is for activity, productivity, and the spending of energy; nighttime is for rest, rejuvenation, and the receiving of energy.

The body cannot perform the miraculous nocturnal task of rejuvenation unless the stomach is empty. Nor can we receive celestial energy at night unless we are empty inside. Food is condensed energy. When you eat, most of your food turns into energy in your body. If you go to sleep too soon after eating, your body will be too full of energy to do its nighttime work. Imagine a roomful of people and then imagine trying to clean, organize, and rearrange that room. Difficult, wouldn't you say? But once the room is empty, it's simple. Can you see from my analogy that your body is in a similar fix if it's not empty? When your stomach is too full, the body is so busy dealing with digestion it can't properly do its normal nighttime job. It's all too easy for the body to fall behind schedule when it can't discharge the toxins that accumulate in our cells and organs each day—which is exactly what happens when it's not allowed to repair itself each night.

HYPOGLYCEMIA

Here's another important point: when we eat, we secrete insulin in order to digest our food. If we eat before sleep, we go to sleep with too much insulin circulating in our bloodstream so that when morning comes, we feel tired and sluggish and have a hard time getting up. This is one of the symptoms of hypoglycemia.

Let me tell you a little bit about hypoglycemia. The food we take before going to sleep is food that the body can't metabolize because it is in a prone position. This food goes to the liver for storage. The liver takes care of fat metabolism, but it also has another important role. The liver neutralizes acidity and therefore helps keep our blood alkaline. When we eat before sleeping, we experience an increased buildup of fat and cholesterol in our bloodstream which, in turn, promotes acidity. And acidic blood is a chief contributor to feelings of fatigue and stress. The excess, undigested food actually exhausts the body, which is unable to process and digest in a reclining position.

Among our vital organs, the liver, pancreas, kidneys, and intestines are particularly overworked. Of course, many people feel they have to eat just in order to sleep. This is a symptom of hypoglycemia. What it means is that your blood sugar has fallen too low for you to fall asleep. Then the body demands that you eat in order to raise your blood sugar level, knowing that it will fall further while you sleep.

Even if what you eat at nine or ten at night is of good quality and healthful, you won't receive the best value from it. It may satisfy your appetite, but without time to digest it properly, you are effectively losing some of its benefits. Foods that are high in fiber and low in fat (e.g., complex carbohydrates) are digested more quickly and easily than animal and dairy foods. They contain less condensed energy and are easier for your body to process and, if you are up and about and active, their energy will disperse more quickly. But even the smallest amount of meat is so laden with condensed energy that it creates an even bigger burden on your body, so much of one that you probably would need more than a three-hour wait before going to sleep.

"A full belly makes a dull brain."

—Benjamin Franklin

CLEANING YOUR BODY AND BETTER SEX

If you are recovering from an illness, you will benefit from allowing three to four hours of not eating before bedtime. Eating has a nourishing, expansive effect on the body. Cleaning or detoxifying is a process of taking out rather than taking in. Waiting more than three hours before bedtime enhances the body's ability to clean and repair itself during sleep. Experiment with the number of hours you allow yourself between the completion of your meal and your bedtime. When you allow more time, I am sure you will feel the difference the next day. For the record, the suggestion to stop eating three hours before bedtime means you should stop eating three hours before getting into bed or stretching out in a chair with your feet up to watch TV or to read. If your body is horizontal, you haven't complied with the suggestion. You will need to wait an additional three hours if you want to have the best digestion and the best sleep. If you reserve the bed exclusively for sleeping and sex, I'm sure you'll find both activities more rewarding.

"Eat little, sleep sound."

—Iranian Proverb

Eating before sleep is a hard habit to break. At the same time, you need to realize that you can't have really good health unless you do break it. If you can't go to sleep without eating for three hours beforehand, the most likely cause is that you're not satisfied with the meals you took during the day. The only way to overcome this habit is to make the day's meals more satisfying. Pay particular attention to breakfast, followed by lunch. People who like to be very active and busy don't often sit down for a complete meal during the course of the day. They can't spare the time and they don't want to be slowed down by food. Often they will eat dinner at a very late hour. Whether they eat early or late, this type of person usually feels more relaxed after dinner, and it is this overdue relaxation that stimulates late-night hunger. Not eating before sleep sounds easy, but it's not. It may require some lifestyle changes.

Key Points:
- To promote the best health, finish your evening meal by eight P.M. Let a full three hours pass before lying down. Stretching out in bed or even on a chaise longue does not allow for good digestion.
- It takes about three hours for your stomach to empty after you finish eating.
- Your stomach must be empty for your body to clean, repair, and recharge itself efficiently while you sleep.
- You will sleep more deeply, need fewer hours, and awake more refreshed.
- Anything you eat before going to sleep—good food or bad—goes to the liver for storage and prevents your liver from getting a rest and repairing itself.

Eat in an Orderly Manner.
Balance has a certain kind of order. You may think what I am about to propose is a very rigid way to eat. A number of older macrobiotic friends have told me just that. My answer is that I'm still here actively counseling

and teaching macrobiotics, and they aren't. So I'll stick with my way. What is my way? Let's take dinner: you can start your meal with soup, followed by a grain and a few different side dishes, and end it with dessert and/or a beverage, if you choose.

TWO TYPES OF SOUP

There are two main types of soup: savory and sweet. Savory soups are well seasoned and mildly salty. Their purpose is to stimulate and activate digestion. Vegetable soup, shoyu soup, and miso soup (vegetable soup seasoned with miso) are savory. Among the three, miso soup has the most ability to promote good digestion.

Sweet vegetable soups are puréed and have a mild, pleasantly sweet and creamy taste—squash soup, onion, cabbage, and leek soup, and carrot soup are some examples. The purpose of sweet vegetable soup is to harmonize, balance, and relax the digestive system.

Savory soup should be started at the beginning of the meal. Whether you finish it before going onto the rest of your meal or continue to consume it throughout the meal, as if it were a side dish, is up to you. There is actually more benefit in taking this type of soup throughout the meal. Sweet vegetable soup doesn't have the same ability to activate digestion but there's no harm in starting your meal with it. Since it lightens, relaxes, and opens up the digestive system, we can enjoy it throughout the meal as well.

Miso soup is a wonderful way to start the day; however, some people who take miso soup for breakfast can't stop eating all day! It makes them excessively hungry. In those cases, I recommend against it. It's better to take it at lunch or dinnertime. But if you're comfortable with it in the morning and it doesn't cause you to overeat, just keep on with it.

GRAIN FROM BEGINNING TO END

Grain is eaten throughout the meal from beginning to end. Now let's talk about vegetable dishes that are interspersed with the grain. As I said earlier, balance has a certain kind of order. To achieve balance, it's best to follow that order. Take some grain, chew it thoroughly, then move on to the vegetable side dishes. Start with the heavier, long-cooked dishes and finish with the lighter, more quickly cooked ones.

Let's go through the order of a meal together. Start the meal with soup. Then take a mouthful of grain, chew it, and swallow it. If you're having a bean (or bean product such as tofu or tempeh), take that next, followed by another mouthful of grain. Then move on to a sea vegetable, such as hijiki or arame, if you're having one. Take a mouthful, chew that, and swallow it. If you're not quite satisfied by one mouthful of sea vegetable, have another, have two or three if you wish. Take some grain, and then go on to whatever other long-cooked vegetable you may be having. Take another mouthful of grain, and then return to the beans, followed by the long-cooked vegetable, then the grain, and then move on to the more quickly cooked vegetable dishes, those that have been sautéed, steamed, or blanched, for instance. My definition of a lightly or quickly cooked vegetable is this: the crunching sound you make while chewing a lightly cooked vegetable should be audible to the person sitting next to you. No crunch means the vegetable is overcooked. Remember to intersperse the grain with the other dishes. Grain is taken consistently throughout the meal. The salad (pressed salad before raw salad) is taken at the end of the meal. Dessert, if you choose to have one, and tea complete the meal.

A meal eaten in this manner has a wavelike pattern. Think of yourself sitting on the beach, watching the tide go out. The tide doesn't go out all at once, does it? No, it waves out. In other words, it goes out but comes back in a bit, out again but back in a bit, and so on. My point is that although the tide continues to come in, overall it's gradually moving out. In the same way, although grain is taken consistently from the beginning to the end of the meal, overall the meal is moving in a certain direction.

Just to avoid confusion, let me say the following: adults generally don't finish one dish before going on to the next, but you can if that is your preference. Generally, most children eat through one dish at a time. They like everything to be as simple as possible. Often, they don't like it if the different foods on their plates are even touching. If you wish to develop direct, simple, childlike thinking, you can eat this way. If, however, you want to think more elaborately, then you should move back and forth, in a wavelike pattern. So you are constantly coming back while moving further and further out—like the tide.

Key Points:
- Orderly eating aids digestion and promotes clear thinking. It will leave you feeling more satisfied.
- If you are having soup, start the meal with it. You may finish your soup before going on to the rest of the meal, or you may eat it throughout the meal.
- Eat grains from the beginning to the end of the meal.
- Gradually move from the heavier, well cooked dishes to the lighter, more quickly cooked or raw dishes. Salads come last and are followed by dessert and tea.
- It is not necessary to finish one dish before moving on to the next. The pattern is a wave-like motion that resembles the tide as it goes out.
- Orderly eating leads to orderly thinking.

Avoid Mixing Foods in the Same Mouthful.
Keep the foods on your plate distinct and separate, not touching. Imitate the child in this respect. To accomplish this, you either have to take smaller portions or put the different foods in small individual dishes as the Japanese do. I don't like to put everything on my plate at once, so I only take a couple of dishes at a time and then go back for the others. It often happens that my children finish the foods I like before I'm ready to refill my plate. It's no different when I'm at the Strengthening Health Institute's residential programs. The Strengthening Health Institute (SHI) is our nonprofit that offers online and on-site personal and professional training programs in the macrobiotic lifestyle. The outcome is that I'm prevented from overeating! Everything is as it should be.

Why do I stress keeping the food on our plates from touching? Digestion is a mechanical process. For instance, if you mix two foods together in the same mouthful, digestive enzymes are going to attach to one food more than to the other. That's their nature. The process works like this: the mouth secretes saliva. Saliva is alkaline. Whichever food becomes more alkalized by the saliva will attract more stomach acid, which, in turn, will attract more alkaline secretions in the duodenum when it arrives there. That food will be well absorbed in the small intestine, and equally so in the large intestine. But the other food will miss out completely. Different foods are digested differently.

If you cook two foods together, such as pressure-cooked rice and beans or stir-fried grain and vegetables, they can be eaten together. They have blended in the cooking process. They are no longer two distinct foods. But if you cook rice and beans separately, eat them separately. Don't put the beans on your rice. There are exceptions. If you cook two dishes separately but mix them together while they're still hot, the residual heat will cause them to blend. In effect, they become one dish. If you want to make a grain and vegetable salad using leftover rice, reheat the rice, then add the vegetables, whether they are raw or previously cooked or freshly cooked. The heat from the rice will allow the ingredients to blend and become digestible. You can let the dish cool down to room temperature before eating it if that is your preference. It is still one dish. Energetically, this is entirely different from mixing distinct foods together on your plate or in your mouth. It's crucial not to mix different foods in the same mouthful. Foods cooked separately should be chewed separately.

As I've already mentioned, children don't like different foods to touch on their plates and, in general, they like simple dishes. But, under some circumstances they do mix everything together. When? When they don't like what they are eating and just want to get it down. When are adults most likely to mix foods together, when they have a healthy appetite and are full of energy, or when their appetite is sluggish and they feel tired?

Here's another question. What stimulates your mind more, eating distinct dishes or eating those that have been mixed together on the plate? The answer, of course, is eating each dish individually. If you eat this way, you will see an improvement in both your digestion and your ability to think.

Set Your Daily Schedule

RISE EARLY AND SLEEP BEFORE MIDNIGHT

Rise early to be more active and discharge more toxins. The time at which you get out of bed in the morning—not your waking time—is what sets the tone for your day. If you want to be more active and productive, get out of bed by seven A.M. at the latest. If you leave your bed at nine, or even worse, at eleven A.M., there's a sense in which you might as well not bother to leave it at all.

Think about this. The sun rises. It rises with a burst of energy that cleans and refreshes everything on earth. When you get out of bed around the time of sunrise, you can take full advantage of this burst of energy. It is at this time that your body has the greatest capacity to discharge excess, to clean and refresh itself. Within an hour or two after sunrise, the sun's movement starts to slow down. By nine A.M., it has slowed down considerably. Let's take a look at exactly what happens when you get up late, as many people do on Sundays. You have a late breakfast—referred to as brunch—usually sometime between ten and noon, a time when we're meant to be active. Now if we eat when we're meant to be active, we get very sluggish. We lie around for the rest of the day, reading the paper, dragging from one thing to another. The effect on us is the same as if we had overeaten, isn't it? Why should this be the case? The answer is that we don't have the ability to digest or process the sun's energy when we're in a horizontal position. The sun's energy is very coarse. We absorb it through the head spiral located toward the back part of the top of the head, and for this to occur we have to be upright.

If you eat a big meal during the day, afterward you feel sluggish, you can't think clearly. Even if you take an afternoon nap in a darkened room, you still feel sluggish when you awake. You don't have to be directly exposed to the sun's rays for this to happen. If we are horizontal when the sun is up, we don't have the ability to process the sun's energy. The immune system is effectively deactivated, and the overall effect on us is the same as that of overeating.

It's just as important for our health to be asleep before midnight as it is to rise with the sun. During the night, we receive very subtle energy from the celestial world, the moon, stars, and planets. As we sleep, we are nourished by this celestial influence. We have to be horizontal for this energy to be most effectively absorbed. Our deepest sleep occurs between one A.M. and three A.M. Celestial vibrations are strongest between midnight and four A.M., at the time when the most stars are visible in the sky, the greatest number being visible at about two A.M. It takes an hour or two to fall into the deepest sleep, so we need to be asleep by eleven P.M. to receive the optimal celestial influence and, therefore, the best results for our health. If this is difficult, given the demands of modern society, try to be in bed by midnight.

> "Early to bed and early to rise, makes a man healthy, wealthy and wise."
>
> —Benjamin Franklin

I have read that we need a certain number of hours of sleep and if we don't get them, we have to "catch up." If you think about this, it doesn't make much sense. How well or poorly we sleep is determined by our diet and activity during the day. If we eat too much or too little, it's hard to sleep. The same holds true for activity. If we sit around all day, we probably will not sleep well. When we work too hard and exhaust ourselves, sleep often does not come easily. The amount of sleep we need is determined by how long it takes our body to clean, repair, and recharge itself. The better our health, the less time we need for the cycle of cleaning, repairing, and recharging. Most people find that they need considerably less sleep within a couple of weeks of adopting the Strengthening Health recommendations. If our diet and activity are not in balance every day, we won't sleep well at night, and if we don't sleep well at night, our body won't be able to clean, repair, and re-energize its organs and nervous system. On the other hand, if our diet and activity are in balance, the sleeping process becomes very efficient, takes less time to achieve, and gives us deeper sleep. The result is that we feel rested and refreshed with fewer hours of sleep. If we are in good health, either a rich, elaborate meal or a light, simple one will satisfy us and provide good energy.

The same principle applies to the subject of sleep. The average person in good health requires five to eight hours of sleep. If we get a little less than that, we will still feel fine and, if we choose to sleep a bit longer, perhaps on the weekend, we'll also feel fine. The bottom line is that when we are in good health, we can be flexible about how much we eat and the amount of sleep we need.

Let's consider the quality of sleep. Deep sleep, undisturbed by dreams, is the most refreshing. If you spend the night dreaming, the mind does not have the opportunity to relax and recharge. If you follow the Strengthening Health suggestions accurately, you will not experience confusing or disturbing dreams and you will awaken with the will and the energy to pursue what you want out of life—to pursue your real dreams.

Everyone is concerned with getting a good night's sleep. If you live in proper rhythm with Nature, eat at regular scheduled intervals, chew your food well, and allow enough time before bed for digestion, you will have no problem with sleep.

Key Points:
- Your rising time regulates your energy and activity for the day. Aren't you less productive if you get up late?
- Rise by seven A.M. to be more active and discharge more toxins. Your body has the greatest ability to discharge and release excess early in the morning.
- Be asleep before midnight to sleep more deeply, awake more refreshed, and be physically stronger.
- Your body can clean and repair itself more efficiently when you are asleep before midnight.

KEEP YOUR MEALTIMES REGULAR

Regular meals regulate all of your body's cycles—physical, emotional, and mental. They make your energy and life more stable. It's important to take your meals at approximately the same time every day. This adjustment alone will greatly improve your health. As easy as this step may sound, the reality is that it takes time and discipline to rethink this aspect of your life. As the world has gotten more complicated, the manner in which we take our most important nourishment is often ignored.

Think about your mealtimes during the past week. Were you able to sit down to your meals at approximately the same time each day? Did you even take the time to sit down when eating breakfast or lunch? If your answer is no, you aren't alone. Most people don't realize the importance of maintaining a regular meal schedule and don't think they are undermining their health by not eating at regular times. But their health is surely suffering.

Even if you still eat meat and potatoes every day, just doing it at regular intervals will let you benefit from your food far more than if you eat these same foods in a disorderly manner. The body responds positively to a set schedule and is very grateful when it is allowed to align itself with Nature—so grateful that it will reward you abundantly with better mental and physical health. This is because the time at which we eat determines how well we digest our food.

When do we have the most active digestion? To answer this question, I have to ask another. Actually, it's a trick question. Should we eat our meals when we're hungry, or should we eat at regular specified times? The answer is that if we eat regular meals and if we don't overeat, then we will be hungry at mealtimes. Why should this be so?

ALIGNING WITH NATURE

Mealtimes are not arbitrary. They are part of the natural cycle of life. Everything in life is governed by the sun's movement, whether throughout the day or throughout the year. The sun has three extreme positions—sunrise, sunset, and the high point in the sky, noon. The extreme angles of the sun indicate what we call mealtimes. The time in between these angles is for activity. Most people are active in the morning and in the spring, less active in the middle of the night or in the dead of winter. Breathing is more active in the daytime and in the summer, and is quieter at night and in the winter.

What breakfast really encourages is rising and separating energy. In the morning, we rise and separate from our families and/or our homes; we all go off in different directions—we separate and enter the larger world. This is the energetic effect of sunrise. We get up, wash, brush our teeth, have breakfast or not, and then leave the house for work, for school, for errands, etc. The usual pattern is one of separating from family and home.

Lunch is a time for either activity or stagnation, depending on when and what we eat. Lunch can give us uplifting, active energy or sinking, stagnating energy. If we want to be active after lunch, we should eat early and the meal should be simple and complete. People who are physically active generally eat a light early lunch. In Spain, lunch is an elaborate meal that is served very late. Since no one can stay awake after such a large and late meal, lunch is quite naturally followed by a long siesta.

Dinner is a time for returning home, a time to gather and unify. Until recently, at least, families ate dinner together, perhaps talking, perhaps arguing, but in any event sharing the events and experiences of the day. Family members communicated, unified, and aligned as a family. This alignment and reunification also follows a natural pattern or tendency.

The nature of energy or of vibrations, as I've mentioned before, is such that vibrations try to align. In other words, they try to become similar in their quality, speed, and direction of movement. Think of a moving merry-go-round. If you want to step on smoothly, you have to be moving in the same direction and at the same speed as the merry-go-round itself. If you are moving faster or slower, your boarding will be jerky because the two different energies are not aligning properly. And, furthermore, should you approach a merry-go-round from the direction opposite to its movement, you will be thrown off even as you attempt to climb on.

Another example of the alignment of energy is this one: imagine a meeting room filled with vegans who have just finished dinner. Generally, vegans have more peaceful energy because they eat a grain- and vegetable-based diet without meat or dairy products. Let's say they drink herbal tea at the end of their meal and as a result are even calmer and more peaceful than usual. In our scenario, these vegans are discussing various types of meditation when someone new enters the room, momentarily disrupting the conversation. Let's say that the newcomer has just left the local sports bar, where he has eaten a dinner of fried chicken washed down with a few beers. The atmosphere in the bar was heated because the local hockey team was losing. You can appreciate that this person's energy would be very strong, perhaps even jarring, compared with the energy of the vegans. The group would no doubt lose its focus and wonder who this guy was and why he was there. Do you see the problem? The newcomer's energy is just too different for it to align quickly with the energy of the others. Either the newcomer or the vegans will feel uncomfortable. Only as time passes will their energy even start to align.

When members of a family come together on a daily basis, they build understanding and communication. So long as they do this, the family will function harmoniously. Each of us goes out every day and encounters many different influences and experiences. We eat different foods, talk to different people, engage in different activities, all of which alter our condition and thinking. We align with individuals outside the family through common or similar points and qualities. This is not a threat to the family, but an asset—as long as we continue to take our evening meal together. Understanding and communication develop as we talk and eat together. We can go out again after dinner, if we choose. As long as the unification process, the aligning process continues at the evening meal, the family's stability and balance will develop and be maintained.

BREAKFAST, LUNCH, AND DINNER

Now that we know that meals are meant to align us with Nature's energy, let's talk specifically about breakfast, lunch, and dinner. As I said earlier, breakfast should give us rising and separating energy so that we can be in harmony with the natural world. The sun rises, the dew evaporates, flowers open. Breakfast the world over has one ingredient in common, and that is liquid. When, for instance, we boil water for tea or coffee, the boiling water evaporates, creating rising and separating energy. Whether breakfast consists of cold cereal with milk, porridge (the difference between a macrobiotic person's breakfast grain and dinner grain is simply the amount of liquid used), miso soup, orange juice, coffee, tea, or simply a glass of water, liquid is the common ingredient. It is what we need to rise and separate. A breakfast consisting of bacon, eggs, and dry toast makes for a difficult day. The food is too dry to create active, separating energy. If we want to get moving, we would have to spread some jam on our toast and have a glass of juice or a cup of coffee. It's the liquid that enables us to be active in the morning. If breakfast is too dry, we're not able to align with Nature's rising and separating energy. On the other hand, we can still function perfectly well if we take just liquid for breakfast.

Breakfast time is also the time to separate from home. If you work at home and don't leave the house before you settle down, if you go from your bed to your office or your studio, perhaps by way of the bathroom and kitchen, I think you'll find that after a while you lose your creativity and your drive. There is simply no polarity. If you work at home, my suggestion is that you go out and do something, then return. Have a cup of tea, buy a newspaper, or just take a walk around the block. Unless you have some degree of separation after breakfast, you'll find that you become tired and stale as the morning wears on.

Dinner is a different matter. Dinner should be more substantial—longer-cooked and not too watery—too much liquid can interfere with sleep. If at dinner we drink too much beer, wine, apple juice, soda, coffee, or tea—the common point being liquid—we can't sleep. (Sugar changes to water in the body, which means we have to watch our intake of simple carbohydrates also.) Dinner should give us settling down and gathering energy since it coincides with the setting of the sun. Dinner is the most suitable meal at which to have a protein.

Imagine your day if you swapped breakfast and dinner. You could no longer align with Nature's energy. Mealtimes are not arbitrary, as I said earlier. The meal is our way of aligning with Nature's energy no matter where we are—even if we live in the middle of Manhattan in a high-rise made of materials that carry an incredible electromagnetic charge, a place where we couldn't be more isolated from Nature. If we have regular meals that consist of appropriate ingredients for the time of day, we will be able to align with Nature's energy. By contrast, if we live in the most pristine setting and eat chaotically, we may be surrounded by Nature but we are not aligning with it. Meals create our connection to Nature. I think of the meal as an anchor that creates stability in our lives, no different from the anchor that keeps a ship from drifting into dangerous waters.

Lunch. Around lunchtime, the sun climbs to its highest point in the sky and appears to hang there motionless for a while before it begins its descent. There are two sorts of energy to choose from at lunchtime: one is active energy, the other is more stagnant. If you want to be active and productive in the afternoon, you would be wise to eat while the sun is still rising. If you wait to eat until it's hanging out at its high point, your energy for the afternoon will be more stagnant.

If we want to be active in the afternoon, at what time should we begin lunch? To answer this question, let's go back to the example I gave earlier. Think about the after-lunch siesta for which Spain is famous. When is lunch eaten in Spain? Usually, from two to four P.M. At twelve, should they even be open, the restaurants are empty. Portugal and Spain are next door to one another, but Portugal has no siesta. In Portugal, lunch is eaten either from twelve to one P.M., or from one to two P.M. During the tourist season, you can distinguish the Spanish from the Portuguese simply by the times they choose to eat. The Portuguese are leaving the restaurants as the Spaniards are entering. The different dining habits of these two cultures are emblematic of their different lifestyles. Nevertheless, in spite of the late hours at which they dine, Spaniards still rise with the sun and therefore enjoy long and productive mornings.

So, if you want to be active in the afternoon, finish lunch by two P.M. at the latest—one P.M. would be even better. The later you start lunch, the less you can accomplish afterward. It's as simple as that. Remember that when you eat, you are aligning with the sun's energy. Try this test. Eat similar lunch food every day for four weeks, but for the first two weeks start lunch at twelve P.M. For the following two weeks, start it at two P.M. You will certainly notice a difference. It's common knowledge that the best way to ensure being useless in the afternoon is to eat a late, rich lunch.

Lunch should be simple yet complete and satisfying. Think of foods that allow you to remain physically and mentally active. The test is whether or not you can work, think, and be productive after eating them.

Here are a few possibilities using grains or grain products and quickly cooked vegetables: vegetable sushi rolls (brown rice and vegetables wrapped in toasted nori seaweed), rice balls, fried rice, fried noodles or noodles in broth, and quick-steamed vegetables or vegetable sautés. What qualifies as a simple and complete meal in our part of the world? The sandwich does. Sandwiches are simple and quick and can be complete and healthful, depending on what's in them. Tofu, hummus, or any vegetable-type spread served on steamed and un-yeasted sourdough bread is an example of a nourishing sandwich. You can complement the sandwich with a bowl of vegetable soup and a vegetable side dish, a salad, for instance. Not so long ago, a lunch consisting of a bowl of soup, a sandwich, and a pickle was a fairly typical meal.

MEALTIMES

Should the main meal of the day be served at midday, or at sunset? Well, there's a good argument for both. Agrarian societies took their main meal at noon and ate lightly in the evening. The advent of the Industrial Age changed that, because a simple meal fit in better with the workday. Both will produce good health; choose what suits your lifestyle.

Try not to skip any meals. How much you eat is up to you; what is significant is the regularity. If you cannot make every meal regular, the most important one is your main meal of the day. Having a regular dinner, the gathering, unifying meal provides the most benefit. When I say a meal should be served at the same time every day, I mean it. A fifteen-minute variation in the schedule is acceptable. Thirty minutes is pushing it. Remember that mealtimes regulate all your body's cycles, so the timing is important for your health.

Your blood-sugar level is one function that follows the sun's movement, as do your activity and energy levels. Digestion, bowel movements, all of your physical and mental cycles—they, too, follow the sun's movement. So if you want regular digestion, regular bowel movements, regular menstruation, regular blood-sugar levels, and more balanced emotions, sit down to regular meals.

When I lived in Portugal, I spent a lot of time in the company of old friends who had been living there for a number of years. We shared many meals together. In some ways, they were more careful about what they ate than I was. Yet that family—both parents and children—did not enjoy good health. I believe there was a single reason. Even though they ate good-quality food, they never sat down to regular meals. They ate when they were hungry, and often they ate standing up.

Nothing has a stronger effect on regulating the body's cycles than regular meals. And nothing has a more disruptive effect than skipping meals, eating chaotically, or eating erratically. The starting times for our three regular meals are as follows: Breakfast, five A.M. to eight-thirty or even nine A.M. Lunch, eleven A.M. to one P.M. Dinner, five P.M. to seven or even seven-thirty P.M. The time at which we eat determines how well or poorly we digest our food. The above are the times at which we have the most active digestion, the times at which we can digest our food most thoroughly. The principle behind this applies to sleep as well. Let's say you need six hours sleep a night. Which schedule will give you more energy: sleeping from eleven P.M. to five A.M., or sleeping from three to nine A.M.? Clearly you are much better off sleeping from eleven P.M. to five A.M., rising when the sun rises to take full advantage of the sun's energy.

Key Points:
- Regular meals regulate all your body's cycles, physical, emotional, and mental.
- You will have better energy and digestion, more regular moods, and clearer thinking.
- The time you start your meal regulates your metabolism. Start your meals earlier to be more active and productive. Breakfast: five to eight-thirty A.M. (nine A.M. at the latest). Lunch: eleven A.M. to one P.M. Dinner: five to seven P.M. (seven-thirty P.M. at the latest).
- Your health will improve more quickly and be more stable.
- Eat your meals at the same time every day.
- Lunch is the most important meal to keep consistent and on time.

The Brief History of Food

Food nourishes us and is necessary to sustain life, but it is also much more than that. A meal is actually about taking the time to receive life. It is the counterbalance to work, exercise, and creative expression. When we take our meals, we realign with Nature and with each other. Most importantly, meals are a time for receiving rather than giving. We exchange ideas and share socially. This is how we return to balance.

How we look at and relate to food itself has changed dramatically over the last 12,000 years of recorded history. The changes have come largely due to the development of an agrarian civilization that eventually gave way to one dominated by science, technology, and industry. It has only been in recent centuries in the West, and now globally, that human beings have begun to feel entirely separate from each other and from Nature.

The word Macrobiotics was first used by German physician Christoph von Hufeland (1762–1836) in his book title translated in English as: *Macrobiotics or the Art of Prolonging Human Life*. Macrobiotics, as we know it today, developed during the 20th century in an effort to integrate the spirituality that developed in the East with the modern science and technology that was developing in the West. George Ohsawa, the founder of modern-day macrobiotics, synthesized these ideas from traditional understanding and chose the word macrobiotics to mean "life according to the largest view." Michio and Aveline Kushi, along with others of George Ohsawa's students, further developed and refined these ideas and then applied them to improving the health and way of life in modern society. Michio Kushi defined macrobiotics as "the universal way of health and longevity."

Macrobiotics is neither a traditional way of eating, nor is it a Japanese diet. It is traditionally based; the modern macrobiotic diet and lifestyle practices developed out of and evolved from the diet and lifestyle practices of the peoples and cultures of the world's long-standing civilizations. The macrobiotic diet incorporates the world's most unique foods from these civilizations (such as rice and miso from Asia, and sourdough bread from Europe, sesame tahini from the Middle East, peanut butter from the West, etc.) and uses them often or daily. Macrobiotic principles are expressed in the traditional cuisines of Asia, India, the Middle East, Europe, and Africa. My understanding and research has shown me that all the world's long-standing civilizations were grain-, bean-, and vegetable-based, all of them had a very strong sense of place, culture, identity, and connection to family and Nature, and therefore were all, in fact, macrobiotic.

As the 21st century unfolds, we continue to increase our involvement in food production and systems. The lifestyle practices of macrobiotics are useful and spiritually fulfilling. They help us learn how to realign with Nature and with those parts of ourselves we feel we may have lost in the past century.

THE BRIEF HISTORY

~12,000 years ago—retreat of the last Ice Age in northern Europe.
Previously, food was scarce and modern agriculture was yet to be redis-covered. Around this time, two noteworthy developments occurred: significant developments in agriculture and strides in boat building occurred over the next few thousand years, which paved the way and made possible our modern society. People could now stay in one place and more easily interact with neighboring people.

~10,000 years ago—evidence of agricultural villages.
The cultivation of cereal grains and the advent of modern grains such as barley, millet, wheat, and rice coincided with the domestication of animals as well as the development of pottery and weaving. The agri-cultural revolution led to the development of villages. All the world's long-standing civilizations cultivated grains as the principal food upon which every meal was based. Over time, people have become synonymous

with and inseparable from their grains: rice in the Far East, bulgur, couscous, pita in the Middle East; chapati in India; bread in Europe; oats in Britain; corn in the Americas. For example, you cannot separate rice from Asia, bread from Europe, or corn from the Americas.

There is a format to a meal. Whereas the United States Department of Agriculture (USDA) food pyramid makes recommendations based on a total daily intake of certain foods, it is much more helpful to plan eating around individual meals. A basic macrobiotic meal includes a grain, and at least one separate vegetable dish. A bowl of soup may be taken at one meal each day. Beans are also included daily. Meals made primarily of grains, beans, vegetables, soup, and pickled and fermented foods remained largely unchanged for thousands of years.

Chiefly supplemental to grains, beans, vegetables, and soups were animal and dairy foods. Historically, in agricultural societies, these foods were eaten in surprisingly small quantities. Meat and dairy were supplemental, not principal foods. Meat was eaten primarily at holidays and celebrations, mainly in the form of roasts and stews. In Europe, before the Industrial Revolution the average meat consumption was 5 to 10 kg (11 to 22 pounds) per person per year. That means for most people only a couple ounces of meat were consumed on a weekly basis. In China, India, and Japan the average was 2kg (4.4 pounds) per person per year. In addition, Japan had no history of dairy consumption, probably due to their consumption of soy products and sea vegetables. In more extreme climates and mountainous regions, dairy products such as cheese and yogurt were often used in ways similar to the use of miso and shoyu (fermented soybean products) in Asia.

~2,000–3,000 years ago—Ancient Greece and Rome began introducing the foods, cuisines, sweets, and spices from their trades with and conquests of tropical and subtropical areas.

~500–600 years ago—age of exploration, trade, and expansion rapidly increased the availability and popularity of exotic foreign foods and vegetables, sugar and spices, plants, and cooking styles.
During the beginning of the age of Western exploration and expansion in the 15th and 16th centuries, foods that were once locally grown and

indigenous to other parts of the world became more widely distributed. Tropical fruits and vegetables became more widely cultivated with their rise in popularity for customary table fare. For instance, the Spanish brought the potato (indigenous to Chile and the Andes) to Europe. Once in Europe, the potato gained wide acceptance over the next two hundred years. This starchy nightshade (related to tomatoes, peppers, and eggplants) began to replace the cereal grains in other cultures. Together with the tomato, these two foods "conquered" Europe more thoroughly than any other. With the age of exploration and Western expansion, many diets lost the important indigenous connection to food, which confused alignment with and created separation from Nature's cycles.

~300–200 years ago—The Industrial Revolution.
Britain, Europe, and the United States began adapting from an agrarian to an industrial society.

~90–100 years ago—World War I.
Advances made in nutritional studies and food science for the war effort.

~80–70 years ago—World War II.
Food science proliferated. The USDA Basic 7 Food Groups recommended that animal and dairy foods comprise about one quarter of the American diet to keep us strong and healthy. Chemicals were introduced into agriculture and the food supply. Modern food preservation also proliferated.

The Industrial Revolution in the 18th and 19th centuries had the greatest effect on changing the eating patterns that led to the modern diet. The industrialization of Britain, Europe, and the United States ushered in technological advances that enhanced the general quality of life as well as agricultural productivity. Industrialization created a demand for people to migrate to cities as well as implementing the widespread construction of factories. Transportation and communication were more mobile, but migration from rural to urban life affected people's eating habits—including dietary proportions.

Daily life became further removed from the natural cycles of the sun, moon, and seasons, and instead began to conform to a business week and a weekend. Nutrition became more imbalanced. With the new pressures of modern, industrialized life, slowly, physical and mental degenerative diseases began to increase.

Refined foods, especially refined grains, became more available on a wider scale (flour, for example, now could be sifted, easily packaged and ready-to-use, whereas, previously, time was needed to prepare the flour at home by hand). Refined foods, however, cause a nutritional imbalance, and many refined foods also cause blood to become more acidic. Minerals create a buffer action to neutralize the acidity. Refined grains lack these minerals. The greatest stores of minerals in grains are in the bran, which is partially or completely removed in the refinement process. Nutrition itself is a fine balance, where one nutrient is needed to absorb and utilize another. Altering this natural balance easily creates an excess of certain nutrients and a deficiency of others.

The combination of the disruption of eating patterns and the addition of refined grains caused nutritional imbalances and deficiencies. Refined grains allowed for the increased use of animal and dairy foods. We crave to supplement the nutrition lost in the refinement process. Increased animal and dairy foods in turn increase our cravings for sweets. These changes largely contributed to the vicious cycle that is the trademark of the modern diet—a diet high in refined foods, animal and dairy fats, and sweets. The strain of modern degenerative diseases began around the beginning of the 20th century and increased following World War II.

In the early 20th century, food began to be broken down into its components: calories, vitamins, proteins, minerals, etc. Judging food based on its components not only perpetuated imbalance, it helped create it. To break down food into its components is to take Nature out of food. Between WWI and WWII, recommendations to increase the consumption of animal and dairy protein only added to the confusion.

WWII paved the way for more devastating changes to our food supply as well to our nutritional guidelines. Modern, commercial food preservation is a by-product of WWII when methods were developed to ensure that foods would last for an indefinite period of time for soldiers overseas. This form of preservation prevents oxidation, enzymes, or bacteria from changing the food in any way. Chemical preservatives take life out of the food, making "dead foods" that cannot sustain health.

The uniqueness of food is that it is always different. The same dish cannot be made twice. Living foods change. Traditional methods of preservation such as drying, smoking, pickling, fermenting, and cold storing maintain and improve the nutrition available in the food, while simultaneously enhancing the natural quality. For example, sun drying increases vitamin D in mushrooms the same way it does in our own skin. Natural pickling and fermentation produces digestive-aiding enzymes, unique and previously nonexistent nutrients, and vitamin B-12. Apples in cold storage increase in both taste and nutrition. Un-yeasted sourdough bread is another example of a traditional preparation that enhances nutrition and satisfaction. Eating naturally preserved foods also enhances our own ability to synthesize nutrients we need. These foods are still living and slowly undergo subtle changes.

Frozen fruits and vegetables also increased during the period after the war. Analytically, these foods may be similar to fresh produce, but our bodies cannot be fooled. Nutrition is more than what can be measured in a laboratory.

Last, but not least, chemicals found their way into agricultural production. The chemical industry developed to create munitions for the war effort. Prior to WWII, natural foods were still commercially available. Whole-grain breads, untreated, local vegetables, natural pickles, and animals raised without hormones and antibiotics were still largely available. However, following the war, the chemical products were immediately applied to agriculture. Petroleum-based fertilizers began their widespread use after WWII. Slowly, the soil changed from living matter, teeming with and supportive of life, to inert matter.

"A nation that destroys its soils destroys itself. Forests are the lungs of our land, purifying the air and giving fresh strength to our people."

—Franklin D. Roosevelt

The excessive use of these fertilizers has destroyed living matter across countless acres of soil and has transformed this soil into inert matter made up of petroleum and its by-products. This destruction causes further soil erosion and ultimately these chemicals seep into our water supplies. The soil on commercial farms is more closely related to plastic, chemically speaking, than soil. This type of soil can only produce lifeless foods. The loss of minerals, unique microorganisms, and other life produces weak crops that need the aid of weed and pest killers in order to live long enough to harvest. These additional chemicals further weaken the crops, and our immune systems along with them.

Note that crop losses have increased each passing year since the late 1940s. This loss is proportional to the increased use of chemicals in agriculture. The soil is not very different from our collective immune systems. Our immunity has further decreased with the excessive use of antibiotics.

We have truly entered the era of modern degenerative illness. We are now expected to die of a degenerative illness, especially heart disease, cancer, or diabetes if an accident does not claim us first. Modern giant food companies have made a science out of food so that it is now possible to create it in a laboratory. It was in the era of WWII that our perception of food as something whole and unique was altered, broken up and transformed into a series of nutrients that could be measured and given out. As a result, food in the modern age is 100 percent consistent, but that also leads to the conclusion that it is not food at all.

~1953 TV became more popular and Swanson introduced TV Dinners.

~1955 First McDonald's opened.

~1956 The USDA modified nutritional recommendations to the Basic Four. The Basic Four recommended animal and dairy foods to comprise as much as 50 percent of our diet, which changed the way the entire world eats.

The diet and food quality in the West further deteriorated after fast foods appeared in the 1950s. Complete meals could simply be heated at home in the oven for a few minutes. The original fast-food restaurants began their spread throughout the United States and Britain. By the 1970s, fast foods had taken over completely. This coincided with the break from the traditional values of the society. Seemingly hundreds and thousands of years of tradition disintegrated overnight.

Most people born since the end of WWII no longer remember what fruits and vegetables are; they have been largely forgotten. Grains were grouped together with potatoes and reduced to starches. The trademark of the modern diet became meat and potatoes. The mythology that complete chains of amino acids could only be found in animal and dairy foods persisted until the 1970s. Although Frances Moore Lappé in her book *Diet for a Small Planet* dispelled this mythology, she still allowed the idea that protein-based nutrition was important.

All food has protein. We do not need to emphasize protein in our diet. The combination of grain, beans, vegetables, seeds, nuts, and fruits gives us the ideal amount of protein to promote lasting health. But the most important thing is that the body runs on glucose, which comes from the complex carbohydrates in our diet. The most important complex carbohydrates are unrefined grains, beans, and land and sea vegetables. What you eat today becomes your blood plasma tomorrow. Our blood plasma renews itself every ten days. We don't need to think of our food combining for complete proteins as long as we eat a variety of these complex carbohydrates within ten days.

"If man's Soul is indeed a kind of Stomach, what else is the true meaning of Spiritual Union but an Eating together?"
—Thomas Carlyle

Sadly, the family meal began to disappear with the new ease of getting quicker and seemingly more efficient meals. It fit in perfectly with the modern technological lifestyle. The family meal is the "glue" of a society. It provides a sense of belonging and stability in life. The dinner meal is very important because it gives everyone a chance to reunite and share the experience of food. Now that the family meal has dissolved, order has begun to change. Recent research has shown that one meal a day that includes talking with each other increases a child's chance of going to college as well as their ability to avoid drugs and alcohol. Cooking with electricity saved time, and getting a meal on the table became even more convenient when the microwave oven was introduced. Both have lessened our sensitivity to food and to cooking.

This is the completion of a cycle. Food that was once natural and shared for proper physical, emotional, and spiritual nourishment and social enjoyment has deteriorated to an almost careless mechanical process or afterthought.

The modern meal as we know it does not fit into a busy schedule. The demands of today's business world are so intense and so overwhelming that we cannot take the time to stop work and eat properly. We have lost touch with Nature and our ability to respond to the changing seasons. We are losing touch with our true human nature, and our feelings are confused. We can no longer enjoy and be guided by the natural rhythms of life.

~2008 The recession and banking collapse.
People are becoming more self-reliant, which includes taking responsibility for our own health.

~2009 to the present day—the continuing development of local food communities.
The 21st century presents us with many choices and opportunities to either continue along a path toward illness or move in the direction of health, both for ourselves and the planet. We are in a unique era when history and science have the opportunity to support each other to create a new medicine for humanity. We can start to move toward health when we reestablish connections to each other, to our communities, to Nature, and to the planet. Now more than ever, science confirms and validates parts of the human experience that have passed the test of time. A healthy future depends on both personal and planetary health.

The recession in 2008 was different from others. For all of my time involved with health, a recession characteristically causes people to spend more time and money on their health. Since 2008, people have been diverted from investing in their personal health. Due to environmental and societal pressures, getting through the day seems to be the main priority of many people. At the same time, there is a counterbalance to this.

"Though an old man I am but a young gardener."
—Thomas Jefferson

We are experiencing a broader collective desire for, and a return to, a local slow-foods culture. Vegetables are in vogue. Farmers' markets and CSAs are gaining momentum and spreading throughout the country.

"Go Green" is a marketing and branding mantra. Artisanal and fermented foods are now becoming a lucrative entrepreneurial niche in some communities. Preserving biodiversity through collecting seeds on small farms and exchanging them with others is now once again an operating prerogative of the true organic agriculture in the country.

In some ways, we seem to have returned to some of the natural philosophies held by the founding fathers. Ben Franklin and our early presidents placed great value in preserving land, seed, and agricultural systems. They were aware of the importance of our connection with Nature and the land. They shared a vision of building a nation and wealth based on an agrarian society, that personal and environmental health were interrelated.

Four understandings are becoming more widely accepted than they have been for decades. The first is a direct relationship between diet and health. It is becoming more and more evident that what we eat is important and that diet can prevent and even reverse serious illness including diabetes, arthritis, cardiovascular disease and many cancers. This means our health is in our own hands. There is no consensus yet on the best way of eating but that will come in time. History and science are confirming that a grain-, bean-, and vegetable-based diet are ideal for personal and planetary health.

The second is that there is a direct relationship between our food choices and the environment, including climate change. These choices determine whether we will preserve or further squander soil, land, water, and air. Modern industrial animal agriculture (CAFO or concentrated animal feeding operations) uses the most water and pollutes the most, followed by chemical and GMO agriculture.

The third is concern for animal welfare. Pets and animals are a very important part of many people's lives today. It is my experience that most people take better care of their pets than they take care of themselves. Many choose to avoid the use of animal testing for pharmaceuticals and cosmetics. There are more vegans today that take it as a moral principle to abstain from animal products than ever before.

And last, the earth is living and evolving. Therefore, it deserves the same care and respect as humans and animals. It does not deserve to be depleted, poisoned/polluted or ravaged through excessive industry, clear cutting, or drilling and mining.

It is becoming increasingly apparent that we are inseparable from each other, animals, and the planet. Now is the time to introduce sustainable and evolving practices that can strengthen and nourish personal and planetary health on all levels. At this point, it comes down to making a choice about how you will live your life. Your daily choices, actions, and attitudes will determine what we leave for our children and future generations. When enough of us embrace these ideals large-scale change will happen.

I see the practice of macrobiotics as a creative hub for the 21st century. A diet and lifestyle that helps to integrate our spiritual perceptions about the world around us, as well as the practical integration of a sustainable agriculture that promotes healthy people and a healthy planet. We all have a vital role in creating personal and planetary health through our daily choices. Step 3 demonstrates some practical applications to make this possible.

DIET: CONTENT AND QUALITY OF MEALS

STEP 3

Eat Two or Three Complete and Nutritionally Balanced Meals Every Day

Grain and vegetable dishes together at the same meal provide the most complete and balanced nutrition.

> "A meal without a grain is just a snack."
>
> —Michio Kushi

PLAN EVERY MEAL AROUND COOKED GRAINS AND GRAIN PRODUCTS

Moses in the Desert

Let's look at the biblical story of Exodus. Moses took the Jewish people out of Egypt to deliver them from slavery into freedom. He wanted the

Jews to build a new life free of the old enslaving concepts. However, the elders preferred what they knew to the possible dangers of the unknown. To fulfill his dream, Moses elected to have his people wander in the desert for forty years until the older generation died off. By then, the young had grasped the idea of living in freedom.

We have reached the end of a long dietary journey into the desert which emphasized animal and dairy foods as the basis of healthy meals.

The largest error was to assume that science was superior to Nature, as you found at the beginning of this section in the Brief History of Food. One significant myth was the notion that cow's milk or infant formula was healthier for babies than mother's milk. I was part of that experiment. My mother didn't nurse me. She fed me commercial baby formula followed by cow's milk. When I was in my twenties and learned about the physiological and psychological benefits of nursing for both mother and child, I asked her why she hadn't nursed me. She answered simply that at the time, doctors thought bottle-feeding was superior. Now we know that nursing develops children's immunity, general health, and thinking ability. It also helps children feel more secure emotionally and promotes a deeper bond between mother and child than bottle-feeding. Maybe your parents and grandparents started the day with a bowl of oatmeal, barley, Wheatena, Cream of Wheat, or corn grits. Compare that practice with today's choice of bacon and eggs with white toast, bagels with cream cheese, or coffee with doughnuts and/or muffins. Many people ate beans and a variety of seasonal fresh vegetables. Vegetable soup was considered essential daily fare. Yes, people did consume some animal and dairy food, but usually in small portions and balanced by all the fresh, natural food in their diets. Even common snacks that people once enjoyed, such as seeds, nuts, and dried fruits have been more or less forgotten. And in many parts of the country anyone advocating healthful food choices is thought to be referring to some foreign diet.

Macrobiotics is a way to help integrate these foods we forgot in the desert.

Today, the current recommendations strongly resemble the Healthful Foods list in the back of this book. This proves that there is a new awareness about healthful nutrition. Hopefully, the government will realize soon enough that plant protein is superior to animal protein and we have no need for dairy food after we are weaned from our mother.

"Healthy citizens are the greatest asset any country can have."
—Winston Churchill

Cereal Grain

There is one major problem, however. Hardly anyone today knows what a cereal grain is (cereal grain was the traditional name for all grains). If you ask people whether they eat cereal grains, the likely answer will be yes. That's because most of us think that dry breakfast cereals such as Cheerios, Rice Krispies, and corn flakes are cereal grains. To avoid confusion, I use the word "grain" to mean cereal grains that have been boiled, pressure-cooked, or used in traditional breads.

So let's talk about grains. Basically a grain is made up of three parts:

- Bran, the outer layer of the kernel, is the part that protects the grain from oxidation. It contains protein, minerals, and vitamins.
- Germ, the heart of the life-giving part, contains oil and vitamins. It is actually the seed of the grain.
- Endosperm, the starchy bulk or center of the grain, is mostly carbohydrate. It is the fruit of the grain, the food the seed uses to grow.

A single grain contains the beginning and the end of all plant food, since it merges the seed and the fruit into one. Grains and grain products are either "whole" or "refined." A grain is whole when all three of those parts are undisturbed and complete. A grain is refined when part or all of the bran or germ has been removed. The more of the bran and germ that is removed, the more refined the grain is. The more refined the grain, the more out of balance it is and the less nutritional value it has. Rice, wheat, and corn are the principal grains grown for human consumption. Rice is used by more than half of the world's population and is seen most widely in one of two types—brown rice and white rice.

Brown rice is whole-grain rice, with only the husk removed; it can be bought in any of three forms—short-, medium-, or long-grain. Short- and medium-grain rice are more natural to temperate climates; long-grain rice is preferable in hotter climates. Short-grain rice has more of a glutinous quality (not to be confused with the gluten in wheat), and when cooked it is somewhat stickier than long-grain rice. Brown rice is the world's most balanced food and is extremely high in nutritional value. It is recommended to be eaten often or daily. Brown rice combines deliciously with all other foods, even foods that are not part of the macrobiotic diet. Amazingly, whatever is cooked in the same pot with brown rice will be thoroughly cooked in the same amount of time it takes to cook the rice.

White rice has had its bran and germ removed, so it does not begin to compare nutritionally with brown rice. You would have to eat seven times as much white rice as brown to ingest the same nutrients!

Referring to a familiar, everyday food such as rice as a "grain" seems to confuse people. Virtually everyone has eaten lots of rice over the years, but probably without ever thinking of it as a grain. Rice is readily available and simple to cook, and it's important that you make it a staple of your daily diet. Another excellent way to ensure that your meal revolves around a grain is to eat pasta or noodles as your main food. Most people tend to like pasta. I am referring, of course, to good quality pasta or noodles, such as Italian durum wheat semolina pasta or Japanese udon or soba. Later in the book you will find a list of other grains, some of which are probably unfamiliar to you. It's best to start by eating brown rice and to develop the habit of making grains the focus of your meal.

When you are ready, visit the natural-food section of your local supermarket or health food store and check out the grains. Incorporate those you are already familiar with into your diet. If they are already part of your diet, use them more regularly as the centerpiece of your meals. My suggestion is that you plan every meal around cooked grains and grain products. Then complete and balance every meal with one or two vegetable dishes. Activate and harmonize your digestion with a bowl of vegetable soup at one or two meals. And always buy the highest-quality organically grown, unrefined, and naturally processed foods you can find.

Grains and Vegetables at Every Meal

Just as we use our mealtimes and rising and sleeping times to align externally with Nature's cycles, so we use the meal itself to align internally with our own biological cycles. Ongoing alignment with both cycles creates a powerful environment for the development of spiritual, emotional, and physical health. We cannot create this important biological alignment without first defining what we mean by the word "meal." A meal consists of a grain or grain product and at least one separate vegetable dish. Even if the grain or grain product has many vegetables in it, such as stir-fried noodles and vegetables, it is classified as a grain dish. This being the case, we are still missing a separate vegetable dish. When we add the vegetable dish, we have a meal. What I'm saying is this: your vegetable dish needs to be a separate dish, not vegetables cooked in or with something else, for example, in soup or in grains or grain products. Any vegetable cooked with grain becomes part of the grain dish. Any vegetable cooked in soup becomes part of the soup itself. To be annoyingly clear about this: the essence of a meal is a grain or grain product and at least one separate, stand-alone vegetable dish.

> "Tell me what you eat, and I will tell you what you are."
> —Anthelme Brillat-Savarin

Principal Foods

The term "principal food" refers to the food that is the centerpiece or core of the meal. In the modern American diet, protein in the form of meat or poultry or fish has been the most common principal food. In today's world, when a meal is planned, the first decision to make is what protein to serve. The rest of the meal evolves from this starting point. Most of the world's long-standing cultures, however, planned their meals around the grain dish, and this is the format we use. The first question to ask is: "What grain or grain product will be the centerpiece of my meal?" We might choose brown rice, barley, noodles, good-quality bread, polenta, or cracked wheat. The choice of grain is the center point around which the rest of the meal—which should include vegetables and other supplemental foods—should be planned.

The point is that natural foods, such as grains and vegetables, which all bestow health benefits, have been out of the mainstream American diet for such a long time that they are now considered weird. If you mention the word rutabaga or parsnip, most people don't know if you're talking about a vegetable or a dance craze. I recently heard of a family in which the children actually used the word rutabaga to taunt and insult each other! We have gotten so far away from wholesome food that we as a nation need reeducation. Paradoxically, although we live in a high-tech world that requires us to master very complicated material, for many of us the thought of having to acquire the simplest, most basic knowledge—how to improve our health through healthful eating—is overwhelming.

Cooking classes are the best starting place for your reeducation. Check the bulletin board of your natural food store for information on cooking classes, lectures, or seminars on natural diet and lifestyle. While you are there, pick up a cookbook or two. Cookbooks are good for ideas and inspiration once you have an understanding and image of healthful cooking and eating.

In the beginning stages, cooking can be learned only through personal experience. This is true of any style of cooking. To learn how to make a dish, we need to know three things—how the dish should look, how it should taste, and how it should smell. We cook from an image, and these factors form the basis of the image of whatever we are making. Once we have an image, we can reproduce the dish. If, when eating out, I come across a dish that I particularly like, I often replicate this dish at home—with slightly different ingredients, if necessary—but the point is that I always work from an image to create a new and healthful addition to my family's diet. In the past, people cooked using their intuition rather than cookbooks; but many years of eating foods that do not properly nourish the brain or the spirit have hampered our intuition.

A Great Way to Eat Food

"Macrobiotics is a great way to eat food." This is the answer given by my son Joe to the question, "What is macrobiotics?" I like the simplicity of his statement. It captures the feeling I have every time I sit down to eat. Once you are eating grains and vegetables on a regular basis, you will be able to understand what Joe meant by his remark. At first, you will begin to feel better and to look younger and brighter. Your thinking and reasoning abilities will become keener. After a short while, you will notice that your taste buds have changed. When this happens, and it will happen quickly, you will stop craving food that is detrimental to your health. The body has its own wisdom, and you will naturally crave healthful food. Hard as it is to believe, sooner or later, bacon and eggs will seem foreign to you!

I want to be clear about this: Americans must change their ideas about the meaning of complete nutrition. The modern practice of eating a lot of protein, especially animal protein, leads to serious illness. There is a real crisis in the healthcare industry because health insurance companies cannot keep up with the huge numbers of people needing medical help and hospitalization. If you accept the concept that we are what we eat and that food can either make us sick or keep us well, then you must conclude that both as a nation and as individuals, we have been making the worst possible food choices for a very long time.

Grains and Vegetables

If we want good health, it is crucial that we return to a diet based on unrefined foods and complex carbohydrates. A grain or grain product and at least one vegetable dish should be eaten at every meal—including breakfast. This may take some getting used to; but after a while, if you aren't able to have a vegetable as part of your breakfast, you will really miss having it. Vegetables complete cereal grains nutritionally, and they will help you to feel more satisfied with your meals. Try to use a variety of cooking styles and a variety of vegetables, because the more you vary both, the better your health will become. Green leafy vegetables, broccoli, and cabbage are all excellent sources of calcium and vitamin C, and they contain a surprising amount of protein.

Most of my children do not like "protein dishes." Some will eat beans occasionally, most like tofu but not tempeh, and only a few of them like seitan (a wheat gluten product). Most of them do like fish, but we serve fish only a few times a month.

In spite of this, they are mostly in the top 50 percent of their grade for height and weight. Where does their protein for growth come from? The only possibility is the combination of grains and vegetables. Fruit, oil, and grain-based sweets are also a regular part of their diet, and I am sure that these foods contribute to their growth as well.

Key Points:
- Grains and/or grain products are the centerpiece of a meal.
- Choose your grain first when planning a meal.
- Soft-cooked grains such as oatmeal or soft rice are best for breakfast.

- Eat brown rice often or daily.
- Brown rice is best when cooked with another grain such as pearled barley, millet, or sweet brown rice.
- Grains have the ideal balance of minerals, proteins, and carbohydrates that our body needs for balance and proper nourishment.
- You do not need to worry about the overall proportion of grains. Just eat a comfortable, satisfying amount.
- Start off with an equal portion of grains and vegetables or more vegetables than grains.

COMPLETE AND BALANCE EVERY MEAL WITH ONE OR TWO VEGETABLE DISHES

"The greatest delight the fields and woods minister is the suggestion of an occult relation between man and the vegetable. I am not alone and unacknowledged. They nod to me and I to them."

—Ralph Waldo Emerson

A Matter of Balance

What do we mean by balance? In order to feel satisfied, our bodies require a certain proportion of basic nutrients. We need approximately seven times more protein than minerals. This one-to-seven ratio represents a balance or an averaging of the numbers between one and ten and is not arbitrary. It derives from the workings of the natural environment. The rotation of the earth on its axis creates a powerful energy that we call earth's force—energy that is released upward from the center of the earth. The movement of the universe also creates a powerful energy—energy that flows downward toward the center of the earth and that we call heaven's force. Heaven's force is seven times greater than earth's force. This is why, in order to escape the earth's gravity and move into outer space, a rocket needs seven thousand pounds of thrust.

Around the world and down the centuries, definitions of balance and beauty have been based on this one-to-seven ratio. For example, classical

Greek statues of the 4th century B.C.E., the Golden Age of Greece, have heads that are approximately one-seventh the size of their bodies. That which is aesthetically beautiful and pleasing to the human eye is not arbitrary either. Rather, it is based on our innate sense of balance, a sense that comes directly from Nature.

Many things conform to the one-to-seven ratio, including the ratio of nutrients necessary to maintain human health and well-being. For example, if you eat a hard-boiled egg (concentrated protein), you will undoubtedly want to sprinkle some salt (minerals) on it. Salt improves the taste of eggs and makes them more digestible. Tofu needs soy sauce to make it tastier and easier to digest.

The human body requires seven times as much carbohydrate as protein. If we eat meat, we quite naturally crave potatoes or beer or sugar—some type of carbohydrate—to balance the meat and make it digestible. Grain is the only food that conforms to these ideal proportions. Grain contains about seven times as much protein as minerals and seven times as much carbohydrate as protein. Meat contains no carbohydrates. Therefore, meat by itself cannot completely satisfy us. Vegetables contain some carbohydrates but not in the one-to-seven proportion. Beans come closer than any food group besides grains.

Fat is a balancing agent between proteins and carbohydrates. The body has no difficulty converting fat into either protein or carbohydrate. If the body needs energy, it breaks fat down into glucose. Glucose provides the energy. Fat is converted to protein all the time. When we work out, we are converting fat into muscle protein. Conversely, protein can easily convert to fat if we eat too much protein or if we are not active.

Here's an important and little-known fact. Refined carbohydrates can produce fat in the body. This means that although many foods do not themselves contain cholesterol, they can create cholesterol. Overeating can also raise cholesterol levels. Craving or eating a lot of fat is a sign that your diet is out of balance. Fat is the nutrient that is most easily converted into protein or carbohydrate in the body. If our diet approximates the one-to-seven proportion of proteins and carbohydrates, we will not crave fat. This is why it is possible to follow a macrobiotic way of eating—which is very low in fat—and feel satisfied. Grain eating is balanced eating.

Simple and Complex Nutrients—Eat One and You Will Crave the Other
There is another element to consider when attempting to balance our diet.
If we eat simple minerals, such as sodium chloride (common table salt), we
will naturally begin to crave complex, or denser, protein—either animal
protein or very dense vegetable protein. When we eat simple minerals, meat
tastes better to us. If we eat complex animal or dairy protein, we will crave
simple (refined) carbohydrates. In practical terms, this means that a hamburger won't taste right on a whole-wheat bun. The complex protein of the
hamburger is not attracted to the complex carbohydrate of the whole-wheat
bun. Or take the example of fish sushi. Of course, it tastes much better
with white rice than with brown because, as we now understand, complex
craves simple. By contrast, vegetable sushi, a simple protein, tastes better
with brown rice, a complex carbohydrate. If you eat white rice, white bread,
sugar, and other simple carbohydrates like potatoes, your body will begin
to crave more complex protein, usually animal and dairy foods. On the
other hand, if you introduce complex minerals into your diet—in the form
of unrefined white sea salt (not Celtic or gray salt, please), seaweed, and
pickles—you will find yourself craving more complex carbohydrates, such
as whole unrefined grains and beans and vegetables. Here's a rewarding
fact of macrobiotic life. Once you are eating whole grains on a daily basis,
you will naturally begin to crave food that is good for you!

Refusing Vegetables
As a child, I refused to eat vegetables. Lettuce and tomato (in a sandwich)
were the only exceptions. My mother was an excellent cook, but I didn't
appreciate her skills. Food was a problem for me. Once a week I was per-
mitted to have dinner out with my friends. These were the meals I liked best.
I ate all the junk food my body could handle. Whether consciously or not,
throughout my childhood I refused vegetables completely. I would eat my
mother's vegetable soup only if she strained out the vegetables. I was that
bad! In light of this confession, it strikes me as highly ironic that I have spent
most of my adult life trying to persuade other people to eat their vegetables.

Within a week of incorporating brown rice into my diet, I started to
enjoy vegetables. I even began to crave them. The very food I had refused
to eat for so long was suddenly appetizing and desirable. Perhaps I have
even caught up with those of you who were smart enough to have eaten

vegetables all along. What I'm trying to convey is the fact that the process of moving from an unhealthful diet to a healthful one occurs naturally, if we follow some simple guidelines. Once we eat brown rice and vegetables on a regular basis, our cravings for unhealthful food tend to disappear.

Seaweed seduced me next. Seaweed amazed me. I remember walking into Sanae, the only macrobiotic restaurant in Boston, on a cold day in February of 1969 and ordering hiziki on impulse. The taste was new to me, neither good nor bad, but the memory of it stayed with me. The hiziki felt right in my body and I wanted to try it again. I have grown to truly love the taste of all seaweed and the way it makes me feel. My observation is that almost everyone grows to love seaweed. For some it takes time, others enjoy it immediately. Seaweed is unique, one of the more primitive foods we have. It provides a kind of nourishment and satisfaction that few other foods offer.

Perhaps it's akin to the love of raw oysters and clams that some of us develop. These are also primitive foods, but seaweed is vegetable-quality and has a wider appeal. My research has shown me that seaweed was traditionally eaten by all major cultures except those in Africa, where people ate river and lake weeds instead. In our own country, some Native American groups traveled great distances to harvest seaweed.

Upsetting the Balance

There are various ways in which we may upset the balance inherent in the macrobiotic diet. One way is by eating too much baked or roasted or toasted food. In essence, baking, roasting, or toasting is carbonizing. If you burn a piece of toast, what you are left with is carbon. Although carbon is a mineral common to all living things, the catch is that once we increase the amount of carbon in our diet through baking, toasting, roasting, or burning, we automatically begin to crave more complex proteins (animal and dairy food) as well as refined grains. Excess carbon throws off the body's entire mineral balance. Cravings for strong foods, such as meat, appear; feelings of guilt and despair occur, and the person to whom this is happening doesn't understand why. Too much baked or roasted or toasted food can be a recipe for disaster.

There are many tempting macrobiotic baked products available in health food stores today; so it's important to keep in mind that if you eat too many of these products, you will find it difficult to resist the lure of other unhealthful foods. Try to limit your intake of baked foods of all kinds, including bagels. It's okay to indulge yourself once in a while, but certainly not on a regular basis.

If a Little Is Good, a Lot Is Not.

The other most common way of upsetting the balance of the macrobiotic diet is by using too much seaweed, especially kombu. Kombu is a type of kelp that is very beneficial to health. It helps lower fat and cholesterol levels, among other things. Seaweed, including kombu, is also a good source of minerals—calcium is one of them—but eating too much kombu over a long period of time can interfere with mineral absorption. To absorb minerals, we need some oil or fat in our diet, and seaweed directly affects how the body utilizes oil and fat.

People tend to think that if a little of something is good for them, then more must be even better; but often that's not true. Excess can lead to serious deficiency. In the case of seaweed, less is more—meaning less is better. Seaweed should be taken in small amounts, but people typically increase their intake over time—often dramatically. As I just mentioned, too much seaweed can interfere with the body's ability to absorb minerals. The following is what can happen if we become mineral-deficient because of an excessive intake of seaweed: in an attempt to regain its ability to absorb minerals, the body develops strong cravings for fat and protein; we begin to eat more fat and protein. Then because we feel better after eating this way, we assume it must be good for us—we must have needed more animal food. Looked at in one way, this is not an incorrect assumption. In order to overcome an imbalance, the body cries out for fat. But you can see that it would be far better not to create an imbalance at all. Be careful with the quantity of seaweed you use. It's important not to upset your body's mineral balance.

There's another problem with eating too much seaweed. One of the things the body does with fat is to convert it into sex hormones. If we decrease the body's fat content too much, in other words, if there isn't enough fat available because its absorption has been interfered with—and an overuse of seaweed and salt can do this—we invite an imbalance of sex hormones.

Key Points:

- Have at least one vegetable dish with every meal, including breakfast.
- Have a variety of vegetable dishes—well cooked, lightly cooked, pressed, pickled, and raw throughout the days and weeks.
- Grains and vegetables together provide the basis of complete and balanced nutrition.
- Do not reheat leftover vegetable dishes. They lose their refreshing and nourishing qualities and leave you unsatisfied. If they have been refrigerated, take them out in advance and let them warm up naturally.

ACTIVATE AND HARMONIZE YOUR DIGESTION WITH A SERVING OF VEGETABLE SOUP AT ONE OR TWO MEALS DAILY

Let's take a closer look at soup. Soup conditions or relaxes the digestive system and readies it to accept the meal. As I mentioned earlier, there are basically two types of soup—savory (what one ordinarily thinks of as vegetable soup) and puréed sweet vegetable soup.

Generally, savory soups, such as miso vegetable, bean vegetable, or shoyu (natural soy sauce) vegetable broth, are taken at the beginning of the meal. Most vegetable or bean soups that we are familiar with are savory soups. Sweet vegetable soups are eaten throughout the meal. If you find this confusing, the safest approach is to eat your soup at the start of your meal.

All savory soups activate digestion. If a naturally fermented seasoning such as miso or shoyu is cooked into the soup, it will further aid the digestive process. Fermentation helps create good bacteria, yeast, and enzymes to form a healthful environment in the intestines.

All sweet vegetable soups, being mild and sweetly creamy, help to relax, harmonize, and coordinate the digestive system and its central organs—the pancreas, stomach, liver, and gallbladder. When these organs are aligned, digestion is smoother. Sweet vegetable soup does not have to be puréed although it is more effective that way.

> "An old-fashioned vegetable soup, without any enhancement, is a more powerful anti-carcinogenic than any known medicine."
>
>   —James Duke, M.D. (USDA)

More Savory than Sweet Vegetable Soup

We all need a combination of sweet and savory soups, but we need about two to three times more savory soup. Serve puréed sweet vegetable soup two to three times in a seven- to ten-day period, and eat a variety of savory soups the rest of the time. Any vegetable soup that has either miso, shoyu, or sea salt cooked in it is a savory soup. For instance, you can turn lentil vegetable soup into miso soup by seasoning it with miso. If you take the same soup and season it with shoyu, you create lentil-vegetable shoyu soup. Both versions qualify as savory.

Relieving Stress

Foods with a creamy texture are more relaxing and consoling, and that soothing quality has a positive effect on the digestive system. During the Great Depression, sales of ice cream skyrocketed. People had no money for anything other than the bare essentials; nevertheless, they bought ice cream. During really hard, stressful times, it seems we seek creamy foods for consolation. If you make sure you have the proper amount of sweet, creamy soup, you will have an easier time controlling the stress level in your everyday life. Stress hardens and tightens the digestive organs. Puréed soup helps them stay relaxed. Remember, if you're feeling nervous or pressured, it's important to take a few minutes to relax before sitting down to eat.

> "Soup puts the heart at ease, calms down the violence of hunger, eliminates the tension of the day, and awakens and refines the appetite."
>
>   —Auguste Escoffier

Miso Soup

Miso soup has always been an important part of the macrobiotic diet. Recently, it's made its way into the mainstream—perhaps because it's so easy to prepare. Please consider restricting your intake of miso soup to what you make at home. The quality of miso paste used by restaurants is often very poor. Traditionally, it took one to two years to age and ferment miso properly. By artificially controlling temperature and using chemical fermentation, commercial miso can be made in one week! As an added insult, commercial miso is often flavored and dyed and may even contain monosodium glutamate (MSG), an unhealthful chemical preservative and taste enhancer. Commercial miso doesn't have any of the benefits that naturally fermented miso, available in most health food stores, has.

More Is Not Better.
It's important to have one or two bowls of soup a day. One bowl is generally enough. If you feel like having a second bowl, by all means have it. If you do have a second soup, try to make it a different type of soup.

For most people however, two soups every day is too much. Eating soup with every meal is definitely a bad idea. As with many other food choices in the macrobiotic diet, more soup is not better. Too much soup, rather than strengthening digestion, will weaken it. As for quantity, a standard cup or small bowl-sized serving is adequate. Please keep in mind that a bowl of soup by itself does not qualify as a meal—even if it contains a grain. It's important to understand that soup, whether it's miso or shoyu or sweet vegetable, does not count as a complete and nutritionally balanced meal—at breakfast or at any other time. Which brings me to my next point. For many years, macrobiotic teaching has recommended taking miso soup at breakfast.

However, it's been my observation that some people are hungry all day long if they do this and, as a result, they overeat. Why? Miso soup has a powerful capacity to stimulate digestion; and when digestion is stimulated, we want to eat. I now recommend taking miso soup no more than once a day at whatever meal works best for you. Experiment. Try it for breakfast on one day, lunch on another and, on another day, for dinner. See at which time it works best for you, at which time you leave the table feeling most satisfied.

Key Points:
- There are two main types of soup: savory vegetable soup is well seasoned and mildly salty; puréed sweet vegetable soup is mildly sweet with a pleasant creamy taste.

- Soup with a savory taste activates digestion and stimulates the appetite.
- Puréed sweet vegetable soup helps relax and harmonize the digestive system. It has a calming and consoling effect.
- Have two to three times more savory than sweet soups, i.e., two to three bowls of sweet vegetable soup in a seven- to ten-day period.

INCORPORATE A WIDE VARIETY OF FOODS INTO YOUR DIET

Natural foods come in an endless variety of interesting combinations, tastes, and textures. If you make an effort to try new foods and new recipes, I can assure you that your taste in food will change quickly.

Greater variety in your diet will make you feel more satisfied and will provide better nutrition as well. Start by adding a few new foods each week. The biggest mistake beginners make is to find a few foods they like and eat them over and over. Although this approach might work for a while, in the end it leads to boredom and dissatisfaction. It is also nutritionally limited. As you become more familiar with natural foods, you will gain confidence in your ability to create satisfying, healthful, and exciting meals. The more new foods you add to your diet, the more your taste for natural foods will return.

I use the word "return" because I believe our taste for healthful food is natural. Years of eating unwisely sap our ability to enjoy natural foods. My proof is that young children love well-prepared natural foods on their first try. From time to time throughout the years, my children have been reluctant to invite their friends over for fear they wouldn't like our way of eating. Usually these friends enjoy the food so much, they ask for seconds. If they don't like our food the first time, they usually come around after a few more tries.

There is far more variety available in a plant-based way of eating than in the modern American diet. The key to success is to consciously increase variety over time. Now that so many supermarkets carry natural foods and organic produce, you can start your education there. Once you feel more confident, make a trip to your local health food store.

Styles of Cooking

Try to use a wide variety of cooking styles when you prepare your meals. The macrobiotic repertoire is extensive. For daily use, I recommend pressure-cooking, boiling, blanching, steaming, steaming with kombu seaweed (called nishime style), soup-making, stewing, quick sautéing with water or oil, sautéing and simmering (kinpira style), pressing and pickling, and raw. On the Styles of Cooking list toward the back of this book (p. 190), you will find baking, broiling, dry-roasting, pan-frying, deep-frying, and tempura (batter-dipped deep-frying) food listed under Occasional Use (p. 197).

When planning your meals, select foods within the following categories: whole grains, soups, vegetables, beans, sea vegetables, and beverages. Use different cooking methods from the above list. Keep in mind that it's best not to pressure-cook vegetables. Start with those cooking styles that are familiar. If possible, take macrobiotic or natural-foods cooking classes. Read cookbooks to inspire and teach you.

Vegetables can be cut in various ways. Try slicing them into rounds or half-moons. You can cut the slices straight across or on the diagonal and you can vary the thickness of the slices. Different methods have subtly different effects on the flavor and appearance of whatever dish you prepare.

Vary the kinds of seasoning and condiments you use. Use different seasonings in dishes you are familiar with and take note of how just a small change in the seasoning of a dish can produce a big difference in taste. Try seasoning that same dish with a little more or less of what you normally use. The type and amount of seasoning will each bring out different aspects of flavor and can subtly alter the consistency of a dish. Some seasonings firm up a dish, so to speak, while others have a softening effect.

It's important to vary the cooking time of vegetables. Most of us could use more lightly cooked vegetables in our diet. What do I mean by a lightly cooked vegetable? It's one that makes a crunchy sound when you bite into it. The sound should be audible to someone sitting next to you. No sound means the vegetable is well cooked. Include a combination of well cooked and lightly cooked vegetable dishes weekly. Experiment with cooking times. Cook familiar dishes a little longer or for a little less time.

And don't forget that raw salad is an important part of the macrobiotic diet. Have a salad at least a few times a week. In most cases, it's fine on a daily basis. Try varying the intensity of the flame when you cook. The same dish can taste quite different depending on whether it's been cooked slowly or quickly. Many people use too much fire when cooking. It seems to be a natural tendency to turn the flame up as high as possible, whether it's needed or not. Excessive use of a high flame in your cooking may make you nervous or irritable. Use a medium flame when you want to bring something to a boil. If necessary, you can always turn it up at the end of cooking. You will feel calmer and steadier as a result.

Vary the combination of dishes you use in meals. Change just one dish and you have added a new meal to your repertoire. And vary the combination of vegetables, grains, beans, and seasonings you use in your dishes.

Cook your food a little longer in the winter for a warming, energizing effect. Cooking food a bit less in the summer will produce a cooling and relaxing effect.

Try to create a variety of color, taste, and consistency in your meals. Variety means using many different ingredients from each of the different categories, changing the method of preparation and changing the combinations of food. Imagine what the meal will look like on the plate, imagine how it will taste. Remember that variety creates interest. Try to surprise your family and friends. Keep them guessing. They are sure to enjoy and appreciate your efforts.

SUGGESTIONS FOR PLANNING MEALS

First considerations
- Grains and vegetables together form the basis of complete and balanced nutrition.
- All food has protein. You do not need to make a special effort to increase protein in your diet. It is nearly impossible to become protein-deficient.
- If you feel that you are craving protein, increase beans, tofu, tempeh, seitan, and possibly add fish.

- A variety of vegetable foods provides the most abundant and well-balanced nutrition available: minerals including calcium, potassium, proteins, carbohydrates, fats including omega-3, and vitamins including vitamin C. Vitamin D comes from exposing your skin to the sun.
- Beans may be included in the same meal or even the same dish as fish.
- Seitan, a wheat gluten product, may be cooked with grains or beans.

When planning your daily meals, try to follow the order below

- Always decide on the grain or grain product first.
- Then choose the vegetable dish and/or dishes that complement and harmonize the grain.
- Next, decide on the soup to further complete the meal.
- Last, supplement with foods from the other categories, specifically beans, sea vegetables, seeds, nuts, fish, fruit, snacks, desserts, sweets, and beverages, if you choose.
- Use these guidelines whether you are eating at home or out.

Questions to ask when planning every meal

- What grains or grain products do I want?
- What vegetable dishes do I want?
- Will they be freshly prepared or leftover?

Questions to ask every day

- What soup will I have today?
- Am I including brown rice in one of my meals today?
- What beans and/or bean products shall I have today?
- Am I including a variety of well cooked, lightly cooked (meaning bright, colorful, and crunchy), and raw vegetable dishes?

Questions to ask when planning your weekly menu

- Am I incorporating sea vegetables into my diet?
- Shall I have fish this week?

- What desserts and snacks shall I have?
- Am I getting enough variety in the other categories, including seeds, nuts, fish, fruit, mild natural sweets, and beverages?
- Are my meals appealing, tasty, colorful, and satisfying?
- Have I remembered to incorporate leftovers to save time on cooking?

ORDER OF PLANNING MEALS

	MODERN DIET	MACROBIOTIC DIET
1. Principal Foods, the centerpiece of every meal	**Protein:** Meat, poultry, eggs, cheese, or fish; For vegetarians: Beans, soy products, textured soy protein, etc.	**Grains or Grain Products:** Brown rice, barley, millet, polenta, pasta, oatmeal, couscous, whole-wheat bread, etc.
2. Main Secondary Foods, they complete, balance, and harmonize every meal	**Starch:** Potatoes, pasta, bread, white rice, or other refined grains	**Vegetables:** Well cooked, lightly cooked, pickles, salad
3. Soup with 1 or 2 meals a day	Infrequent	Miso, vegetable, lentil, puréed squash, etc.
4. Other Foods throughout the week	Salad, vegetables, fruits, snacks and sweets, dessert, or beverages	Beans, seeds, nuts, fish, fruit, snacks, dessert, beverages
5. Essence of a Meal	Protein, starch, and beverage	Grain, vegetable, and soup
6. Typical Meals	Meat, potatoes and coffee Pizza and soda Pizza and beer Hamburger, fries, and soda Omelet, fries, toast, and coffee	Brown rice, steamed kale or collards, and bancha twig tea Couscous, sautéed onion and broccoli, and miso soup Steamed tofu sandwich on whole-wheat bread with tahini and sauerkraut and apple juice Pasta, vegetables, and tea, spring water, or beer Polenta, broccoli rabe, red snapper, and wine

Key Points:

- Create variety by varying the ingredients in each of the categories, changing the method of preparation and the combination of foods in the dishes you create.
- Try not to settle on a few dishes and combinations and then continually repeat them.
- Variety ensures the most balanced nutrition and helps you feel more satisfied.
- All foods contain protein. The vegetable protein in grains, beans, and vegetables is superior to animal protein for health, endurance, and vitality.

BUY THE HIGHEST-QUALITY ORGANICALLY GROWN, UNREFINED, NON-GMO, AND NATURALLY PROCESSED FOODS

High-quality organic food tastes better. It's more nourishing and strengthening to your health. Many people are willing to buy expensive cars, clothes, and houses, but when it comes to buying food they won't spend the extra money for the best quality. Please, don't save money on your food. Try to buy mostly organically grown food, in particular, staples like daily-use vegetables and grains, miso, sea vegetables, shoyu, ume and brown rice vinegars, and umeboshi plums etc., even if you have to travel or mail-order to do it. What is not available, you can certainly supplement with commercially grown food. If most of your food is organically grown, then some unrefined and commercially produced food is not going to harm you and you will enjoy the benefits of increased variety.

That said, it's vital to remember that quality can be adjusted up or down. Here's an example of what I mean: If you think Diet (Content and Quality) is more important than Eating Habits (Format) and you want to eat organically grown, pressure-cooked short- or medium-grain brown rice, but it's not available to you at that moment, then what do you do? Well, many people think if they can't practice perfectly, if they can't have the best food all the time, then they're not good macrobiotics. So they abandon the diet temporarily and proceed to make terrible choices. This is a pretty common response, particularly when traveling. However, if you want to eat well, you can eat well under any circumstances. If you have a health problem, the best thing to do is prepare ahead so you don't get stuck. An understanding of the controlling factors of macrobiotic practice and how to adapt to difficult circumstances is very important.

Adjusting Quality

Let me explain what I mean when I say that quality can be adjusted up or down. Despite what you might think, white rice and commercially made pasta qualify as a grain and grain product. Steamed vegetables without butter are still vegetables. You can order vegan vegetable soup. Will it be macrobiotic quality? No, not exactly. It may be made with potatoes or tomatoes or both but it's still vegetable soup. Remember that as long as you stick to the Format, you will be moving in the direction of health. To tell if you are becoming lax about the Format, watch for danger signals such as reading or watching TV at the table, eating or snacking while standing, not chewing thoroughly, rushing through meals, not allowing three hours between eating and sleeping and so on. If these things begin to happen and you are not alert to them, it's only a matter of time before you create an imbalance, and imbalances tend to perpetuate themselves. So long as you concentrate on the Format of Meals (Eating Habits), over time your diet will become more and more healthful. You will come to understand intuitively what you need to improve and maintain good health. But if you focus on Diet (Content and Quality of Meals), then automatically you will begin thinking in terms of good and bad, right and wrong, calcium and protein, etc., and when we think this way we get off track. It's very easy to fall into this sort of thinking. It's the way we've been taught, and modern education, being so powerful, is hard to overcome.

Our goal is simply this: to have good digestion, good absorption, and good circulation. After all, what is the difference between being young and being old? The answer is good digestion, good absorption, and good circulation. If the food that enters the body can be digested and absorbed and the excess evacuated easily and if the blood can circulate, then we can cure ourselves of anything. We can reverse the effects of illness and unnatural aging, if we practice accurately. We can even wind back our biological clock and become much younger than our biological age.

Vegetarian?

We've found that many restaurants use chicken stock in so-called vegetarian dishes. It is better not to make assumptions. If you're eating away from home, it is best to ask whether meat, poultry, or chicken stock were used in the preparation of the food.

Key Points:
- High-quality food tastes better.
- It's more nourishing and strengthening to your health.
- Quality can be adjusted up or down.
- Buy organically grown food as much as possible. Supplement with commercially grown food when the full variety of organic food is unavailable.
- Make sure to choose non-GMO foods.

LIFESTYLE: APPROACH TO HEALTH

Make Your Daily Life Active

WALK OUTSIDE FOR THIRTY MINUTES EVERY DAY. LIFE-RELATED EXERCISE PROVIDES THE MOST BENEFIT FOR LASTING HEALTH

I want to encourage you to make your daily life as active as you can by incorporating what I call universal exercise. Universal exercise means life-related exercise—activities directly connected to life. These are the activities that provide the most benefit and balance for all of us.

When do you think people were generally healthier—in the past when they led physically active daily lives, or today when they are so exercise-conscious? I always ask this question in seminars and the audience almost always responds: "In the past."

Healthy people rarely think about exercise. Their lives are so active that there's no need. They play; they enjoy and challenge themselves; they may garden, do home repairs, dance, or engage in sports. In other words, they are active but they are not formally exercising. We've been educated to think we need structured exercise. We don't. What we need is to move our bodies, to play, to enjoy ourselves physically, to challenge and stimulate ourselves. Structured exercise has a kind of hardness and rigidity about it; play has a soft and flexible quality.

Here's an analogy I like. Who is healthier—the person who eats a healthful diet or the person who eats an inadequate diet and takes supplements? My point is that since healthy people are clearly getting all the nourishment they need from their diet, the idea of taking supplements never occurs to them.

Let's apply this observation to exercise. Structured exercise is nothing more than a supplement for those people who have inadequate daily activity. In order to feel well, those who lead sedentary lives have to compensate with some kind of regular program of exercise.

Exercise versus Play

Healthy children never think about exercise until they go to school where they are taught that they need to exercise. Before that they simply played and were healthy and happy. Children lose their energy only when they're told to do something they don't want to do, such as cleaning their rooms. A child's natural need to move is changing now because of poor diet. It's not natural for children to want to sit around all day and watch television. My children enjoy television but they know it's self-limiting. After a while they are always running off to do something else. Only on rare occasions do I have to say, "That's enough TV."

The best exercise for your health is the exercise that human beings were designed to do, exercise that doesn't require machinery, gyms, or classes. Like the air we breathe, it's free of charge. I refer to walking. Walking outside at a comfortable pace with an unforced stride is the best exercise on the planet.

Don't worry about cardiovascular rates and, please, don't engage in "power walking." The value of walking comes from the rhythmic movement—not the pace. A somewhat brisk half-hour walk every day (or two fifteen-minute ones) will keep the body fit and the spirits high. Walking increases flexibility and improves digestion, energy, and cardiovascular health. It strengthens the bones and helps clear the mind and balance the nervous system. Walking is the ideal activity for everyone.

It is the brown rice of physical activity, so to speak. It's best not to think of walking as "exercise" per se. You can think of it as a way to get from point A to point B, if you like; you can think of it as a period of time to clear your mind and let your thoughts come. The more open your mind is when you walk, the more benefit you will receive. The people who get the least out of walking are the ones who are trying to accomplish something, such as getting their heart rate up or listening to music or a podcast on their phone. Why? When we have an agenda, the mind closes to other possibilities. Take children as your model. Children have the best activity; they play and enjoy themselves. They don't think they're exercising or getting healthy. As long as they're playing and enjoying themselves, their minds are open.

If strenuous exercise were the panacea it is said to be, then professional athletes would be among the healthiest people in the world. Yet this is not the case. Many, perhaps even a majority, of them suffer from serious chronic injuries and other health problems. Many die young. Modern nutritional thinking says that large amounts of animal food are necessary for building stamina and keeping a competitive edge. As a result, the diet of athletes is usually high in meat, dairy products, and refined carbohydrates. Athletes are given to believe that their health will not suffer since participation in strenuous sports compensates for dietary excess. Now, you don't have to be a genius to understand that if you eat excessively, your body will suffer the effects regardless of how much you exercise. It's a matter of common sense.

Not too long ago, I saw the results of a research study on the immune system of professional athletes as compared to that of the average person. According to this study, the immune system of the professional athlete is weaker than that of the average person. Apparently, professional athletes are more likely to come down with colds than are those who don't compete professionally. When the body is overworked, immunity is impaired. Pushing the body beyond its natural limits in any way is not a healthful thing to do.

> "The sovereign invigorator of the body is exercise, and of all exercises walking is the best."
>
> —Thomas Jefferson

Walking and Balance

It's not necessary to walk briskly for a full half-hour at one time. Two fifteen-minute walks are also effective. Keep in mind that the benefits of walking come from the balancing effect of rhythmic movement on the body. We derive the greatest benefits from walking when our arms are free to swing like a pendulum. The alternating movement of arms and legs has a balancing effect on the body as a whole, and on its functions as well. To be specific, this is what happens: both parts of the digestive system, the ascending and the descending colon, coordinate with each other; the left lung and the right lung do the same as well as the kidneys and adrenals. Both branches of the autonomic nervous system—that part of the overall nervous system that regulates breathing, digestion, and, in fact, all of the body's automatic functions—are coordinated and brought into balance.

At the same time, walking helps balance the mind. When you feel anxious or worried, try taking a walk. After a short time, you will find yourself thinking more clearly and, in general, feeling better. If you are depressed, taking a walk will refresh your spirits. If you are overtired, a walk will renew your energy. If you have too much energy, a walk will settle you down.

The feet and legs have two roots, one is the heart and lungs and the other is the brain. Each step is activating and coordinating the two chambers of the heart and both lungs. At the same time walking activates and harmonizes the left and right hemispheres of the brain. The bottom of the feet especially correlate with the brain. The greatest benefit comes from walking barefoot on the grass or beach by the edge of the water.

"Today I have grown taller from walking with trees."

—Karl Baker

Walk Outdoors

Walking outdoors is far more beneficial than walking indoors. We need to be outside for one simple but compelling reason. Nature has the best circulation. Anything we do outdoors helps our circulation more than anything done inside. A walk outside in pleasant surroundings, in the woods or in a park, for example, amid grass and trees, is ideal; but even a walk on a busy city street is better than walking inside on a treadmill or track. When you walk, the quality of the air you take in is important and, as a rule, outdoor air is less polluted than indoor air. One of the most important benefits of walking is exchanging your internal environment with the external. Walking outdoors harmonizes, cleans, refreshes, and renews you in every possible way—physically, energetically, emotionally, and mentally. With this in mind, try to keep your home or office well ventilated. Open your windows.

Do Healthy People Exercise?

Let's consider an earlier statement of mine: healthy people rarely think about exercising. The fact is that the most valuable exercise occurs as we go about living our daily lives. When we walk, shop, clean, or do other things around the house, we are exercising without really thinking about it. And when we are active while doing what we enjoy—whether it's dancing, tennis, martial arts, swimming, mountain climbing, or biking—we are exercising without having to force ourselves. It's important to find activities that are satisfying, challenging, and stimulating. The thought should not be, "I have to do this, it's good for me," but rather, "I can't wait to get out there and do this." It's simply common sense that if you engage in activities you enjoy, you will keep on doing them and never think of them as "exercise." I want to be very clear about this. I am not saying don't exercise. What I'm saying is this: make your life active. Do whatever stimulates and challenges you. If you think it's "good" for you, don't do it.

Again, take healthy children as a model. Observe them. See how they always try to challenge and stimulate themselves. When they've had enough of something, they move on to something else.

Many people find daily exercise combined with a healthful diet to be the easiest Strengthening Health recommendation to follow. Walking is an enjoyable way to keep physically fit. If you are not already in the habit of walking, you will be surprised by the deep sense of well-being that a daily walk gives.

"All truly great thoughts are conceived by walking."

—Friedrich Nietzsche

A Barometer

If our exercise is appropriate, our appetite for healthful food will be enhanced. Appropriate exercise helps us eat less and feel more satisfied. We can tell that our exercise is inappropriate if our craving for rich food and sweets increases, if we overeat but feel less satisfied.

Cleaning

In more traditional times, even as recently as fifty years ago, cleaning was valued in proportion to its benefits. Cleanliness, of both person and surroundings, was said to be next in importance to godliness. Like walking, the benefits of cleaning are universal—unless you have an attitude about it! We feel better physically and mentally when we clean. Cleaning clears the mind as it activates the body. It helps harmonize and balance our condition. Try it and you'll see.

Obesity in Children

Obesity is a major problem in the United States. Approximately two out of three adults are overweight and more than one in six children are overweight or obese. "Morbidly obese" is the term used to define that degree of obesity that is considered life threatening. There are so many obese children that even the government has been forced to take notice. Obesity in children is the cause of the current epidemic of Childhood Onset Diabetes. Obesity starts with diet. Children who are fed too many high-fat foods and sweets are less inclined to run around and play because their young bodies are too busy trying to metabolize all the excess. These children are most comfortable slumped in front of a TV set or computer for hours at a time.

Many of my children's friends are not from macrobiotic families, so at our birthday parties we usually serve ice cream and other sugared foods to make their friends feel comfortable. Of course, there are always plenty of macrobiotic goodies as well. Over the past decade, I've noticed that often these children hardly touch the cake and ice cream, although my children usually eat their fair share. My explanation of this seemingly odd behavior is that these children don't find party foods to be anything special. These foods are special for my children because they don't have them very often. For their friends, however, cake and ice cream are actually everyday foods. The result is an ever-increasing rate of obesity among children.

A healthful diet creates a natural craving for activity. It's a kind of chain reaction. We need a good diet in order to be active. If we are active and if we are satisfied with our food, chances are we won't find ourselves overeating.

War and Nutrition

If we use history as a guide, we can see the effects of the decline in nutrition and activity levels by analyzing the health of the soldiers who fought in various wars. Roman soldiers were hired mercenaries. They were paid in grain, primarily an ancient type of barley, and this grain was their principal source of nutrition. Fueled by a grain-based diet, Roman soldiers conquered almost half the world. Roman generals maintained a strict daily regimen that kept their legions fit for the task of conquering strong foes, sometimes armies far larger than their own. It was not unusual for a legion to march twenty-five to thirty miles a day, each man carrying full weaponry and daily food supplies on his back. The fall of the Roman Empire followed on the heels of widespread changes in eating habits and daily activity. The Roman legionnaires, by eating the foods of the lands they had conquered and occupied, grew lazy and gluttonous, often gorging themselves until they vomited. Banquets, at which huge amounts of food were consumed, became a daily feature of life. A downfall was inevitable.

Autopsies of young soldiers who died in action in the Korean War revealed badly clogged arteries and signs of advanced cardiovascular disease. The medical community was shocked. The question asked was whether the government's policy of feeding soldiers a high-protein, high-meat diet had caused the disease. Autopsies of soldiers who died in the Vietnam War presented similar findings. In light of the evidence, it's difficult to understand why the government took so long to change its food recommendations.

Key Points:
- Walk outside to get the maximum benefit. Walking outside aligns you with the natural environment. Contact with the earth, exposure to trees and grass and to the natural circulation of air are crucial to good health.

- Walking is not exercise. It is natural movement. It creates harmony between body and mind, improves circulation and digestion, and increases flexibility and bone strength.
- Walking outside renews you in every way—physically, energetically, emotionally, and mentally.
- Walk once a day for a minimum of thirty minutes or twice a day for fifteen minutes. A natural, comfortable stride is recommended.
- Imitate children and try to play rather than exercise.
- Life-related activities such as cleaning, gardening, dancing, etc., provide the most benefits.

GIVE YOURSELF A DAILY BODY RUB

Gently rub your entire body with a hot, damp cotton washcloth for ten to fifteen minutes every morning and/or night. Do the rub before or after your bath or shower. Do it separately from either at the sink or in a dedicated body rub basin. The body rub is the secret of the fountain of youth. In effect, it winds back the body's biological clock. If you do a daily body rub, walk outside for thirty minutes, and chew your food thoroughly, day by day you will become younger in body and mind. Others will remark and ask what you have been doing!

The body rub is one of the world's best beauty treatments. People come to me for counseling with a variety of skin problems—brown liver spots, white patches, blemishes, and skin that is loose, dry, or sagging. Often they blame these conditions on age, but I believe they have unhealthy skin because they don't know how to care for themselves.

Within a few months, sometimes as little as a few weeks, these blemishes begin to disappear. Beautiful new and younger-looking skin comes shining through. Of course, your progress depends on what you eat and how well and faithfully you do the body rub. Everyone wants to look younger and healthier. Billions of dollars are spent every year on beauty creams, remedies, and treatments, most of which don't work. The body rub is free and it does work.

New Skin in Twenty-Eight Days

The skin completely renews itself every twenty-eight days. In essence, your skin is no more than a month old at any given moment. Cells in the skin are continuously dying and replacing themselves. We can renew our skin in a healthy or unhealthy way. How the skin renews itself depends on what we have been eating over the previous days, weeks, and months. One of the benefits of eating well is that fresh blood is drawn continuously to the surface areas of the body, stimulating the skin. If we eat healthful foods and do the body rub, we can nourish our skin on a daily basis and, as a result, our skin will become younger-looking and more beautiful. Once past puberty, people of all ages can benefit from the body rub. Healthy skin is slightly shiny and moist. If your skin is healthy, your entire body perspires lightly and easily. Such skin is smooth, soft to the touch, and resilient. If you push or pull it, it bounces back energetically. Healthy skin looks fresh without the aid of creams and moisturizers, and is free of blemishes and pimples. The skin is an excellent barometer of overall health. I always use skin diagnosis in counseling. It tells me about the client's diet, past health problems, and ability to maintain good health in the future.

Most of us take our skin for granted. We all want skin that looks young and healthy, yet few of us give a thought to the skin's function. Skin is our largest organ, containing oil, sweat glands, blood vessels, nerve cells, and immune cells. It has innumerable functions. It protects us from the environment, helps to keep us warm and to cool us down, produces vitamin D, excretes toxins, and, most importantly, keeps us in one piece!

The Skin Is Our Largest Organ.

The skin is a large, hard-working organ, and one of its more significant jobs is to discharge toxins from our bodies.

However, certain foods clog our skin—fatty meat, dairy products, tropical fruit, sugar, eggs, chicken, baked flour products, etc. Clogged skin means that moisture and oil cannot pass through the pores. If we eat the above-mentioned foods on a daily basis, our skin becomes dry. Most people think that dry skin is caused by a lack of oil, so they turn to the common remedy for dry skin—moisturizer. Applying such a remedy will temporarily moisten the skin, but then what happens? Where does the moisturizer go? It is absorbed into the fat layer of the skin, further clogging it, especially if the moisturizer is petroleum-based, like mineral oil and such saturated-fat products as coconut or palm oil.

The skin's tiny capillaries are connected to the body's large main arteries and veins through a vast network of blood vessels of ever-increasing size. It stands to reason that if these capillaries become clogged, the functioning of the circulatory system will be adversely affected. If the skin becomes so clogged that it can no longer discharge oil or moisture, then the excess fat and fluid go back into circulation through the blood vessels, looking, so to speak, for another exit. Over time, circulation will become sluggish, often to the point of putting a strain on the heart.

To help understand this process dynamically, it's useful to look at the mechanism of an event that occurs all too often in our daily lives—the traffic jam. A traffic jam on one road often clogs traffic on other nearby roads. It takes only one backed-up highway exit to slow the flow of traffic and overload the entire system. Most of us have experienced, to our discomfort, what happens on a late Sunday afternoon in the summer when several exits are blocked by traffic.

Nervous System, Immune System, and Meridians
There are peripheral nerve cells in the skin that govern sensitivity and sensory perception. Since the peripheral nerve cells also send messages to the central nervous system, they influence our emotions as well. In fact, the body's entire system of nerves is affected by the condition of the skin. Imbalances in the skin affect how we respond to heat, cold, touch, pressure, and vibrations. Depending on the condition of our skin, we may become over- or under-sensitive to any of the above.

The skin also contains lymphocytes, cells that are an important part of the immune system. Lymphocytes protect against viruses, bacteria, and parasites. When the skin is clogged, its ability to provide immunity is weakened.

Acupuncture Meridians
Acupuncture meridians run under the skin and are connected to the body's internal organs. Meridians are not vessels or containers. They

are energy streams, somewhat analogous to mountain streams, and, as such, they have precise paths. Meridians nourish the organs and allow them to discharge excess pressure. They help the internal organs regulate themselves and adjust to the environment. Although Western science does not acknowledge the existence of meridians, they have been known and used for thousands of years in the Far East. The ancient arts of acupuncture and shiatsu massage are based on and use the extensive system of meridian points.

I use meridian diagnosis extensively. It is one of my main methods for assessing someone's state of health. Meridian diagnosis gives me more information about the functioning of the body's organs and systems than any other aspect of traditional Far Eastern diagnosis. It allows me to determine how well or poorly the body's energy is flowing along its meridians. The quality of energy flow is what tells me how the corresponding organ is functioning. The meridians actually become clogged as fatty deposits collect under the skin and as organ function weakens. When the organs are not able to adjust, they lose their ability to maintain a healthy condition. They are either losing energy or building up excess pressure.

The Pressure Valve

The skin is the body's largest organ; it is also the body's largest opening. The skin functions as a kind of pressure valve. There are many ways to release pressure. Talking, writing, physical activity, urination, bowel elimination, menstruation, and sex are just some of them. Obviously, when the skin is clogged, it cannot release pressure smoothly or easily. One of the criteria of healthy skin is that its pores can open at will to release excess pressure from the body—in the same way that they open to release excess heat from the body. Our skin continually interacts with the environment in an attempt to keep the body's temperature and pressure balanced between the internal and external environments.

The body rub helps the skin function more efficiently. Clogged skin loses its ability to release internal pressure, leaving us much more adversely affected by stress. Once the skin is no longer clogged, we can release fluids and toxins the way Nature intended—by perspiring freely over our entire body. It's a commonly held belief that excess energy can be released only through exercise and activity. Not true. We all know people who talk more than seems appropriate.

What is not understood is that excessive talking is somewhat involuntary. It's the body's way of trying to rid itself of excess energy and stress. However, if the skin is open, internal pressure is released continuously. Once you are doing the body rub every day, you will be amazed at how much calmer you are and how much better you feel.

The Kidneys, Intestines, Lungs, and Liver

The kidneys are our main excretory organs. They work together with the intestines to eliminate excess from the body. The liver aids this process by detoxifying the blood. The body's normal way of discharging excess is through urination and bowel elimination. As long as the kidneys, intestines, and liver are functioning efficiently, the body will not send excess to the skin. But if these organs become tired, sluggish, or stagnated, the body's only choice is to send that excess to the surface—that is, to the skin or possibly to the lungs—for discharge.

One of the great benefits of the body rub is that it takes some of the strain off the kidneys, intestines, lungs, and liver. By helping to clean the body, the body rub gives those organs a chance to rest and repair so they can function more easily and efficiently. It is vitally important to concentrate on the health of your skin. If the skin is unable to aid in the elimination of toxins and if the kidneys, intestines, and liver are clogged and sluggish, the body has no choice but to store the excess waste, which then increases the strain on your health.

Perspiration

If you don't perspire easily, this may be an indication that your skin is dry and clogged. Perspiration is natural. Many of us perspire only from certain parts of the body, like the armpits or the forehead. If your skin is functioning properly, you should perspire from your entire body. When, for instance, you take a sauna, your pores should open easily. You should soon be covered in perspiration from head to toe. After the body rub becomes part of your daily routine, your skin will open and you will perspire freely, releasing those fluids and toxins that have been trapped inside.

Doing the Body Rub—Gently Rub, Not Scrub

I have explained the dynamics of the skin's structure and function in some detail in order to help you understand the importance of the health practice that I call the body rub. The body rub is deeply cleansing to the skin. It draws out the fat that has been collecting beneath the surface and clogging your pores. A word of warning: if your skin looks and feels drier at first than it did before you began doing the body rub, take heart. This is good news. It's proof that you are doing the body rub accurately. Fat must gather under the surface of the skin before it can be discharged, and as it gathers, the skin becomes drier. I have one client who characterized the skin on her arms and legs as reptilian during the first month. Please, be patient and you will see your skin improve steadily from this point on, as she did.

The body rub is easy to do and brings immediate gratification. Some of my clients call it their morning cup of coffee—the ones who do it before bedtime report an improvement in their sleep. The body rub is easy to do. Fill your bathroom sink or a dedicated body rub basin with the hottest tap water possible—though not scalding. The washcloth should be 100 percent cotton, preferably organic, and unbleached or white. Fold it in half once and then in half again, making four layers. Dip the cloth in the hot water and then squeeze out the excess. The cloth should be damp but not dripping. Re-dip it in the hot water as often as necessary. Rub your skin in a back-and-forth motion, gently and systematically. A useful image is that of the tide coming in and going out. Progress in an orderly way over your entire body. You can work from the face down to the feet or from the extremities in toward the center (just below the navel).

The Areas of Importance Are as Follows:
1. Hands, wrists, fingers (and between the fingers), feet (tops and bottoms), ankles, toes (and between the toes)
2. Face and neck
3. Armpits and groin
4. Centerline of the body, from tip of the chin to pubic bone; chest and abdominal areas
5. Bottom of rib cage zigzagging from right to left
6. Back, including sacrum and coccyx (tailbone)

7. Elbows and knees
8. All other areas of body

IF YOU ARE PRESSED FOR TIME, DO STEPS 1 AND 2 OR 1, 2, AND 3

Do not attempt to redden your skin by using a lot of pressure. Use only the weight of your hand without pressing. Keep in mind that this is a rub and not a scrub. Your back-and-forth movement should be vigorous but gentle; light yet not too light. If there are parts of the skin that don't turn red, don't worry, just spend a bit more time on them. Eventually, when the overall condition of your skin improves and your circulation is responding to the treatment, your skin will redden quickly. A word of caution: many people have very delicate, weak skin. If your skin is thin and weak and you apply too much pressure, you can literally rub your skin off. You can think of the scabs that result as your battle scars! If you are very gentle in the beginning, your skin will become stronger more quickly. The initial process is similar to starting an exercise program. Begin slowly and build up gradually for the best results. Please be very careful when doing your face, especially the forehead and bridge of the nose. The skin along the spine is also exceptionally sensitive.

Keep Your Bath or Shower Separate

When you do the body rub, please do it separately from your bath or shower. Do it right before or right after. If you remain under the shower or in the tub water when doing the rub, you will lose too many vital minerals. Hot steam relaxes the body, but since steam has the capacity to draw out minerals, too much steam can be dangerous. Five to seven minutes is safe. I recommend two methods for keeping warm if you become chilled while doing the rub, usually in winter. One is to fill the tub with hot water to just below your ankles. Then sit on the edge of the tub and proceed with the rub. The second method, the one I prefer, is to start with a very short hot shower, then turn the water off and do the rub. This allows the steam and heat from the shower to keep you warm. The bathroom will have begun to cool down by the time you are through with the rub, at which point you can finish with another very short hot shower.

Other Benefits

Another benefit of the daily body rub is that it encourages you to become more open and accepting of your body. If you really dislike doing the rub, one possibility is that you are uncomfortable with your body. In time, if you do the rub on a daily basis, your self-image will improve. You will learn to appreciate your uniqueness and you will grow to genuinely care for and respect your body. If you spend a little extra time on areas you particularly don't like, your self-image will change more quickly. Done regularly, the body rub will improve every aspect of your physical, emotional, and mental health. A word of caution: using a loofah or dry brush is not the same practice as the body rub. The purpose of the rub is to coax the pores of the skin to open in order to draw out stored fats and toxins. If you combine hot, damp heat with the softness of a washcloth, you can easily achieve your goal. A loofa, however, even if damp, will only impede your progress. Yes, it can remove the dead outer skin, but its very coarseness causes the pores of the living skin to close tightly, thus sealing in those fats and toxins. A dry brush may be very effective for abrading dead skin and tightening your pores, but by using one you will accomplish exactly the opposite of what you want. The body rub takes longer, but it is much more effective if your goal is to create healthy, resilient skin.

I have spent years trying to determine the best way to do the body rub, and my conclusion is that strong pressure is not as effective as light pressure. As I said earlier, the body rub is a rub, not a scrub. Light pressure applied by the natural weight of the hand is what best stimulates the circulation of energy and the opening of the pores of the skin. Once the pores can open easily, they can also close easily, and it is this easy opening and closing in response to both internal and external environments that is one of the hallmarks of resilient skin. If you do a daily body rub with a damp cloth and light pressure, you will discover this for yourself.

When you eat well and do the rub, in effect what you are doing is to draw a continuous supply of fresh blood to any given area. As for the face, one of the effects of improved circulation is the reduction and possible elimination of fine lines and wrinkles. Also, the rub improves muscle tone as well as skin texture, so that when the facial muscles are strengthened, wrinkles tend to fade or vanish.

If you've eaten a lot of cheese and other fatty and baked foods in your life, you no doubt have deposits of cellulite in your legs, hips, and buttocks. Some of my clients tell me that these parts of their bodies literally look like cottage cheese! The body rub will help break down these deposits and allow them to leave your system. Of course, if you continue to eat foods that cause cellulite, you will find yourself in an endless cycle of frustration. Now that you know the cause of cellulite, the next time you are tempted to eat cheese, just picture where it will end up. Maybe that will help you resist the temptation.

If you have very rough, red skin and feel you have to use a moisturizer, use it sparingly before going to sleep. Please don't use it in the morning. Just do the body rub. After a while, even very rough, dry skin will soften and regenerate. Except for extreme cases of very dry skin, it is unnecessary and hinders rather than helps. If used habitually, even the best-quality moisturizer can clog the skin. If you must use a moisturizer, select one made with liquid vegetable oil, such as sesame or olive; avoid any oil that becomes solid at room temperature, such as coconut oil.

Key Points:
- Use a medium-weight cotton washcloth. Fold it in half twice.
- Organic cotton is best.
- Fill your sink or your basin with hot water, dip the cloth, and wring it out. Re-dip the cloth frequently to keep it hot and fresh.
- Rub gently in a back-and-forth motion. Do not rub in circles.
- Rub gently; don't scrub. Gentle pressure yields better results.
- Do the rub separately from your bath or shower.
- The purpose of the rub is to open your pores and draw out fats and toxins. This will allow your skin to breathe naturally.
- Years of animal and dairy food, fruits, sweets, baked and fatty food clog the skin and prevent it from breathing naturally.
- The skin needs to breathe freely just as the lungs do.

Doing the Body Rub Results In:
- An increase in the circulation of blood, lymph, and energy that will improve the nutrition, oxygen flow, stimulation, and health of all your organs.

- Better energy all day after a morning rub and deeper sleep after an evening rub.
- More effective release of stored toxins.
- Improved immunity to disease.
- Clearer thinking, keener memory, and more optimistic outlook.
- Improved self-image.
- Increased sensual awareness.

CULTIVATE AND TAKE TIME FOR HOBBIES

Hobbies are very, very important for good health. Yet these days how many of us have a hobby? Not many, I suspect. Hobby is a rather old-fashioned word, so I'm often asked what I mean when I use it. To me, a hobby is something that brings an aspect of completion or fullness or balance to our lives, something we do for enjoyment—a favorite activity (not passivity)—but not what we do day to day for a living.

> "To insure good health: eat lightly, breathe deeply, live moderately."
>
> —William Londen

Let me give you an example from an older time. The samurai of Japan were professional warriors, rigorously trained in the martial arts, who spent their lives fighting. To make sure their development wasn't overly one-sided, they also studied tea ceremony or poetry or brush painting, something very different, very highly refined, in order to make balance.

Now let me give you an example from modern life. I ask, "Do you have a hobby?" You answer, "Yes, reading." But if your job is mental, reading doesn't meet my definition of a hobby. A hobby has to be different from work, something that brings polarity and interest to your life.

I like this example: years ago, in *Science News*, I came across a piece about a scientist with very interesting ideas. What struck me was the fact that a couple of times a week he and his brother got together and played guitar and sang just for the fun of it. His work was technical, highly skilled, demanding, and precise. His hobby released him, balanced his work. In my view, the reason he had such interesting ideas was because he spent his free time doing something he enjoyed that was very different from his work.

"Dare to err and dare to dream. Deep meaning often lies in childish play."

—Johann Friedrich von Schiller

Hobbies are a kind of self-reflection, a way of maintaining balance, a way to develop different sides of our nature. They are for our enjoyment, pleasure, and satisfaction. My advice is, if you don't have a hobby, choose anything you think you might enjoy. If you find you don't like it, try something else. Often clients will tell me they don't have time for a hobby. My answer is always the same: "You don't *not* have time for a hobby, because a hobby will enrich your life. Your practice and your health will improve if you have a hobby." Everything needs polarity. We add chopped parsley to sweet vegetable soup. The garnish brings the soup to life. The garnish is the hobby, in a manner of speaking.

Key Points:
- Hobbies make balance for the more structured and pressured areas of life.
- Hobbies help relieve stress and promote physical and mental flexibility.
- Hobbies keep your mind more open and flexible and can bring a deep sense of satisfaction.
- Have fun with your hobbies.

Create a More Natural Environment

Recharging Station

What is a home? In the macrobiotic way of thinking, home is a charging station, a place to relax, return to balance, and enrich life. Therefore, we must create the healthiest environment we can so that we are nourished rather than depleted by our surroundings. The more natural the environment around us, the brighter, more refreshed, and positive we feel. Then, automatically, we make better choices in all the other areas of life.

Let's say you go on a picnic. The food tastes especially delicious and you sleep more soundly that night. Why? You're out of doors in the country with congenial company, the air is fresh, and usually you engage in some sort of physical activity. All this contributes to improved circulation. Whatever you do that improves your circulation creates a healthier appetite and a deeper, more restful night's sleep.

The direction modern life is taking is well beyond our control, but there are steps we can take that will reverse many of its worst effects. Most of us worry about those things over which we have no control, yet ignore those things we can change, things we can do every day to improve our lives. We have a choice. We can take time for our meals of grains and vegetables, stick to our daily schedule, walk, do the body rub, and surround ourselves with green plants and natural materials, on our person and in our home. Each of the first five steps, if done regularly, strengthens the effect of the others. Together, the first five steps form the essence of good health. Whether we apply these principles to the life of one person, to a family, to a community, or to a society, east, west, north, or south, they work. They are simple; they are unique. They worked in the past, they work today, and they will work in the future. Why? Because they are based on the common sense of our ancestors but adapted to modern life.

SURROUND YOURSELF WITH GREEN PLANTS

There was a time, not so long ago, when houseplants were considered merely decorative. Walking into a house or office filled with green plants was a pleasant, even soothing, experience, but hardly a life-enhancing one; not so any more. Plants are a necessity these days. We depend on them to clean the air we breathe, having discovered that green plants are far more efficient at removing pollutants than any machine.

Plants absorb many harmful contaminants, such as formaldehyde, benzene, and carbon monoxide. Formaldehyde, one of the worst, is considered to be a contributing factor to the high cancer rate in the United States. Formaldehyde is found in many of the materials used in home building and furnishings, including plywood, particle board, decorative paneling, floor covering, and carpet backing. It is also found in items we regularly bring into the house, such as grocery bags, waxed bags, facial tissues, common cleaning agents, fire-retardant and permanent-press clothing, tobacco, and cooking and heating gas.

Among the most efficient air cleaners are spider plants, golden pothos, and elephant ear philodendron. Dr. William Wolverton, formerly a senior research scientist at NASA, has calculated that fifteen to twenty of these common houseplants can clean and refresh the air in an average-sized house. Interestingly, NASA has concluded that plants become more effective at cleaning the air as pollution levels increase. It seems that in areas of low-level pollution, fewer molecules come into contact with the leaf's surface, so the benefits are not as great. Why are green plants so effective? They are natural generators of the negative ions in the air we breathe. Negative ionization promotes a feeling of well-being, of fresh-ness, and of rejuvenation.

Negative Ionization

Negative ionization increases with movement. If you walk by a waterfall, if you walk in the woods, you feel refreshed and exhilarated. The natural circulation of the water as it falls and the wind as it blows through the trees increases the amount of negative ionization in the air. When you clean a room, when you do the body rub, you are also increasing it.

An ion is a particle that can carry either a negative or a positive electrical charge. In this case, negatively charged ions are the ones we want around us. Negative ionization occurs when ions move away from the earth. It's helpful to think of negative ions as moving up and out, cleaning and refreshing everything as they go. Positive ions are those that move toward the center of the earth. Think of them as moving down and in, bringing heaviness and stagnation with them.

Any room that's not cleaned for a while will take on a dark, heavy feeling. When you open the window and pull up the shades to let in air and sunlight, when you clean the space, what you are actually doing is changing positive ions to negative ones. Fresh air, sunlight, and thorough cleaning can transform any room by infusing it with refreshed energy. Being in such a room feels wonderful. Negative ionization is big news these days. Many people are buying ionizing machines for their homes. Green plants are far cheaper and far more effective. They play a significant role in promoting good health.

Large, strong plants that grow upward are more effective than hanging plants for changing the energy in your house or office. Buy potted plants that sit on the floor. If space permits, make sure a few of them are large. A hanging plant is better than no plant at all, so, if you have a space problem, resort to using one. Use as many plants as you care to, making sure there are not so many that the room looks overcrowded or movement is hampered. You don't want your guests to feel they need a machete!

Noise Pollution

One of the unsung virtues of plants is that they protect us from noise pollution. Have you ever spent time in an evergreen forest? In 1985, I was invited to teach at a macrobiotic summer camp that was held in a pine forest north of Oslo, Norway. One day, during my free time, I went for a walk in the woods. For some reason, it felt eerie being there. It took a while for me to realize that this was the first time I had ever experienced complete quiet. There was simply nothing to hear.

Plants have the ability to absorb sound. All plants can do this, but evergreens are especially adept at soaking up noise. If you keep a lot of plants in the house, they will help keep the noise level down. It's easier to maintain good health in a quiet house. Doors slamming, television or music blasting, and people shouting all take their toll on our health.

> "One must be out-of-doors enough to experience wholesome reality, as ballast to thought and sentiment. Health requires this relaxation, this aimless life."
> —Henry David Thoreau

Green Plants in the Bedroom

The most important places in the house to keep plants are the bedroom, the kitchen, and the bathroom. Many people think plants should not be kept in the bedroom. I disagree. During the day, plants give out oxygen and take in carbon dioxide. At night, they give out carbon dioxide and take in oxygen. We need more oxygen during the day, less at night, more in summer, less in winter. This natural cycle of taking in and giving out leads to greater overall oxygen intake. Having plants in the bedroom at night helps us sleep more deeply and that means we can take in more oxygen over the course of the next day. Plants in the bedroom serve to regulate the oxygen ratio so that we receive the right amount of oxygen while we sleep. As I said earlier, the body cleans and repairs itself during the night and our plants will be right there to aid in the nocturnal rejuvenation.

It's essential to have green plants in the kitchen. Ideally, the kitchen should be sealed off from the rest of the house so that cooking fumes and odors can be vented outside. Gas fumes generate a lot of pollution that spreads easily throughout the house. Green plants will help minimize their effect on our health. Water is one of the main sources of pollution in today's houses, so it's best to keep green plants in the bathroom as well.

Because green plants work so diligently night and day to clean the air we breathe, they deserve proper care. Actually, houseplants require only minimal attention, but they do have certain needs. They require the right amount of water at regular intervals, and they must have the appropriate light. If you place a plant in direct sunlight, make sure it's meant to have a strong exposure. Different species have different needs, so be sure to get some advice from the florist or consult a book. Keep your plants in clay pots so that their roots can breathe. Check every couple of seasons to see whether they require larger pots.

Key Points:
- The most important places for green plants are the bedroom, kitchen, bathroom, and any other room in which you spend time.
- Green plants generate negative ionization that creates a calmer, more peaceful, and refreshing environment.
- Green plants enable us to be clearer, brighter, and more active during the day. Their presence promotes quiet, restful, deep sleep at night.
- Green plants are the most efficient air filtration system known, especially spider plants, golden pothos (devil's ivy), snake plants, peace lily, and elephant ear philodendron.
- Choose strong, upward-growing plants overhanging ones.
- Choose plants that are hardy and easy to care for.

WEAR PURE COTTON CLOTHING NEXT TO YOUR SKIN

The body runs on electrical impulses. Nutrition, digestion, immunity, and our nervous system all depend on electrical impulses to do their work. Because pure cotton carries less of a static electrical charge than other material, when worn directly against the skin it helps neutralize imbalances within the body. If you have an imbalance in your nervous, immune, or digestive system or in your meridians, pure cotton will help counteract that imbalance. Wearing pure cotton next to your skin is one of the quickest and easiest ways to improve and maintain your health.

Synthetics carry the strongest static electrical charge. Think of the fireworks display that occurs when you make a bed using synthetic sheets or blankets. Try making the bed with the lights off! The strong static electrical charge in synthetics interferes with the body's functioning.

Synthetic fabrics make imbalances worse. Some materials that are natural to begin with go through chemical processing that produces the same effect on the body as synthetics. Rayon is a good example.

Cotton is the most neutral fabric, followed by linen, silk, and wool. Silk is natural, but its animal quality gives it a strong static charge. Wool is also natural, but it carries a much stronger charge than cotton or even silk. It's best not to wear wool directly against the skin.

Everyone, but especially people living in modern houses or high-rise apartment buildings, has an electromagnetic imbalance in his or her environment. Natural materials help lessen all imbalances. Synthetics increase, amplify, and enhance imbalances. Whatever the condition of your body or your environment, it will worsen if you wear synthetics directly against your skin. If you are feeling tired, wearing a synthetic next to your skin will increase your fatigue. If you are feeling anxious, it will make you feel more anxious. Your health problems will worsen quickly if you wear synthetics against your skin.

It is especially important to wear pure cotton underwear, bras, socks, and pajamas and to use pure cotton sheets, pillowcases, towels, and wash-cloths. Organic cotton is even better. If you follow this simple suggestion, you will feel more refreshed and enjoy better resistance to illness. Start by replacing your underwear and socks. It's often difficult to find all-cotton goods. Shop carefully and make sure to read the content labels. These days, even items advertised as cotton often contain a small percentage of synthetic. When you do find what suits you, keep a record of where the item was purchased. This is helpful when it's time to reorder.

Key Points:
- Cotton is a buffer that helps neutralize imbalances in the body and environment.
- Woolens and synthetics can amplify imbalances in your body and environment.
- Underwear, socks, bras, sheets, pillowcases, and towels should be 100 percent cotton.
- Wear cotton against the skin under clothing made from other materials.
- Try to find organic cotton.

USE NATURAL MATERIALS, WOOD, COTTON, WOOL, ETC. IN YOUR HOME

Think of your home as a recharging station. We leave home to go to work, to shop, to go to school, or to play. We return to refresh, re-nourish, and rebalance so we have the energy and the will to leave again. If our homes and furnishings are made from natural materials, we can recharge more effectively.

It's best to have furniture made of real wood, to choose cotton for your upholstery, drapes, and curtains and wool for your carpeting. Wool carpeting is far better for your health than synthetic which, like imitation wood and plywood, is processed with formaldehyde. If you can replace the man-made materials in your home with natural ones, you will feel much more comfortable in your day-to-day life.

Natural Bedding

Try to buy 100 percent organic cotton sheets. They can be expensive, so keep your eye out for sales. Avoid sheets that do not require ironing. They have been treated with formaldehyde. It's far better for your health to sleep on high-quality, wrinkled but non-toxic sheets than on smooth toxic ones. It's all a matter of priorities. Reasonably priced, high-quality, pure cotton towels and washcloths are relatively easy to find. Still, it's necessary to read the content labels carefully.

A futon is a good possible choice for a mattress. Futons are generally made of cotton and their frames of wood. Make sure the futon you buy is all-cotton or cotton and wool. If you are not ready to change your entire bed, you can buy just the futon mattress and place it over your existing mattress or box spring. Organic rubber/latex mattresses are also a good choice. You can also buy an organic latex topper to place over your existing mattress. Conventional mattresses are made with synthetic materials (and metal as well, in the case of innerspring mattresses), so the sooner you can replace yours with a futon or natural bed, the faster your health will improve. You will enjoy the experience of having natural materials close to you. In the beginning, it may take some effort to replace all your synthetic belongings; but after the initial outlay of energy and money, it will be easy to replace items as they wear out. Surrounding yourself with cotton is a good health habit that will help you feel and look your best.

Transparent Building

Years ago when teaching at a seminar in Switzerland, I had the privilege of spending time in a house built of completely natural materials. The concrete was free of iron so it gave off no electromagnetic charge, and the wood had been specially treated. When you were inside this house, you felt almost as if you were outdoors. It was the most transparent building environment I have ever been in. Teaching at that seminar was effortless because I was being energized all day.

Contrast that environment with that of department stores, for instance, where you are surrounded by synthetic materials and relentless fluorescent lighting. In such an environment, I very quickly become irritable. Being in man-made surroundings exhausts your body and shatters your thinking. I always feel sorry for the salespeople who have to endure this discomfort on a daily basis. Often, nowadays, there's also loud music playing. I sometimes wonder if these stores are uncomfortable on purpose. Maybe the idea is to get you to buy quickly and leave.

It's best that whatever you bring into your home be as free of chemicals and toxins as possible. Avoid using household cleaning products with high chemical content. They create their own pollution. A wide variety of excellent chemical-free cleaning products are available in health food stores, most of which are not tested on animals.

Natural-food stores also have a large selection of self-care products, including cosmetics. Use these instead of conventional products that are full of chemicals detrimental to health, chemicals that are absorbed through the pores and into the body's organs, where they create an additional burden on the immune system. Natural products are just as effective as—and in most cases superior to—those laced with chemicals. If you are unable to find what you need in your area, you can order from any number of catalogue companies that specialize in natural products.

Fooling the Compass

I often carry a compass with me to check out different environments. I have been amazed by some of my findings. In certain apartment buildings, my

compass was a full ninety degrees off! The concrete used in these buildings carries such a strong electromagnetic charge that when I was facing
north my compass said I was facing east. Imagine how this distortion
affects our health. If a compass can be thrown so severely out of balance,
then we certainly can be too. The heart of our blood is hemoglobin, an
iron-containing protein. Iron is magnetic, so our blood is profoundly
affected by electromagnetic fields of energy.

Many studies have shown that electromagnetic fields are detrimental
to health. Older homes, generally built with more natural materials,
tend to have weaker electromagnetic fields than new ones.

At one time, I lived in a hundred-year-old Victorian farmhouse that
had a very comfortable feeling. It was simply decorated, with old furniture that we liked and had gotten used to. The quality of the house and
the decorations helped create a feeling of comfort and well-being. When
friends visited, they often remarked on this. My point is that if we surround ourselves with natural materials, we can create a harmonious and
balanced environment in which we can refresh and recharge ourselves.

How many times have you found yourself in physical surroundings
that make you feel uneasy, even fidgety, without being able to understand
why? It could be that you are sensitive enough to be adversely affected by
unnatural surroundings. The excessive use of synthetics and chemically
toxic materials is what creates this discomfort. Natural materials can
help. Natural materials, such as wood, cotton, and wool, act as a buffer,
helping to lessen and balance electromagnetic interference.

Things We Can Control

Certain things are within our control. It's best not to use microwave
ovens. Their so-called acceptable levels of radiation pollute our homes.
Electric blankets are very harmful. We want to rest and recharge naturally, without interference. Electric stoves are another major source of
electromagnetic radiation. I recommend that you cook with gas. If natural
gas isn't available where you live, switch from electricity to propane gas.
It's easy to do and convenient to use. Cooking with electricity affects the
taste and consistency of food. The flavors don't harmonize naturally, and
it's difficult to achieve the desired crispness. Professional chefs always
choose to cook with gas.

If you have any fluorescent light bulbs in your house, replace them with incandescent or full-spectrum ones. You and your house will look much better in the glow of incandescent lighting. And your state of mind will improve. Fluorescent lighting has been proven to cause depression.

Television sets also emit harmful rays, so try to avoid spending hours sitting in front of yours. Remember that the farther away you sit from the television set, the less exposure you will receive. It's best to turn the TV off when you're not watching it, as electromagnetic fields pass through walls. Lastly, please don't put a television set in your bedroom.

I am aware that the beginning of anything can be overwhelming, and the practice of macrobiotics is no exception. Let's say that you have begun to eat good food in an orderly way, and have started your walking program and are doing the body rub and reaping its benefits. The next step is to surround yourself with materials that will enhance your sense of well-being and contribute to your overall good health.

Key Points:
- Choose natural materials when replacing home furnishings.
- Use natural wood, cotton, and wool instead of synthetic materials in your home.
- Try a natural futon, a cotton and wool mattress, or a natural rubber/latex mattress for sleeping.
- Use natural cleaning products, soaps, and cosmetics.
- Stop using microwave ovens and electric blankets.
- Cook with natural, propane, or even butane gas. Please do not cook with electricity.
- Watch television sparingly.

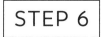

Make Your Macrobiotic Practice Work

KEEPING TO THE FORMAT OF MEALS IMPROVES YOUR ABILITY TO MAKE HEALTHFUL FOOD CHOICES. GOOD EATING HABITS, STEPS ONE AND TWO, ARE THE CONTROLLING FACTORS IN GOOD HEALTH.

The Biggest Mistake

The sixth step incorporates the essence of each of the five previous steps. The point here is that by keeping to the Format of Meals, we automatically have clear guidelines as to wise food choices under any and all circumstances, whether we're eating at home, in a restaurant, or on an airplane. As I said earlier, the biggest mistake most people make is to focus on Diet: Content and Quality rather than on Eating Habits: Format of Meals. Eating Habits are what keep us on track.

Eating at Home versus Eating Out

Food choices that are clear when we eat at home can seem murky when we eat out. When we're at home, we can choose the highest-quality organically grown brown rice, organic vegetables, the best-quality miso and so on. If we are at the mercy of a mediocre restaurant, we might order white rice and steamed broccoli (possibly even frozen). The quality is lower, yes, but the Format is intact. We have a grain and a vegetable on our plate. Quality can always be adjusted up or down depending on where we find ourselves. Of course, the degree of the adjustment depends on our condition. We must ask: "What can my health afford at this time? How liberal can I be?"

As simple as this might sound, most people see little or no connection between meals at home and meals outside the home. At home they take care to make good choices but when they eat out they often throw away the guidelines, meaning the Format of Meals, and choose whatever appeals to them. This is a serious mistake. The Format is what helps us maintain our direction toward health. If, however, we believe Content and Quality are more important than Format and we can't get organic short-grain rice, the temptation is to abandon the Format as well. Once we create a separation in our minds between what we eat at home and what we eat outside, it follows that we begin to see food in terms of black and white. We think, "I ate something I shouldn't have, I'm off the diet, I'm in trouble, I can never eat out, this is too hard." But, really, if we focus on the Format wherever we are, we will automatically make the wisest choices possible and we will continue to move in the direction of health.

The Second Biggest Mistake

Let's look at maintaining the direction toward health from another angle: structure (another word for Format) versus variety. The second biggest mistake most people make is to allow the structure, which should be tight, to become loose. Once that happens, the need for variety diminishes and eventually changes to a pattern of repetition, a pattern that directs us away from health. If the legs of a table are loose, the table can be said to have a wobbly structure. It can barely support itself. If we remove the legs altogether, the table will collapse completely. Or to use Nature's model once again, the sun rises and sets every day, a phenomenon that is part of the structure of the universe. If the sun doesn't rise or set, it's all over for the planet. In the same way, once we let the structure or Format go, we set ourselves on a path away from health.

Here are the main danger signals:
- You don't sit down and take time for your meals.
- You start to read, watch TV, or listen to the radio during meals.

- You eat quickly and forget to chew well.
- You do other things while eating.
- Your mealtimes become irregular.
- You stop having a grain and vegetable with every meal.

How does this work? Let's say you want to have lunch at twelve-thirty, no later than one o'clock, but you're too busy to eat. By the time you do eat, your appetite is completely altered because your blood sugar has fallen. Low blood sugar means that in order to feel satisfied, either you have to eat more than usual—in other words, overeat—or you have to have something sweet. It follows that, once having eaten a late lunch, you have no appetite for dinner at the regular time. If you keep to your regular dinnertime but eat less than usual, an hour or two later you'll want a snack. Or, instead of dinner at six, let's say you decide to eat at eight-thirty. Either way, you won't have three full hours between dinner and bedtime since you have to go to bed at a reasonable hour in order to get up early the next morning. You don't sleep very well that night (no one sleeps well on a full stomach). It's difficult to get up the next morning and, when you do drag yourself out of bed, you don't feel refreshed. You can see how one change in the structure or Format inevitably leads to another and how, in the end, these changes will lead you away from health.

Although having a grain and vegetable with every meal comes under the heading of Diet, there is an overlap with Format. The meal you sit down to eat must qualify as a meal, meaning it must contain a grain or grain product and a vegetable. When you stop having both a grain and a vegetable with every meal, most commonly that meal is breakfast and it's the vegetable that disappears from the plate. If you've reached this stage, you can pretty much assume you've begun to lose your direction. You're getting way off track.

Balance and Imbalance Perpetuate Themselves.

One of the guiding principles of life is that balance perpetuates itself. And, as you might suspect, imbalance perpetuates itself as well. As you let go of more and more of the structure, you start to feel more and more pressure. You might believe the buildup of pressure comes from having to market, prepare, and cook the food or from the pressure of having to eat at a regular time—but I don't think so. I think the reverse is true. The usual pattern is that you feel rushed, so you begin to rush your meals. The more we rush our meals, the more rushed we feel. Sitting down and taking time for meals actually eases pressure. If you think of a meal as a time for recharging, reorienting, and regaining balance, if no matter how stressed you feel you take the time to sit down, eat slowly, and chew well, when you finish eating you will feel refreshed and calm. Any decisions you make in this frame of mind are bound to be wiser than those made under pressure.

Some people find it helpful to think of chewing as a form of meditation, somewhat like breathing practices. The result in both cases is heightened mental and emotional clarity and a feeling of deep calm. Remember, it's important to come to the table prepared to chew. Before you sit down, ask yourself, "What are my priorities?" If good health is one of them, then take time for your meal, eat your food slowly, and chew it well.

Structure versus Variety

Let's go back to structure versus variety. I said earlier that when the structure becomes loose, the need for variety diminishes—or we could say, tightens—and eventually repetition replaces variety altogether. In effect, polarity is reversed. What do I mean by this? Let me start with a basic premise: the more we seek variety, the more nutrition we get from our food. If we eat the same few foods over and over again, eventually not much happens. If someone repeats the same thing over and over again, eventually you stop hearing what is being said. It goes in one ear and out the other. It's no different with food. In one end and out the other—without much benefit.

Unfortunately, often we don't notice that this is happening. It's difficult to be aware of what we're eating day to day. Food is the closest thing to us, so we don't have the advantage of perspective. We think we have variety—we eat blanched, steamed, and sautéed vegetables daily; we eat different grains, oatmeal, brown rice, millet, barley—where's the repetition in all this? Every morning we have oatmeal and steamed kale; for lunch we have rice and blanched broccoli and cabbage; for dinner miso soup, rice with sesame seeds, sautéed mixed vegetables, pressed salad with napa cabbage. Isn't that variety? No. It's repetition. Taking several dishes and repeating them day after day after day is repetition. Having blanched broccoli and cabbage every day for lunch is repetition. Having oatmeal for breakfast every morning is repetition.

Appetite is stimulated by variety. Variety also creates satisfaction. If we lack variety in both ingredients and preparation, we don't feel satisfied with our food, and so we overeat at mealtimes and snack before bed.

Key Points:
- Good eating habits, steps one and two, are the controlling factors in good health.
- Good eating habits automatically lead to healthier food choices.
- When traveling or eating out, keep to the format of grains and vegetables as the basis of a meal. Quality can be adjusted up or down. White rice or commercial pasta is a better choice than going without a grain.
- Vegan commercial vegetable soup is a better choice than no soup at all.

KEEP A DAILY MENU BOOK TO HELP YOU BECOME MORE OBJECTIVE ABOUT YOUR MACROBIOTIC PRACTICE

Underlying everything in this book so far is the basic question, how do we keep moving in the direction of health? Keeping a menu book—or a journal, if you prefer to call it that—is the best way I know of. It's very difficult to be aware of what we're doing day to day, especially with regard to diet. As I've said before, food is the closest thing to us, so it's hard to be objective. The power of a menu book is that it lets you see if you are really getting enough variety.

Enter the date, time, and menu for every meal, snack, or nibble that passes your lips, along with a brief comment on how you felt that day. Review your menu book every so often and reflect on its contents. It's difficult to be objective when you are entering information. Objectivity comes later. In this way, you will know whether or not you are getting variety. Keeping a daily menu book takes the guesswork out of tracking the changes in your health. (It's not necessary to include recipes, although you may if you wish.)

Your menu book can be as simple or as detailed as you care to make it. Some people keep track of their daily functions as well as their daily food—bowel movements, bedtime, sleep patterns, moods, and so on. Looking back, you can see how you were feeling physically, mentally, and emotionally on any given day. Then you can begin to correlate what you ate or did on a particular day with how you felt that day. For instance: I did this and I felt really good—my thinking was clear, I ate this and I didn't feel very well, I did this and I was irritable, I did that and I was really tired. You can't learn this sort of thing in school. How certain foods, patterns, and behaviors affect you can only be self-taught. If you write just a sentence or two every day, that should be enough to jog your memory and help you discover whether you are really doing what you think you're doing. I can't stress enough the importance of keeping a menu book. It's one way to measure how serious your commitment is to improving and strengthening your health.

I must confess that I've never really kept a menu book; but in the past, during the years when I was teaching several times a week, I kept a kind of journal. I entered the outline of every lecture I gave along with some comments, no matter how often I lectured on the same topic. It's interesting to look back over these journals. There are times when I thought my condition was good and my thinking orderly, but my journal shows otherwise. Or, looking back at other periods when my notes indicate that my condition was off, I can see by the outline of my lecture that my thinking was very clear and orderly. The point is that when you're in the throes of doing something, it's nearly impossible to be objective. But when you look back, you can often see the truth.

One final comment on this point: you might think you don't need to do this, you're an experienced cook, you don't need to improve your cooking. Let me assure you that even experienced, longtime macrobiotic cooks keep menu books. I can guarantee that if you keep one, your practice will improve, as will your cooking. Objectivity is the key. You can see where you've fallen short or gone overboard.

Key Points:

- Keep a hard or spiral-bound book in your kitchen to record your menus and snacks.
- Keep notes on your activities, symptoms, and general feelings.
- Refer back to previous days, weeks, and months to see any patterns that emerge from your practice.
- Keeping a daily menu book is one of the best ways to improve your practice and discover your mistakes.
- Such a journal allows you to evaluate your practice and its benefits more objectively.

Cultivate the Spirit of Health

"In order to change we must be sick and tired of being sick and tired."

—Author Unknown

The seventh step is the one that completes the other six, the one without which the other six remain mechanical and, in a sense, external to us, animated by willpower rather than love. What is too often missing from current macrobiotic practice is the spirit of health itself. It's taken me a long time to work out how to convey the essence of this spirit—one that is inseparable from the theory and practice of macrobiotics. Lacking this spirit, we can never make the transition to lasting health. Please bear with me as I repeat once again: health is a direction, a condition we move toward day by day throughout life. Sickness is also a direction. Depending on the totality of our eating habits, diet, and daily lifestyle practices, we move in one direction or the other. It should be no surprise then that if we follow the macrobiotic guidelines accurately, we move toward health. If we ignore them, we move toward sickness. Let me state something unequivocally: health is a condition we grow into throughout our lives. This is a very important point. Today, the most commonly held belief is that we start out in life with a certain amount of health—call it our capital—that we spend as we age until, in a manner of speaking, we are bankrupt. Now, to believe that aging is a fate that brings, among other things, the loss of bones, teeth, beautiful skin, flexibility, memory, and the ability to enjoy and fully participate in life—that this fate is as sure as death and taxes—is a very heavy burden to bear. Yet this belief is so strong that everyone who can afford to carries the financial burden of a lifetime of health insurance.

Is this kind of deterioration really the human fate? I don't think so. Is the aging process I have just described based on a natural model of aging—of living in harmony with Nature—or is it simply the experience of those who live an anti-natural lifestyle? I think you know the answer. Let me assure you that it is not natural to deteriorate with age. If you look at Nature's model—take for instance, trees—what do you see? Once the aptly named "mighty oak" has grown to fullness, then seedlings sprout and when these seedlings need more light and more space to continue growing, the oak passes on. In other words, when the oak has fulfilled its destiny, it moves on.

> "A wise man should consider that health is the greatest of human blessings, and learn how by his own thought to derive the benefit from his illness."
>
> —Hippocrates

In the past, people readily moved on when they had had enough of life. It was that simple. (In fact, the novels of the 19th century are filled with death-bed scenes involving characters who, having reached this point, put their affairs in order, paid their debts, said their farewells to family and friends, and either sat down or lay down and died.) They chose the time and place of their death. They died not of sickness but because they had had enough of life. Some of you might have had parents or grandparents who were able to do this. Odd though it might seem to us, it's really no different from anything else we've had enough of in life. No matter how much we enjoy something, eventually we reach a point of satiation where more isn't going to add to the experience. In fact, it may well detract from it. We can have the best conversation, the best meal, the best vacation, whatever. Still, sooner or later, we get to the point of fullness and satisfaction. We've had enough. It's time to move on. It's a sign of spiritual maturity to know when that time is.

For the first eighteen to twenty years after birth, we grow our bodies. At that point, the body should stop growing—in terms of weight as well as height. Our natural weight is achieved somewhere between the ages of sixteen and twenty. People new to macrobiotics are sometimes quite heavy. The prospect of losing weight appeals to them, but often they lose more than they are comfortable with. I always ask, "How much did you weigh when you were sixteen? How much did you weigh when you got your first driver's license? That's your natural weight, and that's probably what you'll end up weighing." They become alarmed. "That's too thin," they say. No, it's not too thin. Let me explain. As I said, we spend the first part of life growing the body. At birth, the body is not completely formed. The nervous system is not fully developed, nor are the lungs, immune system, or bones. We take the next sixteen to twenty years to grow these, after which we stop growing physically and begin to grow mentally and spiritually. That is, we begin to grow our consciousness.

"Dwell not upon thy weariness, thy strength shall be according to the measure of thy desire."
—Arabian Proverb

Health itself has three aspects: physical, mental, and spiritual. Physical health is the foundation of mental and spiritual health. When we have good vitality, good energy, then we sleep well. If we sleep well, then we are alert and our memory is excellent. We don't anger easily. We are filled with a deep sense of joy and appreciation. On the other hand, with limited physical vitality, sleep isn't usually sound or refreshing, memory is unreliable, and there is a tendency to become easily irritated. Worst of all, joy and alertness are lost, along with feelings of gratitude for life itself. As I said, the first part of life is devoted to the growth of the body and the creation of a high degree of physical health. Physical health is the foundation for the growth and nourishment of mental and spiritual health. When you look at traditional societies, you see that they valued their elders for their life's experience and their ability to guide younger people. Think about it, if the elders were incapable of guiding their own lives because of impaired memory and physical debilitation, how could they guide anyone else? Why would anyone seek them out? The answer is that the memory of the elders didn't deteriorate. On the contrary, it increased with age. Their patience with life itself, their joy, their appreciation for all of life, their understanding of the relationship between difficulty and happiness—all these increased and flowered as they aged. Just as the flower represents the culmination of the growth process of a plant, the final maturation before passing on to the next stage, in the same way old age should be the flowering of our life on earth.

What we refer to when we talk about health these days—health being merely an absence of serious illness—is a very recent model. The world's health began to deteriorate at the time of the Industrial Revolution, but the definitive turning point was World War II.

It's most important that we reexamine our definition of health itself. We must ask ourselves what health is and what we need to do to develop it so that old age is once again a flowering. One thing that does change with age is that we become less interested in sensory experience and more interested in social matters. We become more interested in discovering for ourselves the meaning of life—that is, in discovering what we came here to do so that we can complete the task, so that one day we can honestly say we are satisfied, we have had enough of this life.

> "And man dies and is buried, and all his words and actions are forgotten, but the food he has eaten lives after him in the sound or rotten bones of his children."
> —George Orwell

I'd have to say, based on my years of counseling so many seriously ill older people, that most of them never did what they really wanted to with their lives. They were waiting until retirement to make their dreams a reality, but once retired they found they didn't want to do anything. Almost inevitably what followed was a very rapid physical and mental deterioration. It's almost axiomatic that doing what we really want to do day to day is what nourishes life and health. Those activities that we never grow tired of, that we don't want to retire from, that, in effect, never end for us, are life- and health-giving. Work we love is a form of play. If we live this way, then, like the elders of traditional eras, when we are ready to hand the baton off to someone else we will do it with gratitude and in the spirit of adventure.

Let's start here: we are all guided by our consciousness. If our consciousness keeps telling us that we are going to get sick and die, then that's generally what happens. But if our consciousness is constantly guiding us toward health, health is what we get. A genuinely healthy person has more energy, more vitality, and a greater interest in life as he or she ages. I have seen it over and over. We all have this capacity.

I have spent the greater part of my adult life trying to create the guidelines that will help those who are interested achieve the kind of health I have been describing. Let's examine the seventh step or last guideline in more detail.

> "Dream lofty dreams, and as you dream, so shall you become."
>
> —James Allen

BE OPEN AND CURIOUS AND CULTIVATE AN ENDLESS APPRECIATION FOR ALL OF LIFE

Everyone likes to look at healthy children. Why do you suppose that is? For one thing, their faces are open and clear, not closed and clouded with conceptual thinking, bad experiences, and heavy responsibilities. Since they don't have to get up in the morning and work at jobs they hate, their faces reflect an incredible openness and sense of curiosity. This openness is the source of their energy. When you look at a child, you see bright freshness. The same sort of freshness you see when you look at a healthy plant. A healthy plant is one that is getting the proper nourishment. The soil, water, sunlight, breeze, temperature—everything is suitable. We can say the plant has good nourishment and good circulation. When we look at a healthy child, we see the same thing. Healthy children can eat very, very little or they can eat a lot, or they can eat very simple food and still grow very well. The reason for this is that they have good digestion, meaning they are able to absorb nutrition very efficiently from whatever amount of food they eat. At the same time, they have excellent circulation. They can go out in the coldest weather with almost no clothing on and they don't feel the cold. Their circulation is so good that they have no hardness in their bodies. You can bend children, twist them like pretzels, and the more you do this the funnier they think it is.

"Gratitude is the heart's memory."

—French Proverb

We can see this very clearly by looking at plants. If their nourishment, temperature, or circulation is off, plants react very quickly by losing their freshness. If you over-water, they become limp and lifeless; if you under-water, they become hard, dry, and inflexible. What I am trying to convey with this analogy is that openness or freshness, curiosity, and appreciation mean that we are connected to Nature, connected to life itself—or to God, if you prefer to say it that way. The benefits of a good connection are good nourishment and good circulation.

Experts today are concerned about children's lack of activity. As I mentioned earlier, we are in the midst of a nationwide epidemic of juvenile obesity as well as juvenile diabetes. Parents are being urged to take their children outside and play with them. Isn't this a strange idea? When I was a kid, our parents couldn't get us to come indoors, even for meals. It was a constant battle. There is something really wrong when kids don't want to play. Before children were told that they had to exercise to be healthy, they had the best exercise in the world—play—but once they were introduced to it as a concept, they no longer wanted to exercise at all. Today, children's minds are infected with unhealthy ideas from many sources. Their minds are full of junk ideas, their bodies full of junk food. The inevitable result is a loss of openness and circulation. All of a sudden, it's too cold or too hot to go outside. Minds and bodies close and become inflexible and our children no longer have the openness, freshness, and curiosity they had just two or three years earlier.

"Plant a kernel of wheat and you reap a pint; plant a pint and you reap a bushel. Always the law works to give you back more than you give."

—Anthony Norvell

The way for anyone to recover openness and curiosity is to consciously practice gratitude and appreciation. This practice opens the mind and the heart. When we complain, blame, and criticize, we close our minds. You can say we close ourselves off to life itself or to Nature or to God. Let me give you an example of what I mean. In the early years of my practice, I had a client with colon cancer who had refused surgery. This man, who was a concentration camp survivor, had an iron will. For a year and a half, he ate everything I recommended. After the first nine months, he went to have a checkup with the doctor who had diagnosed him. When the doctor couldn't find any trace of the cancer, he assumed he had misdiagnosed the case. My client continued to practice macrobiotics for another nine months. Then one day I got a phone call from his son. He told me his father had begun to eat other sorts of food and was having health problems again. I suggested that his father return to my original recommendations. The son called back and told me his father was refusing to eat the macrobiotic way, that he would rather die than continue to eat the food. And that's what happened. He ate the macrobiotic way for eighteen months, but during all that time he failed to develop a sense of gratitude or appreciation for what had been given to him. I know it sounds harsh, but I have seen this kind of response again and again in my thirty-odd years of counseling. The man with colon cancer was so strong-willed that he would have eaten sawdust for a year and a half if I had recommended it. Yet because he didn't develop a deep sense of appreciation, the food that gave him back his life never became delicious to him.

> "To speak gratitude is courteous and pleasant, to enact gratitude is generous and noble, but to live gratitude is to touch heaven."
>
> —Johannes A. Gaertner

Let's say there's a man you like, someone you appreciate, and that person does something you're not too crazy about. You don't drop him. Since you're fond of him and appreciate his qualities, you don't give too much weight to what he's done. You cut him some slack. However, if you aren't open to him to start with and, as a consequence, can't appreciate his finer qualities, then what he's just done becomes a huge impediment and chances are you'll drop him altogether.

What I'm getting at is this: appreciation shows openness. If we're open to someone, we see more and more of their good qualities. If we're closed, we see more and more of their negative ones. Appreciation is an expression of our openness to life, our willingness to receive life itself. And that openness manifests itself day to day in a deep interest in and curiosity about life, about everything—food, friendship, love, sex, adventures, travel, history, and so on.

"Take only memories, leave nothing but footprints."
—Chief Seattle

BE FLEXIBLE AND ADAPTABLE IN YOUR PRACTICE

There are only two ways I know of that will help you keep your practice flexible and adaptable. One is to establish a deep connection with the source of life and renewal that is the natural world. You can do this by practicing the 7 Steps really well. The other is to keep in touch with new developments in macrobiotic thinking. Everything changes over time. Everything adapts or dies. Nothing is fixed in cement, including macrobiotics. In today's rapidly changing world, adaptability and flexibility are more important than ever before. Those people who have been practicing for five, ten, twenty years and haven't adapted their ways of cooking and eating to the changing conditions of life inevitably get into trouble. We have to look carefully at what we're doing on a daily basis. If we can't recognize an imbalance in ourselves—and it's very hard to see in oneself—then we should seek guidance.

Of course, the degree of flexibility you can permit yourself depends on your health and the circumstances in which you find yourself. Health is freedom. The better your health, the more relaxed you can afford to be socially. If your health can't afford it, then no matter what the situation or circumstance is, it's better not to mess around. If you're healthy, one binge won't harm you; but if you have a serious health problem and you've been practicing well, one binge can cause devastation. If health were money and you were making five hundred dollars a week, then a thousand-dollar car repair would represent serious damage to your financial health. But if you were making ten thousand a week, it would be no big deal.

Ideally, of course, it would be wonderful if everyone could eat very carefully day to day and be adaptable and flexible socially when appropriate.

To be able to do this depends on your degree of health. My hope is that you make yourself healthy as quickly as possible so you can do what you want. Let me repeat that health is freedom. People think that freedom produces more freedom, but I don't agree. I prefer to use words like order or structure rather than discipline, but the meaning is the same. Freedom rests on and comes out of discipline.

"When you're finished changing, you're finished."
—Benjamin Franklin

Where is it most important to exercise discipline, in our Eating Habits or in our Diet? Do we exercise discipline by making sure we sit down to eat, take time for meals, have a grain and vegetable with every meal, etc., or do we exercise it by thinking, I can eat this, I can't eat that? The answer, of course, is we apply discipline with respect to our Eating Habits. For most people, diet is not discipline. If we enjoy the food, we look forward to eating it. In my book, that's not discipline. One last point: please try to be flexible and adaptable not only in your own practice but also in your dealings with your children, partners, relatives, and friends.

DEVELOP A STRONG WILL AND THE DETERMINATION TO CREATE YOUR OWN HEALTH

The will to create enduring health has to come from within. No matter how loving, generous, and helpful family and friends are, this is a gift they cannot give us. My longtime observation is that people who want to become well do just that. I am always being asked, "Can macrobiotics help cure my illness?" But the question should be, "Can macrobiotics help me cure myself?" It's the person who determines the outcome, not the disease, just as it's the person who determines what illness he or she will get. Have you ever wondered why it is that we get one sort of illness and not another? Based on my counseling experience, I can tell you that we get only that type of illness or disease that perfectly fits our nature. Why should this be the case? Think about it. Becoming ill is an indication—an alarm-bell, in some cases—that we've gotten way off track, that we are seriously out of balance. And we each get out of balance in our own particular way. The type of illness we contract tells us what we need to learn about ourselves in order to get back on track.

"Valor consists in the power of self-recovery."
—Ralph Waldo Emerson

If we are open and appreciative, then we can understand the significance of the illness in our lives, and we can change. If not, then we will just go on repeating the behavior that brought us the illness in the first place. Those who have overcome a terminal illness all say the same thing. "My illness was the best thing that ever happened to me. It changed my life."

"It is idle to say that men are not responsible for their misfortunes."
—Samuel Butler

Some years ago, I invited a young couple from Philadelphia to be part of a panel discussion I led after a lecture I gave at a natural-foods convention. The husband had had testicular cancer many years before and had refused to have his testicle removed surgically. In the beginning, he didn't practice macrobiotics consistently well. He'd visit me, practice well for a while, and then ease up. Well, the cancer spread, it put pressure on his kidneys, and he nearly died. He had to have serious, heavy-duty chemotherapy. He recovered, but his doctors claimed that the spread was due to my interference in his medical treatment. He said, "No, he gave me good advice but I didn't take it. This was entirely my fault." At any rate, his doctors told him he would be sterile. It's important to know that throughout this long ordeal, he never gave up practicing his version of macrobiotics. I assured him that if he could bring himself to practice really well, he could overcome the sterility. I'm happy to tell you the couple has three strong, healthy children. During the panel discussion, his wife said, "My husband's cancer was the best thing that ever happened to us. Without it, we wouldn't have found the macrobiotic way of life and we wouldn't have had such wonderful children," one of whom is a highly gifted pianist. I was used to hearing such remarks from the person who'd been ill, but this was the first time I had ever heard—and from a spouse—that macrobiotics was the best thing that had ever happened to an entire family.

"Who is strong? He that can conquer his bad habits."
—Benjamin Franklin

BE ACCURATE IN YOUR PRACTICE

Accuracy is a spiritual practice, plain and simple. If we are accurate in our practice, it means that we have the ability to devote ourselves to something, to be with something completely without any separation, without any distraction. It means that we understand the value of small things and how the small relates to the large, how the part relates to the whole. So often, it's the little things in life that make a difference. It's been said, and rightly so, that God is in the details. For example, we can make the most wonderful dish in the world, but if we don't season it properly, it won't come to life, it won't taste delicious even though everything up to the point of seasoning was done well. The point at which we add salt to a dish determines the degree of flavor the dish will have, whether it will taste salty or sweet. In this case, accurate timing is crucial.

To practice the macrobiotic way of life accurately means you must pay attention. You must give your undivided attention to sitting down to eat, to chewing well, to getting variety, to doing the body rub, and so on. To pay attention means to be there, mind, body, and spirit—with no separation—in the moment you are doing these things. Accuracy is something that is learned by example and training very early in life. If we haven't had the good fortune to learn it then, we have to work hard to recover our ability to be accurate. And this ability is often the deciding factor in whether or not we recover. Accuracy is a condition of body, mind, and spirit. It is a spiritual practice, not a mechanical one.

"When walking, walk. When eating, eat."
—Zen Proverb

My father was a diamond setter. He taught only two people, my cousin and myself, although there were many others who wanted to learn the trade at that time. When you apprenticed yourself to him, your first job was to sweep the floors, sweep them well and sweep them endlessly, because the bits of precious metals and gems that had fallen to the floor in the course of the work had to be recovered. Almost everybody failed the sweeping test. They couldn't or didn't want to learn to sweep accurately. If they couldn't be accurate when sweeping, my father wouldn't teach them anything more. He'd say, "They're not worth teaching. They can't even sweep the floor." His thinking was, if you're going to do something, do it well or don't do it at all.

Accuracy regarding the seemingly smallest and most meaningless tasks—that is, the willingness, the patience and the ability to do the most meaningless thing fully and completely—is a quality that fewer and fewer people seem to value. Yet those living in spiritual communities, such as monasteries, willingly undertake the most menial chores and do them with appreciation and joy, understanding that it is through this work that they will grow spiritually. If you find it difficult to be accurate, then perhaps one way to develop this quality would be to take on more and more menial tasks and do them with a full heart. Try it and see. The more accurate and precise you can be in your practice, the more you will receive from your efforts—across the board.

Now, although I use the word "accurate," often the client will substitute the word "strict." I want to be clear about this—accuracy and strictness are two entirely different qualities. For one person, to eat simply is accurate. For another, to eat widely is accurate. For some, to eat in restaurants is accurate. For others, to stay away from restaurants is accurate. Accuracy and strictness are not connected in any way; but often when people hear "accuracy," they interpret it as strictness. Strictness is a straight path to rigidity, and rigidity is a condition of hardness.

> "Good timber does not grow with ease. The stronger the wind, the stronger the trees."
>
> —J. Willard Marriot

Please, think about the meaning of the word accuracy and about how to be accurate. Accuracy implies flexibility and adaptability according to the circumstances. It's impossible to be accurate if you don't know what the requirements are. Part of learning to be accurate is to find out what the requirements are. They might involve attending classes, reading books, and so on—in other words, taking the time to find out whatever it is you really need to do to develop that quality of mind, body, and spirit we call accuracy.

CREATE A GOOD SUPPORT NETWORK.

The need to create a good support network is greater than ever. So much of what we have to learn can only be transmitted personally. In the old days, serious students had the attractive option of living in study houses. Most of us who are still actively teaching macrobiotics spent time living in study houses—six months, a year, five years—where we lived and breathed the subject. We roomed together, studied together, played together, cooked for each other, and ate together. The focus of life in the study house was to deepen one's understanding of all aspects of the macrobiotic way. The sort of education we got was very different from what most people have access to today.

Short of a study house, what can you do to create a support network? All of us need to find ways to be around healthy macrobiotic people. If among your friends or acquaintances there's a macrobiotic family that knows how to practice well, try to spend time with them. If you live in a major city, chances are you can find a macrobiotic community there. Information of this sort is sometimes posted on health food store bulletin boards. If you live in a more remote area, the best thing you can do is to attend major macrobiotic programs at least a few times a year—even if you have to travel great distances to get to them. Doing this will make all the difference in your practice and your health. Being in a group of people who are healthy really picks you up. There's a group dynamic that works to everyone's benefit. Your health will improve more rapidly than it would on your own, no matter how well you are practicing. And if your practice has deteriorated because of isolation, you will be inspired to clean up your act.

When I first established my school, the Strengthening Health Institute, the program consisted of two non-residential weekends. I soon realized that for the program to become more effective, it had to be residential. Students need to feel they are part of the school; they need to be involved at every level. I wanted to recreate the experience I had had of living and breathing macrobiotics, and that's very difficult to achieve if students arrive in the morning and leave in the evening. Macrobiotic study programs generally offer a traditional learning structure. As with martial-arts schools, there is usually a mix of new and experienced students, something along the lines of a one-room schoolhouse where different grades are taught together and a bit like the structure in large families where the older children typically help the younger ones.

Please do whatever it takes to create your network. Without one, it is much harder to move in the direction of health.

LEARN TO COOK WELL

Finally, learn to cook well. I can't emphasize this enough. Macrobiotic food has a bad reputation. Many people think the food is terrible. Well, it all depends on your experience. If your first macrobiotic meal is bad, it's easy to dismiss all macrobiotic food. It's useful to remember that the world is full of bad cooks—no matter what sort of food they are preparing. And macrobiotics is no exception. However, a bad macrobiotic meal may be worse for you than an ordinary meal! Unrefined, organic grains and vegetables carry more ki (energy) than their counterparts. They store more energy and vitality. If macrobiotic food is well prepared, it nourishes you more than ordinary food. The downside is that if it's poorly prepared, the effects stay with you longer. We can say that macrobiotic cuisine has the potential to be the most delicious or the most dreadful of any cuisine.

> "Good cooking does not depend on whether the dish is large or small, expensive or economical. If one has the art, then a piece of celery or salted cabbage can be made into a marvelous delicacy; whereas if one has not the art, not all the greatest delicacies and rarities of land, sea or sky are of any avail."
>
> —Yuan Mei

Please remember that no one's cooking is perfect. Perfection is not the point and it's not our goal. Even the best cooks falter. What we strive for is the ability to express ourselves accurately through our cooking, in the same way that artists express themselves accurately through their art. I don't think anyone will dispute that cooking is an art. What's more, cooking is a form of art that creates life. And what is art, if not the expression of one's personal vision of life on earth? Our ability to stay with macrobiotics—and not just to stay with it but to embrace it with a full heart, to choose it enthusiastically over all other ways of life—depends a lot on how well we learn to cook. Whether we cook every day or periodically, we should know how to cook well. The more we know about what it takes to put a delicious macrobiotic meal on the table, the more appreciative we can be of the efforts of others.

I've observed over the years that there seem to be two different takes on the subject of macrobiotic food. The basic one, and the one I subscribe to, is that the food itself is delicious. Our job is to learn how to bring out its natural taste, color, and texture, using simple ingredients and traditional techniques. Simple ingredients and proper techniques are all we need to produce a delicious, satisfying meal. In this style of cooking, modeled after Japanese temple cooking, seasoning, spices, and oil are used sparingly but to great effect.

Then there's the other approach. The thinking behind it goes something like this: "I'll put up with this food for now, but once I get healthy I'll be able to eat the good stuff. I'll be able to eat more widely." There's nothing wrong, per se, with eating widely or with eating simply. It all depends on our condition. What's wrong is the implication that once we can use more oil, once we can cook with herbs and spices, once we can eat tropical fruits and vegetables, then we'll be practicing the "real" macrobiotics and our food will be truly delicious. This is simply not true. Furthermore, what's particularly unsettling about this approach is the belief that the simple meals we eat day to day are not the most delicious, satisfying, nourishing, or fulfilling ones we can have. I think this is a dangerous approach. There is nothing more delicious than well-prepared brown rice or miso soup or blanched, steamed, or sautéed vegetables. On what do I base my assertion? The test for me is how many days in a row, how many years in a row I can eat a particular food and continue to find it delicious, satisfying, and nourishing. Now, we've all gone to fine restaurants and thought the food was incredible and said, "That was one of the best meals I've ever had." I translate such a statement to mean that if we eat such a meal once a year, it does taste that delicious. But if we eat it once a month, it tastes a bit less delicious. And, if we eat it weekly, well—you get the picture. If we eat such a meal every day, it's a safe bet that we won't be able to stand the sight or smell of it after a while. It's just too much. It's an assault on our senses. What this means to me is that such a meal is not truly delicious. Of course, from time to time, it's wonderful to have such a meal. It's a bit like describing someone as a great person and then saying you can only take that person in limited doses—which is quite different from saying, "This is a great person, someone I really want to spend lots of time with."

> "Cook it with pleasure—eat it with joy."
> —Clarissa Dickson Wright

The problem is that learning to bring out the truly delicious natural taste of food without relying on such things as herbs and spices to take up the slack takes more time, patience, sensitivity, and skill than other sorts of cooking. Here's a generalization I think is valid: since I've been involved in macrobiotics, I've observed that you can divide people practicing macrobiotics into two groups. Those who, when they come up against a problem, look inward and those who, in the same circumstances, look outward. The ones who look outward don't last. (Actually, they don't last at anything.) Let's say they become dissatisfied with one or more aspects of the macrobiotic way of life—the philosophy, the healthcare, the spirituality, the cooking, whatever—it doesn't really matter. Eventually we all meet with resistance. We come up against the brick wall of ourselves, so to speak. It's part of living. And then we have two basic choices. We can look outward and think, "Someone out there has got to get me past this, someone has got to help me or I'm out of here." Or we can look inward and think, "I already have the means to help myself. If I just stick with this, I'll get through it." Inevitably, we all arrive at that point of resistance in our cooking. We find ourselves thinking, "Is this all there is, no more ingredients, no more choices?" I can guarantee this will happen to you. When it does, if you stop and ask yourself, "What can I do to make my food more delicious and exciting?" a new dimension will open up and you will be able to take your cooking to the next level. This is how the process of growth works.

If we look outside ourselves for the answer, then we relinquish the ability and the power to create or change our lives. This doesn't mean that we have to do everything by ourselves, that we can't ask for help. At one time or another, we all need guides; but we are the ones who choose them. We are the ones who decide when we need help and for how long a time. We might decide we need shiatsu massage or that we want to improve our cooking or that we have to learn more about macrobiotic philosophy so that we can better help ourselves. This frame of mind is the polar opposite of someone who thinks, "This person is going to help me" or "that person is going to save my life." That's dependence. We are moving toward freedom.

Everything I've been saying comes down to this: a healthy person is self-reliant and self-sufficient. My approach to life has always been that if we're here, we already have what we need to take care of all our problems. We might require help from time to time to get past a rough spot or to have something pointed out to us or to give us a little push. But, still, it's up to us to choose what we want to do and how much energy we want to give it. It's up to us to take the initiative in our own lives. In other words, it's up to us to behave in a self-sufficient manner, and that means not waiting around for someone or something "out there" to come to our aid. Modern life encourages dependence. Part of the macrobiotic journey or adventure—for it is an adventure—is to free ourselves of that dependence by learning to develop our own healing ability and, through struggle, to gain the power to create the life we want.

"A good cook is like a sorceress who dispenses happiness."
—Elsa Schiaparelli

For many of us today, the principal issue is one of health. The challenge is how to create good health so that we are free to live our lives. But let's not forget that health is guided by spirit. And it is in the spirit of macrobiotics to look at the challenges and difficulties that come our way as gifts. For it is in meeting challenges and in overcoming difficulties that we begin to develop the power to heal ourselves, the power to build the life we want. To be truly healthy, we have to embrace the spirit of health.

Which brings me to my final point. Although the spirit of health has many components, it would be a grave mistake to forget the totality. We cannot separate one part from any of the others without destroying the whole. For instance, leaning to cook well requires accuracy, but it also it requires flexibility and openness. You see what I mean. Macrobiotic thinking differs from modern thinking in both its ability and its willingness to look first at the whole, and only then at the parts out of which that whole is formed. If we look at life through the lens of macrobiotics, it becomes clear that each part of life is dependent on all the other parts. It follows then that if we destroy any part of life, we contribute to the destruction of all of life. On the brighter side—or what used to be called "the side of the angels"—if we enhance any part of life, we help to refresh all of life.

Benefits

"Health is like money, we never have a true idea of its value until we lose it."

—Josh Billings

When we practice the 7 Steps, we can improve conditions ranging from high blood pressure to obesity to cancer.

GOOD SLEEP

Our sleep is regulated by our eating habits, diet, and activity. Sleep problems are the result of an imbalance in diet and activity. It's understandable that sleep problems are common because overall we have poor eating habits, low-quality diets, and a lack of outdoor activity. In today's world, the time we need to sleep is actually increasing as a result of poor diet—too much liquids or sweets, animal foods including meat, poultry, eggs, and hard cheese and other dairy products, hard baked goods, chips, salty foods, and cold foods and iced drinks.

Tips for Healthy Sleep
- Eat on a regular schedule (p. 77).
- Stop eating three hours before bedtime.
- Walk outside for at least a half hour a day. It can be a combined half hour. All outdoor activity is helpful especially in a park or natural setting (p. 119).
- Minimize use of televisions, cell phones, and computers before sleep.

- Don't watch disturbing news programs or television shows before going to bed.
- Your bed is for reading, sleep, and sex only—not for working like paying bills.
- Have organic cotton bedclothes, sheets, pillowcases, linens, and comforters.
- Keep the colors and textures in your room quiet and soft.
- Eat a plant-based diet including a variety of unrefined grains and grain products, beans, vegetables, soups, and naturally pickled and fermented foods. This will help even if your diet is not exclusively plant-based (p. 95).
- Keep green plants in your bedroom (p. 140).

GOOD ENERGY

One of the biggest complaints in modern life is fatigue. That is because without regular eating and sleeping schedules and the lack of nutritionally dense foods and outdoor activities, the body cannot naturally detoxify, neutralize acidity, and eliminate toxins. As the toxins and acidity accumulate, the amount of oxygen combining with hemoglobin diminishes and there is less oxygen available for the brain and other vital organs. (Hemoglobin is the iron-containing protein in red blood cells that binds with and transports oxygen throughout the body.) Causing lack of energy, headaches, muscle weakness, and negativity. In addition, the lymph system uses an enormous amount of energy. When our eating and lifestyle practices are poor, a good deal of our energy goes toward cleaning and balancing our body and is not available for daily life activities.

We recommend the best way to feel more energized is to eat less processed foods and move toward a plant-based diet. A plant-based diet has the most energizing foods because they are high in fiber, nutrients, and minerals. The high fiber helps the body to detoxify the gut and digestion. Also improves the ability to absorb nutrients. The foods to eat for energy are whole grains, beans, vegetables, fruits, nuts, seeds, and naturally pickled and fermented foods. The combination of these foods will improve the nutrition and balance in your body and eliminate toxins.

GOOD APPETITE

The most important aspect of these practices grows from a desire to be healthy. The approach that we take helps people rediscover their natural appetite that leads to lasting health. We stress eating habits as much as food choices so we can experience deeper satisfaction from our meals and greater enjoyment of our food. Introducing one healthy food develops our appetite for other healthy foods. Healthy people have a total enjoyment and satisfaction from healthy foods, which continually grows over time.

HEALTHY WEIGHT

Healthy weight is natural. It is like breathing; we don't need to think about it. Weight itself is an indicator of our overall health and the balance of our diet and physical and mental activity. Trying or struggling to lose weight, count calories, or extremely restrict food choices or quantity rarely leads to long-term success. The most effective long-term way to get to your natural, healthy weight is through adding healthy diet and lifestyle practices. Base your diet on a variety of cooked grains, beans, and vegetables and eat a comfortable amount so that you feel satisfied. Your body will naturally adjust the amount of food over time as your digestion improves.

There are four general conditions that indicate that you have a healthy weight. First, you find healthy, plant-based foods delicious and satisfying. Second, you have natural (without the use of any laxatives) bowel movements once or twice a day. Third, you are physically and mentally strong with a "can-do" attitude. Fourth, you are energetic enough to live a creative, active, and engaged life.

Tips for Healthy Weight
- Try to create a regular eating and sleeping schedule. Lunch is the most important meal to keep consistent. Try to start lunch no later than one o'clock (p. 79).
- Sit down to eat without doing other things (p. 55).
- Focus on satisfaction, not restriction.

- Satisfaction can grow endlessly, whereas restriction leads to excess over time.
- See food as food, not as calories, ingredients, or nutrients. A few simple ingredients that are easy to understand are the best indicators that the food has been simply or naturally processed. A variety of plant-based foods and cooking styles provides all nutrients that we need abundantly. Breaking up food into its nutritional constituent parts deters us from finding our sense of taste, natural appetite, and satisfaction.
- Choose the most delicious and satisfying foods from the Healthful Foods List (p. 189).
- Enjoy and appreciate the value of daily activity in your life. It adds up when you think about it, and also nourishes your appetite for healthy food.
- Take a walk after eating.

BLOOD SUGAR

The macrobiotic way of eating is high fiber, balanced, and nutritionally dense. Meaning the foods are composed of complex carbohydrates (grains, beans, vegetables, etc.) that break down slowly and go through your entire digestive system before being absorbed into your blood. This process keeps your blood sugar, moods, and energy even and stable. Unlike a diet rich in sodas and soft drinks or processed and refined foods that are absorbed into your blood quickly causing your blood sugar to spike. White sugar quickly raises blood sugar and high fructose corn syrup and agave nectar tend to create insulin resistance where the insulin becomes ineffective in lowering blood sugar.

There is an extreme polarization in our society between people who have hypoglycemia or low blood sugar and people developing type 2 diabetes or high blood sugar. This problem has worsened over the years as our meal times and daily schedules have become more chaotic and people eat more processed animal and dairy foods, poultry, eggs, cheese, tuna fish, shellfish, refined baked foods, and cold foods and iced drinks.

Over time hypoglycemia causes us to feel pressured, stressed, highly impatient, aggressive, and emotionally up and down. In the case of type 2 diabetes we tend to lose our will power, discipline, and drive over time to improve our health.

Interestingly, these two types of blood sugar problems tend to stabilize and improve quickly through dietary, activity, and lifestyle changes.

Tips for Healthy Blood Sugar

- Try to create a regular eating and sleeping schedule. Try to not skip lunch and to start eating your lunch no later than one o'clock. This alone helps to stabilize your blood sugar (p. 148).
- Eat slowly and chew well (p. 59).
- Have a cooked grain and separate vegetable dish at every meal.
- Eat beans, lentils, or chickpeas daily.
- Eat a variety of sweet tasting vegetables and leafy greens.
- Walk outside at least thirty minutes daily.
- Give yourself a daily body rub.

BLOOD PRESSURE

High blood pressure is also caused by unhealthy eating habits and lifestyle practices. Following the 7 Steps will help balance and stabilize your blood pressure. The combination of fats, salt, and liquids cause the blood pressure to rise and become erratic. Salt alone will not necessarily raise blood pressure as in the traditional Japanese diet. In the past the Japanese had a high salt diet with little high blood pressure. Now that they have adopted the modern diet, blood pressure is a serious problem. The fat is mainly from the excessive consumption of poor quality animal and dairy foods that are naturally high in fat and lack fiber and minerals to digest and eliminate properly. Simple and refined sugars (white sugar, high fructose corn syrup, and agave nectar) can also turn to fat in the body. These products also break down into water and carbon dioxide further compromising the blood quality. Refined flour products further contribute to the problem. This combination makes the blood vessels, veins, and arteries rigid and lose their natural flexibility over time and further contributes to high blood pressure.

Tips for Healthy Blood Pressure
- Try to create a regular eating and sleeping schedule.
- Stop eating three hours before getting into bed.
- Eat slowly and chew well (p. 59).
- Have a cooked grain and separate vegetable dish at every meal.
- Eat beans daily.
- Eat quick steamed greens everyday.
- Eat a wide variety of vegetables from the Healthful Foods List.
- Walk outside at least thirty minutes daily.
- Give yourself a daily body rub for ten to fifteen minutes.
- Minimize hard baked flour products, chips and salty nuts, and seeds.

ANTI-INFLAMMATORY

The modern diet lacks fiber and vital nutrients, has refined salt and sugar, and is highly acidifying, making it tough on the kidneys, liver, spleen, and intestines to naturally eliminate harmful toxins, neutralize excess acidity, and produce vital nutrients for the body. When this happens, the intestines and kidneys become weak and the excess acidity moves to the joints and muscles to be neutralized. However, as you continue eating highly acidic foods, the acidity and toxins start to build up, causing inflammation and eventually arthritis and physical limitations. Remember, joint and muscle health are directly related to our diet, lifestyle, and gut health.

Practicing macrobiotics improves strength, movement, digestion, and flexibility. Eat a plant-based diet of whole grains, beans, vegetables, soups, nuts and seeds, and naturally pickled and fermented foods. These foods are alkalizing instead of acidic. And have fiber and nutrients to nourish the body, improve gut health, and reduce inflammation. The most effective fiber in reducing inflammation is grains, followed by beans and vegetables. Fruits are less effective. On top of it, when you find joint and muscle pain relief, you feel better emotionally as well. Dealing with inflammation is tough, as you feel restricted in what you can do and over-sensitive or drained emotionally. So getting back that independence and physical ability leaves you feeling positive, inspired, and ready to go.

Anti-Inflammatory Tips

- Minimize or avoid the most inflammatory foods: refined flour products, fried fast foods, processed meat and dairy products, margarine, and sodas or soft drinks.
- Experiment to see if the nightshades—potatoes, tomatoes, eggplants, and bell peppers—affect your inflammation.
- Eat a variety of leafy greens, cruciferous vegetables (broccoli, cauliflower, cabbage, arugula, daikon, watercress, etc.), and naturally pickled and fermented foods including miso soup, sauerkraut, kimchi, umeboshi plums, and oil-cured olives.
- Body rub—Gently rub your entire body with a hot, damp cotton washcloth for ten to fifteen minutes at night or in the morning to activate circulation and deeply clean the skin. Do the body rub before or after your bath or shower.
- Topically bruised cabbage—take whiter leaves of cabbage and gently go over with rolling pin. Then place on joints to reduce arthritis inflammation and alleviate pain. Found to be better than ice for joint pain.
- Take a walk every day—important for joggers who have knee joint pain (p. 119).
- Do yoga—to increase flexibility and movement.

STRONG IMMUNITY

Following the 7 Steps will provide you with plenty of prebiotics and probiotics. Prebiotics are the fiber in your food especially in grains, beans, vegetables, and fruits. They act as food for probiotics to grow on. They also carry out toxins and maintain a healthy environment in your intestines. Probiotics are the microbial life that you continually supply through your food and environment. Probiotics are found in naturally pickled and fermented foods. Eating probiotics regularly nourishes and supports gut and overall health.

Having a diet full of prebiotics and probiotics creates a healthy gut with beneficial microbes that naturally keep unhealthy ones out and defend against sickness. Conversely, if you do not have enough healthy gut bacteria, the unhealthy ones can take over. A loss of diversity in your gut environment can also reduce the presence of healthy bacteria. Influences that decrease this diversity are animal and dairy foods, processed foods, chemicals in food and water, and frequent reliance on antibiotics.

Because we've largely destroyed the natural balance of our microbiomes with the modern diet and loss of contact with nature, we have often chosen instead to resort to artificial means to protect ourselves from germs and the environment. It is a self-protective, defensive measure that keeps us from connecting fully with nature, and further weakens our immunity. However, you can always rebuild healthy microbes in the gut with healthy eating and lifestyle practices.

Strong Immunity Tips
- Have a variety of grains, beans, vegetables, seeds, nuts, and fruits.
- Use organic foods as often as possible.
- Consider installing or buying a high-quality water filtration system for cooking and drinking.
- Have naturally pickled and fermented foods. The healthiest fermented foods are naturally prepared miso soup, sauerkraut and kimchi, umeboshi plums, naturally cured olives, and vinegar (apple cider, brown rice, balsamic, and umeboshi).
- Create a healthy home environment by bringing in natural materials and green plants.
- Allow for plenty of sunshine and fresh air to circulate.
- Garden and interact with nature and healthy soil.

FOOD SECTION

About Chef Susan Waxman

I grew up in Richland, Pennsylvania, a small town in the heart of Pennsylvania Dutch country. Coming from a small town had its benefits. As a child, I spent lots of time playing outdoors and had the opportunity to spend a lot of time with my grandparents and family. Almost everyone in my family cooked well. My parents prepared fresh food almost daily and our requirement was to be on time for meals, use good manners, and help clean up afterward. They recognized the importance of a family meal and saw it as an opportunity to spend time together. Of course, at times it was an infringement on playtime, but overall I felt appreciative for the meals and values my parents provided. I was quite fortunate for the stability this brought me, and those experiences continue to help me today.

I began to cook when I was young. The first cooking class I gave was in second grade when we were required to give some type of demonstration.

Being a bit of a procrastinator I was not prepared.

At breakfast I got the great idea to teach the class how to make oatmeal, so I got my father to teach me. I headed off to school armed with my ingredients, a pot, hot plate, and wooden utensils. My class was a success and the oatmeal I made was both delicious and vegan!

When I was in my teens, my grandparents and relatives began to develop degenerative health problems. Diabetes, high cholesterol, high blood pressure, and breast cancer were touching the lives of my family.

I became concerned that the same health problems could become part of my future, since science at that time indicated that many of these health problems were hereditary. Throughout my high school years I led quite an active life. I could pretty much eat whatever I wanted and not gain a pound. While I was not a huge fan of meat, I did love cheese, ice cream, pretzels, and pizza. During my freshman year of college, my unhealthy lifestyle of bad food and bad beer caught up with me and I started to gain weight. I wasn't happy with my body so I decided to make some changes like taking regular walks and eating more vegetables. I also eliminated refined sugar from my diet.

Over the next couple years, I continued to watch the health of my family members decline. I saw how they struggled with their effort to diet and make changes later in life. I decided I would rather make changes to my lifestyle while I was young.

At the age of twenty-two I became more and more interested in health. I began exploring vegetarian cooking both for better health and ethical reasons; I like animals. A number of years later I discovered macrobiotics when my friend, Ralph, invited me to attend a lecture on macrobiotics given by Patrick Riley, a macrobiotic teacher and shiatsu practitioner. That lecture changed my life. The philosophy made perfect sense to me and I liked the idea that we are in control of our destinies. Transitioning to a macrobiotic diet was pretty easy for me as I was already a vegetarian eating grains, veggies, and beans. This was the beginning of my lifelong study of macrobiotics and my passion, food.

Susan's Philosophy on Food

"True healthcare reform starts in your kitchen, not in Washington."

—Anonymous

We need food to live. Many things in our lives are beyond our immediate control. The single thing that is within our reach, of which we can obtain the most control, is our daily food. This is a wonderful opportunity because our food choices have the most ability to determine our destiny. At any given time we are either moving toward health or away from health by the food and lifestyle choices we make. The way we choose to fuel our bodies has the most lasting influence on all aspects of our lives from physical health to emotional and spiritual well being.

There is more hype around food these days, whether it is to cure an ailment, prevent disease, or enhance a physical quality for optimum strength and beauty. In fact there appear to be so many options it has become confusing. In the past few years, there has been increased awareness of the benefits of plant-based diets. Once considered strange and unhealthy, plant-based diets have been welcomed into the realm of popular culture, thanks to a growing cognizance of the environmental, economic, and personal benefits to be reaped from adopting a plant-based diet. I like to describe the macrobiotic diet as the most well thought-out plant-based diet because we use a variety of cooking styles, a variety of grains, vegetables, and beans. We choose foods that are indigenous, which helps us to align with nature and better balance with our immediate environment.

Finally, we include plenty of natural probiotics through the use of fermented foods and beverages. This is in alignment with the dietary practices of the world's centenarians. When we have our health we have no limitations. For me that is pretty cool, and it makes the animals and plants happy too.

OVERVIEW

The recipes in our book are all vegan and based on a variety of world cuisines. The unique aspect is that I use macrobiotic philosophy and the principle of balance in all aspects of the recipes, from the ingredients used to the order of preparation.

The term "macrobiotic" was first used by Hippocrates, the father of Western medicine, to describe people who led long, healthy lives. Aristotle, Herodotus, and Galen also used the term to describe a lifestyle based upon a balanced diet that resulted in good health and longevity. Dr. Christophe Hufeland, a 18th-century German physician, also used the term "macrobiotic" in his book, *The Art of Prolonging Human Life*. Like the Greeks before him, Dr. Hufeland made the connection between diet and a long and healthy life. Dr. Hufeland also referenced a "life force" that he claimed was present in all things, and could be influenced by and changed through diet and lifestyle. The idea of a life force is universal: energy, ki, chi, and prana are all synonymous.

The belief that the food we eat provides not only sustenance but is also a governing factor in our overall health and happiness has long been a part of Eastern culture, even before the term "macrobiotics" became part of the lexicon. This philosophy is in line with my belief that we have the ability to create our own health and, ultimately, become the master of our own destiny. Looking at the world from an energetic perspective in which all things possess an energetic quality enables us to look at our lives through the same lens and create change where we want it. When this perspective is put into practice in our diet and lifestyle, macrobiotics can be defined as an intentional, conscious approach to living. Good food and good living are the keys to lasting health.

In the recipe section, I provide the reader with the practical tools for cooking and menu planning from an energetic perspective. Each cooking style has its unique energetic quality, meaning the dish itself has the ability to activate or stabilize our circulation. Every recipe is created with an image and intent in mind, which determines the energy of the resulting dish. When creating a dish or a recipe, good taste depends on what is put together and how it is put together.

An orderly approach to cooking allows the natural flavor of the ingredients used to come through, instead of relying on heavy seasonings. Combining all of these elements in cooking is what ultimately creates lasting health. The good feelings and energy you receive when you eat my food is proof of a well balanced, healthy recipe.

Macrobiotic philosophy and food energetics is a life-long study of mine. Cooking and creating healthy dishes is my art. As a macrobiotic teacher, counselor, and chef, I have spent most of my life helping people attain and maintain optimum health. It is my hope that more people will be inspired to cook and make the connection that what we put into our bodies affects all aspects of our physical, emotional, and spiritual health.

To me, cooking is a creative form of expression. It is about developing a relationship with food and all good cooks have a love of food. I believe that the essence and true spirit of the cook shines through in the food they make. Food is life-sustaining, healing, spiritual, and fun. It is one of the ultimate expressions of love for oneself, family, and friends.

Susan Waxman is an internationally recognized macrobiotic teacher, counselor, and health educator. She is also the codirector of and executive chef at the Strengthening Health Institute (SHI) in Philadelphia, Pennsylvania, a center dedicated to macrobiotic education, whose goal is the promotion of personal and planetary health. Widely recognized for her culinary expertise and understanding of the energetic properties of food, she has taught throughout the United States and abroad. Susan's innovative style and attention to detail show through in the flavor and healing power of her food.

As a teacher and health educator, Susan has worked with everyone from mothers hoping to improve their families' eating habits to well-known celebrities and people with serious illnesses.

Before dedicating her life to macrobiotics, Susan worked with children and young adults in the field of social services. She holds degrees in Psychology, Sociology, and Anthropology from the University of Pittsburgh.

Suggestions for Getting Started

Try to use:
- Organically grown, seasonal foods where possible.
- Whole and partially refined grains and grain products instead of refined grains, and brown rice instead of white rice.
- Un-yeasted sourdough bread.
- One fresh vegetable dish for every meal.
- Unrefined white sea salt.
- Unrefined oils, such as light sesame oil, organic extra virgin olive oil, or safflower oil.
- Jams without added sugar.
- Fruit juices without added sugar.
- Rice syrup, maple syrup, and barley-malt syrup as natural sweeteners instead of sugar, honey, stevia, or agave nectar.
- Wild white-meat fish or salmon over meat and chicken.
- Proteins such as beans, tofu, seitan, and tempeh instead of meat and cheese.
- Non-stimulating teas and organic black coffee.
- Sea vegetables for your cooking. These vegetables are sources of valuable nutrients, including calcium, potassium, and beta-carotene that help reduce cholesterol, rid the body of toxins, and strengthen immunity.
- Foods from the Foods for Regular Use list (p. 191).

Healthful Foods List

CREATING VARIETY IN YOUR COOKING

Variety is the key to enjoyment, satisfaction, and balanced nutrition. Other foods included on a regular basis are:

- Select foods within the following categories: grains, soups, vegetables, beans, sea vegetables, condiments, pickles, beverages, and occasional foods.
- Use different cooking methods: boiling, steaming, sautéing, etc. (see Styles of Cooking below)
- Cut vegetables in different ways.
- Vary amount of water used.
- Vary kinds of seasoning and condiments.
- Amounts of seasoning and condiments.
- Vary cooking time: don't overcook or pressure cook vegetables.
- Use higher or lower flame in cooking food.
- Combination of foods and dishes.
- Adjust your cooking according to seasonal changes.

COOKING IN ADVANCE

- Grains, beans, sea vegetables, dried daikon, squash, kombu, azuki beans, and other well-cooked dishes can be cooked for two to three days at a time. These dishes may be reheated.
- Try to make at least one vegetable dish and soup fresh each day. The lightly cooked vegetable dishes are best consumed within one to two days.
- Soup may be reheated gently.
- **Do not reheat leftover vegetable dishes.** Take out the vegetable dishes that need refrigeration in advance and allow them to warm up to room temperature naturally.

STYLES OF COOKING

Use often

Pressure cooking
Boiling
Blanching
Steaming
Steaming with kombu (Nishime)
Soup making
Stewing
Quick water sautéing
Quick oil sautéing
Sautéing and simmering (Kimpira)
Pressing
Pickling
Raw

Use occasionally

Baking
Broiling
Dry roasting
Pan-frying
Deep-frying
Tempura (batter-dipped and deep-fried)

FOODS FOR REGULAR USE

These are the most important foods for everyone.
They are essential to a healthy, balanced, and nutritious diet.

GRAINS AND GRAIN PRODUCTS

Use a variety with every meal. Eat brown rice often or daily.

WHOLE GRAINS

Use often

Short-grain brown rice
Medium-grain brown rice
Barley (pearled)
Millet
Wheat berries
Farro (pearled)
Corn (corn on the cob)
Whole oats
Rye
Buckwheat
Long-grain brown rice: for hot
climates
Whole, Cracked, and Flaked
Grains

WHOLE, CRACKED & FLAKED GRAINS

Use occasionally

Sweet brown rice
Mochi
Hato-mugi barley,
Pearl barley, Job's Tears,
Barley grits
Bulgur
Cracked wheat
Couscous
Rolled oats
Steel-cut oats
Corn grits
Corn meal (Polenta)
Rye flakes, barley flakes, or
other flakes
Other traditional grains
including amaranth, quinoa, etc.

FLOUR PRODUCTS

Use occasionally

Whole-wheat noodles
Italian pasta (unenriched)
Japanese wheat noodles (Udon)
Japanese thin wheat noodles
(Somen)
Japanese buckwheat noodles
(Soba)
Bread: un-yeasted, sourdough
wheat, spelt, or rye
Puffed wheat gluten (Fu)
Boiled wheat gluten (Seitan)

VEGETABLE SOUPS

1 to 2 servings every day with a meal.

Mildly season soups with barley miso, brown rice miso, shoyu, or sea salt.
Use barley (mugi) miso or brown rice (genmai) miso.
Garnish soups often with chopped scallion or parsley.

Miso vegetable soup: with wakame seaweed, a variety of vegetables, and miso.

Clear shoyu soup: with kombu seaweed, dried shiitake mushroom, a variety of vegetables, and mild shoyu.

Puréed sweet vegetables soup: seasoned with sea salt.

Puréed sweet vegetable soup with millet or barley: Cook in a small amount of grain to make a creamy soup. Season with sea salt.

Other types of vegetable soup: with a variety of vegetables, sea vegetables, beans, grains, or pasta.

Bean vegetable soup: Cook leftover beans in vegetable soup until creamy.

Grain vegetable soup: Cook leftover grains such as brown rice, barley, or millet in vegetable soup until creamy. Season with miso.

Noodle vegetable soup: with wheat or buckwheat noodles.

Fish vegetable soup: with white meat fish.

VEGETABLES

Eat one or more vegetable dishes with every meal.
Do not reheat leftover vegetable dishes.

Use often

[1] Green Leafy:

Arugula
Bok choy
Carrot tops
Chinese cabbage (napa)
Collard greens
Daikon greens
Dandelion greens
Kale
Leek
Mustard greens
Parsley
Romaine lettuce
Scallion
Turnip greens
Watercress

[2] Round:

Acorn squash
Broccoli
Brussels sprouts
Buttercup squash
Butternut squash
Cabbage
Cauliflower
Hokkaido pumpkin
Onion
Pumpkin
Red cabbage
Rutabaga
Turnip
Shiitake mushroom (dried)

Use often

[3] Root:

Burdock
Carrots
Daikon
Dandelion roots
Jinenjo
Lotus root
Parsnip
Radish

[4] Sweet vegetables:

Sweet vegetables are a combination of round and root vegetables, these vegetables become sweet when cooked. *Broccoli and cauliflower are not usually considered sweet vegetables, however, they add a richness and freshness to puréed soups when combined with the sweet vegetables.

Broccoli*
Cabbage
Carrots
Cauliflower*
Daikon
Leek
Onion
Parsnip
Pumpkin
Sweet potato
Winter Squash

Use occasionally

Artichoke
Asparagus
Avocado
Beets
Broccoli Rabe
Celery
Chives
Cucumber
Endive
Escarole
Fennel
Green beans
Green peas
Iceberg lettuce
Jerusalem artichoke
Kohlrabi
Lambsquarters
Mushrooms
Patty pan squash
Purslane
Salsify
Snap beans
Snow peas
Spinach
Sprouts
Summer squash
Taro potato (albi)
Tomato (fresh or sun-dried)
Wax beans
Zucchini

BEANS AND BEAN PRODUCTS

Have 1 to 1½ servings per day.

Cook beans with a 1-inch piece of kombu seaweed to make
them more digestible.
A serving of beans or bean products is ½ to 1 cup.
Beans may be cooked with vegetables, with grains, or in soups.
Season beans at the end of cooking with sea salt or shoyu.

BEANS	BEANS	BEAN PRODUCTS
Use often	*Use occasionally*	*Use occasionally*
Azuki beans	Black-eyed peas	Dried tofu
Black soy beans	Black turtle beans	Fresh tofu
Chickpeas (Garbanzos)	Cannellini beans	Natto Tempeh
Green or black lentils	Great Northern beans	
	Kidney beans	
	Lima beans	
	Mung beans	
	Navy beans	
	Pinto beans	
	Soybeans	
	Split peas	
	Whole dried peas	

SEA VEGETABLES

Use small amounts daily in cooking.

Nori, wakame, and kombu are used as a part of daily cooking.
They are used in a variety of dishes including: soups, vegetable,
bean, and grain dishes.

Use often	*Use occasionally*	*Optional use*
Toasted nori sheet	Arame	Agar-agar
Wakame	Hiziki	Dulse
Kombu		Sea palm

PICKLED VEGETABLES

Use as a garnish often or daily.

Wash or soak the pickles if they taste salty.

Use often	Use occasionally
Sauerkraut (white or red)	Beet pickles
Kimchi	Bran pickles
Quick shoyu pickles	Brine pickles
Quick ume-vinegar pickles	Daikon radish pickles (Takuan)
	Shoyu pickles

TABLE CONDIMENTS

Try to use one to two condiments every day.

Condiments are used on foods at the table—not in cooking.
Make a condiment tray and keep it on the table as a reminder to use them.
Condiments with an (*) can be bought—it is best to make the others at home.

Use often	Use occasionally
Toasted sesame seeds: 1–2 tsp.	Apple cider vinegar**
Green Ao nori flakes*: 1/2–1 tsp.	Brown rice vinegar**
Ume Shiso powder*: 1/4 tsp.	Umeboshi vinegar
Umeboshi (Pickled plums)*: 1/2–1 plum	Lemon juice: from fresh lemon**
Nuts & seeds	Boiled nori condiment: 1–2 tsp.
*Sprinkle on food.	** Not recommended in water or tea.

SEASONINGS FOR COOKING

Use the full variety to make your food tasty.
Seasonings are used in cooking—not at the table.

Use often	Use occasionally
Unrefined white sea salt: Si brand	Apple cider vinegar
Barley miso (Mugi): aged at least 24 months	Balsamic vinegar
Brown rice miso (Genmai): aged at least 12 months	Brown rice vinegar
	Chili peppers
Shoyu (naturally fermented soy sauce): aged at least 18 months	Ginger
	Harissa
Light sesame oil	Horseradish
Extra virgin olive oil	Wasabi horseradish
	Umeboshi plum
	Umeboshi paste
	Umeboshi vinegar
	Garlic
	Lemon
	Saffron
	Soybean miso (Hatcho)
	Mirin (sweet taste)
	Toasted/dark sesame oil
	European herbs

BEVERAGES

Drink a comfortable amount for thirst.

Use often	Use occasionally	Use occasionally
Bancha twig tea (kukicha)	Roasted dandelion root tea	Black coffee or tea
Bancha leaf tea (green tea)	Kombu tea	Microbrewed beer
Roasted barley tea	Mu tea (mild)	Natural sake
Roasted brown rice tea	Carrot or carrot-greens juice	Red or white wine
Filtered water	Carrot, apple, and greens juice	Sweet vegetable drink
	Carrot, apple, and orange juice	Soy milk: with kombu

FOODS FOR OCCASIONAL USE

These foods are good for creating a more varied and satisfying diet.
They are not essential.

FISH

1 to 3 times a week.

Choose from non-fatty, wild white-meat fish or wild salmon occasionally.

Cod	Porgy	Salmon
Flounder	Red and other snapper	Sea Bass
Haddock	Scrod	Sardines
Hake	Sole	Turbot
Halibut	Other non-fatty, white-meat	
Ling	fish	

SEEDS AND NUTS

½ to 1 cup seeds, and 1 to 2 cups nuts a week (lightly roasted-unsalted).
Seeds and nuts may be used in cooking, as garnishes with a variety of
dishes, and as snacks.
Seeds and nuts may be eaten boiled, blanched, lightly dry, or oil-roasted.
Pumpkin seeds and occasionally sunflower seeds and walnuts may be
eaten raw.

Seeds	*Nuts*
Pumpkin seeds	Chestnuts
Sesame seeds	Almonds
Sunflower seeds	Peanuts
Caraway seeds	Walnuts
Flax seeds: freshly ground	Pecans
Roasted tan tahini	Hazelnuts
Roasted black tahini	Pistachios
Tohum tahini	Peanut butter
	Almond butter

SNACKS

Can be used almost daily.

Snacks may be eaten in moderate amounts.
Try not to let them interfere with your regular meals.

Leftovers
Pounded sweet rice (Mochi)
Amasake
Noodles
Nuts
Seeds

Puffed whole cereal grains
Popcorn: homemade,
unbuttered
Rice cakes
Corn Thins
Rice balls

Nori, brown rice and vegetable
rolls (Sushi)
Steamed sweet portatoes
Sweet vegetable jam
Soy milk: with kombu

SWEETS AND SWEETENERS

Can be used almost daily.

Use often

Sweet vegetables
Sweet vegetable drink
Sweet vegetable jam
Chestnuts or chestnut purée

Use occasionally

Amasake
Barley malt (pure)
Brown rice syrup
Pure maple syrup
Hot apple cider: diluted with bancha twig tea or
filtered water
Hot apple juice: diluted with bancha twig tea or
filtered water

FRUITS

3 to 7 times a week.

Cooked, dried, or fresh, seasonal Northern climate fruits.

Ground Fruit

Blueberries
Blackberries
Cantaloupe
Honeydew
Raspberries
Strawberries
Watermelon

Tree Fruit

Apples
Apricots
Cherries
Dates
Grapes
Figs
Raisins

Peaches
Pears
Plums
Tangerines
Oranges

USE SPARINGLY OR AVOID

These foods depend on your health.
Many are very acidifying or affect blood sugar.

BAKED FLOUR PRODUCTS AND REFINED GRAINS

Muffins
Crackers
Cookies
Pancakes
Chips
Baked pastries
White rice

BEVERAGES

Green magma
Whiskey (natural quality)
Rice milk
Frozen Rice Dream

SEASONINGS AND SPICES

Tropical spices
All commercial seasonings

VEGETABLES

Bamboo shoots
Curly dock
Eggplant
Ferns
Ginseng
Green or red pepper
New Zealand spinach
Okra
Plantain
Potato
Rhubarb
Swiss chard
Yam

PICKLES

Dill pickles
Herb pickles
Garlic pickles
Spiced pickles
Vinegar pickles
Apple cider vinegar pickles
Wine vinegar pickles

BLUE SKINNED FISH

Herring
Tuna

ALL TROPICAL NUTS

Brazil nuts
Macadamia nuts

ALL TROPICAL FRUIT, INCLUDING:

Mango
Papaya
Pineapple
Grapefruit

AVOID AS MUCH AS POSSIBLE

These are the worst foods for everybody.

RED MEAT

Beef

Lamb

Pork

POULTRY

Chicken

Duck

Turkey

BLUE SKINNED FISH

Tuna

Blue fish

Swordfish

DAIRY FOODS & EGGS

Milk

Butter

Cheese

Yogurt

Frozen yogurt

Ice cream

BEVERAGES

Artificial beverages

Cold drinks, iced drinks

Distilled water

Hard liquor

Herbal teas

Mineral-bubbling waters

Regular tea

Stimulant beverages

Sugared beverages

Tap water

Carbonated waters

SWEETENERS

Agave nectar

Artificial sweeteners

Brown sugar

Carob

Chocolate

Corn sugar

High-fructose corn syrup

Concentrated fruit sweeteners

Honey

Molasses

Stevia

Sugar substitutes

White sugar

OTHER FOODS

Bananas

Coconut

Coconut oil

Palm oil

Palm kernel oil

Palm fruit oil

Cashews

Lard

Margarine

Artificially processed foods

All foods containing trans fats

Recommended Cookware

- Stainless steel saucepans and stock with lids in various sizes
- Stainless steel skillets, medium and larger size
- Pressure cooker
- Stainless steel or bamboo steamer basket
- Colander
- Metal flame deflector, ideally two
- Japanese donabe pot—this is an earthenware pot used to cook grains.
- Cast-iron skillets
- Deeper style cast-iron pot used for sautéing, stews, and deep frying
- Enamel coated cast-iron Dutch oven to cook beans, grains, or stew
- Hand immersion blender for puréed soups
- Blender or food processor
- Juicer
- Porcelain grater
- Vegetable knife and paring knife
- Wooden cutting board
- Wooden spoons, spatulas, rice paddles, and cooking chopsticks
- Metal spoons
- Fine mesh vegetable skimmer
- Medium and large wire spider
- Wet and dry measuring cups specific to the ingredient being used
- An assortment of prep bowls stainless or Pyrex
- Glass bottles with pouring spouts for oil and liquid seasonings
- Water filter

Note on Seasoning

The use of salt and seasoning is relative to taste. A certain amount of salt is necessary to balance a dish but eating too much salt can contribute to undesirable symptoms and potentially harm your health. In each recipe I give a range starting with the least amount to the highest amount needed. This is a suggested guideline for the use of salt and salty seasonings. I recommend that you try to stay within the range. If you are accustomed to more seasoning it may take some time for your taste to adjust. If you desire simply add a little more salt.

RECIPES AND MEAL PLANS

BREAKFAST GRAINS

There are many theories surrounding the benefits of eating breakfast. When I was growing up, my parents would often say, "start your day off right by eating a good breakfast." Many people say that breakfast is the most important meal of the day. While I don't necessarily consider breakfast to be the most important meal of the day, I do think that eating breakfast is beneficial to most people for several reasons.

Eating breakfast activates our metabolism and keeps our blood sugar stable. When our blood sugar is stable, we have better overall energy and are better able to focus throughout the morning. Breakfast does not have to be a large meal—just enough food to lightly raise your blood sugar and get your motor running will do the trick. I do think that breakfast is important for children and teenagers, because eating breakfast will help them focus in school. If you want to shed a few pounds or maintain an appropriate weight, then breakfast is very important because it will help to keep your metabolism more active throughout the day.

Note: When planning your breakfast, choose a grain-based dish and complete the meal with a light vegetable side dish, such as steamed or blanched greens.

SOFT RICE

You can easily make soft rice out of any leftover rice dish. You are simply adding water and cooking the rice until it reaches a soft and creamy consistency. I think that you will find this dish to be both nourishing and satisfying.

Preparation time: 30 minutes
Serves 2

Ingredients
- 1 cup leftover brown rice
- Water as needed, approximately 2 cups

Preparation
- Pour ½ cup of water into a pot, and begin to heat on a low flame.
- After 1 minute or so, add the rice to the pot. As the rice begins to cook it will absorb some of the water. Use a wooden spoon or rice paddle to break up any clumps of rice.
- Add a little more water and bring to a very gentle boil.
- Place a flame deflector under the pot and partially cover.
- Gently fold the bottom to the top every few minutes to prevent sticking.
- Continue to add water and cook on low until the rice is soft and creamy in texture.
- Soft rice needs to simmer 20 to 30 minutes.

Variations
- Add a little umeboshi plum toward the end of cooking. Umeboshi soft rice strengthens our digestive system and is the universal cure for flu and cold symptoms.

- Add a little of fresh or frozen corn toward the end of cooking time. This variation is helpful when trying to relax a tight condition and for prostate problems.
- When making this dish for kids, trying adding a little rice syrup or barley malt to sweeten the soft rice.

—◇—

STEEL-CUT OATS

Steel-cut oats take a little more time and planning than rolled oats, but they are much more nourishing.

Preparation time: 45 to 50 minutes
Serves 4

Ingredients
- 1 cup steel-cut oats
- 4 to 5 cups water
- 1/16 teaspoon sea salt

Preparation
- Place steel-cut oats and 2 cups water in a saucepan.
- Bring the water and oats to a boil, then add the sea salt.
- Lower the flame and allow the oats to begin to absorb some of the water, about 5 to 7 minutes.
- Add another 2 cups of water and partially cover the pot. Bring the water to a boil, then lower the flame and cover. Place a flame deflector under the pot and simmer on low for 20 minutes.
- Uncover the pot, fold the bottom into the top to help the oats cook evenly and prevent them from sticking.
- Simmer another 15 minutes and serve.

Note: If you like a creamier consistency, you can add a little more water to the dish while it is simmering.

ROLLED OATS

Rolled oats come in various textures and thickness. I prefer the "thick-cut" rolled oats for their heartier texture.

Preparation time: 10 to 15 minutes
Serves 2

Ingredients
- 1 cup thick-cut rolled oats
- 2 cups water
- $\frac{1}{16}$ teaspoon sea salt

Preparation
- Place 1½ cups of water and the oats in a pot. Let the oats sit in the water for 2 to 3 minutes.
- Turn the flame on a low setting and bring to a boil, uncovered.
- Add the sea salt.
- As the oats begin to absorb some of the water, add more water and gently fold the bottom into the top to blend the ingredients.
- Cook uncovered for a few minutes, stirring occasionally.
- As the oats continue to cook, the consistency will thicken and the texture will become more creamy. Continue to cook for another 5 minutes.
- Cover completely, turn off the flame, and let sit for another 4 to 5 minutes before serving.

SOFT MILLET

Soft millet with sweet vegetables is a very stabilizing porridge. By that, I mean it has a natural balancing effect on our blood sugar so it is helpful for both hypoglycemia and diabetes.

Preparation time: 1 hour
Serves 4 to 5

Ingredients
- 1 cup millet
- ½ cup diced onions
- ½ to 1 cup chopped sweet vegetable of your choice (carrots, winter squash, cabbage, etc.)
- 1/16 to 1/8 teaspoon sea salt
- 5 to 5½ cups water

Preparation
- Place the onions in a pot with ½ cup water and bring the water to a boil.
- Add a few grains salt and cook the onions for 2 to 3 minutes.
- Add the other vegetables, the millet, the remaining water, and the salt.
- Partially cover and bring to a boil.
- Lower the flame, cover completely, place a flame deflector under the pot, and cook for 40 minutes.
- Remove the lid and fold the top into the bottom to blend the vegetables with the millet. The texture should be creamy. Add more water as needed to reach the desired consistency.
- Replace the cover and cook for another 10 minutes.

Note: Soft millet can be made using leftover millet. Just add a little water to the bottom of a pot. Add the millet and slowly begin to heat (this is very similar to the preparation for soft rice). Add additional water as needed and continue to cook until you reach the desired consistency.

SWEET COUSCOUS

Breakfast couscous cooks very quickly and is a time-saver for busy mornings.

Preparation time: 10 minutes
Serves 2 to 3

Ingredients
- 1 cup whole-wheat couscous
- 1 cup organic apple juice
- 1⅓ cups water
- ¹⁄₁₆ teaspoon sea salt

Preparation
- Pour all wet ingredients into a pot and bring to a boil.
- Add the couscous and a pinch of salt.
- Lower the flame, cover, and place a flame deflector under the pot.
- Cook for 1 to 2 minutes on a low flame.
- Turn off the flame and let the pot sit for 5 to 7 minutes.
- Remove the cover and stir the couscous with a wooden spoon before serving.

STEAMED SOURDOUGH BREAD

Bread is a staple among all European cultures. Good-quality bread is satisfying, nourishing, and a good source of protein. When shopping for bread, read the ingredients label. There should only be a few main ingredients; flour, salt, and water. Real sourdough bread does not contain any commercial yeast but makes use of "wild yeast" in the environment. Steaming bread makes the bread more digestible and makes the nutrients in the bread more bio-available.

Preparation time: 2 to 4 minutes

1 to 2 slices per person

Ingredients
- Sourdough bread
- A small amount of water for steaming
- A stainless steel pot and a steamer basket. I prefer using a steamer basket that sits on top of the pot (not the collapsible ones that fit inside). You can use either a stainless steel or bamboo steamer basket; both work well.

Preparation
- Add an inch of water to cover the bottom of the pot and place the steamer basket on top of the pot.
- Place the bread inside the basket, turn on the flame, and cover.
- When the bread gives off a "fresh-baked" aroma, after 2–5 minutes, it is ready.
- Remove the bread from the basket, place it on a bamboo mat that is on top of a plate.
- Allow the bread to cool a bit before adding your favorite topping.

Topping Suggestions: tahini or peanut butter and sauerkraut, tahini or peanut butter and fruit spread, hummus and sauerkraut with cucumbers, onion, or squash butter.

LUNCH AND DINNER GRAINS

BROWN RICE

As the most balanced of all cereal grains, brown rice has many unique qualities. Unlike other grains, it grows on both dry land and in water. Brown rice is also very flexible and adaptable in that it combines well with other grains, beans, and vegetables. Of all the whole-cereal grains, brown rice has the greatest ability to bring our bodies into balance and strengthen our overall health.

Despite its numerous benefits, it is possible to eat too much brown rice! For most people, a serving of brown rice five to seven days a week is enough to create a good condition and maintain strong vitality. Eating too much brown rice creates an overly contracted internal condition which can lead to other health problems. Personally, I like to combine my brown rice with other grains and beans. This combination gives us strength and vitality while also providing more variety in our diet. Below is a recipe for basic brown rice and some helpful hints on how to prepare rice combinations, including how to vary the proportions to create a balance that suits your personal needs.

Brown rice needs to washed and soaked before cooking. Soaking the rice makes it more digestible, allowing the grain to open up and release more nutrients. For best results we recommend soaking the brown rice overnight, up to twenty hours and cooking the rice in the soaking water.

Preparation

- Wash the rice by placing it in a bowl and covering with water. Use your hand to gently swish the grain around several times, then pour the water off. Repeat this process two more times, for a total of three rinses.
- Whole grains may be washed and soaked together with the brown rice.
- Partially refined (pearled) or cracked grains are not soaked and are added right before you are ready to cook your rice.
- Place washed grain in a bowl along with the pre-measured water to soak, then cover with a bamboo mat.

⊷◈⊶

PRESSURE STEAMED BROWN RICE USING A DONABE POT

This is my favorite way to cook rice. The energetic quality is more relaxed, with the texture and consistency in between pressure-cooked and steamed rice, while still maintaining plenty of flavor. It is perfect for people making a small amount of grain. In addition it is easy to determine the exact amount of water so almost everyone can make the perfect pot of rice.

Preparation time: 50 minutes
Serves 4 to 5

Ingredients

- ⅔ cup brown rice
- ⅓ cup other grain
- 2 cups water
- ¹⁄₁₆ teaspoon sea salt or 1-inch piece kombu

Cookware

- Earthen Japanese-style donabe pot

Preparation

- Place the soaked rice and soaking water in a pot.
- If you are adding any partially refined or cracked grain, add it at this time along with any additional water needed to keep the 1:2 grain-to-water ratio.
- Add a pinch of sea salt or a piece of kombu.
- Place the inside lid on the pot, aligning the 2 holes with the handles.
- Place the domed lid with a hole on top of the inside lid, aligning the hole between the handles.
- Bring the water to a boil over a medium-high flame.
- When steam emerges from the hole in the lid, place a flame deflector under the pot, and reduce the heat to the lowest setting.
- Simmer on low for 40 to 50 minutes.
- Remove the rice using a moistened wooden paddle and place the rice in a serving bowl. Cover the rice with a bamboo mat until serving time.

Note: To care for your pot; do not put the pot on a flame if the bottom is wet. It is okay to soak the rice directly in the pot, just make sure not to get the bottom wet. This pot is not to be used on an electric stove. When cleaning remove the lid and set to the side allowing it to cool completely before washing. Allow the pot to cool completely before soaking. Do not put the lid back on the pot until everything is completely dry. I know this sounds like a high-maintenance pot but it actually cleans up easily and really makes delicious rice.

PRESSURE-COOKED BROWN RICE WITH GRAINS

Preparation time: 50 to 60 minutes

2 cups of dry brown rice yields 5 to 6 servings

Ingredients

- 1⅔ cups organic brown rice
- ⅓ cup grain, such as sweet brown rice or barley
- 2½ to 2⅔ cups water
- ⅛ teaspoon sea salt or 1 square inch kombu

Preparation

- Place the rice and the soaking water in a pressure cooker.
- Add any additional grains and additional water.
- Add the sea salt or kombu, cover, and bring to full pressure on a medium flame.
- Place a flame deflector under the pressure cooker and reduce the flame to low.
- Cook under low pressure for 45 to 50 minutes.
- Turn off the flame and remove pot from the stove.
- Let sit, allowing the pressure to come down naturally.
- Remove the rice from the pressure cooker using a moistened wooden rice paddle.
- Place the rice in a bowl and cover with a light bamboo mat until ready to serve.

PRESSURE-COOKED BROWN RICE WITH BEANS

Preparation time: 55 to 60 minutes

2 cups of dry rice and beans yields 6 to 7 servings

Ingredients
- 1⅔ cups organic brown rice
- ⅓ cup beans
- 3 to 3¾ cups water
- 1 square inch kombu

Cookware
- pressure cooker
- rice paddle

Preparation
- Wash the rice by placing it in a bowl and covering with water. Use your hand to gently swish the grain around several times, then pour the water off. Repeat this process two more times, for a total of three rinses. Soak overnight.
- Azuki beans may be washed and soaked together with the rice. Use the soaking water.
- Lentils do not need to be soaked; sort and wash before cooking.
- All other beans soaked separately.
- Sort and wash the beans. Soak at least 6 to 8 hours.
- When you are ready to cook, discard the soaking water and add the beans to the rice along with additional water.
- Place the rice and the soaking water in a pressure cooker.
- Add the beans and additional water.
- Add a piece of rinsed kombu, cover, and bring to full pressure on a medium flame.
- Place a flame deflector under the pressure cooker and reduce the flame to low.

- Cook under low pressure for 50 minutes.
- Turn off the flame and remove pot from the stove.
- Let sit, allowing the pressure to come down naturally.
- Remove the rice from the pressure cooker using a moistened wooden rice paddle.
- Place the rice in a bowl and cover with a light bamboo mat until ready to serve.

Note: The amount of water you use will vary slightly according to the bean you are cooking. For example, lentils are not soaked so they require more water when cooking.

POT-BOILED BROWN RICE

I like to boil my rice in warmer weather, since boiling is a lighter style of cooking than pressure-cooking. I sometimes choose to cook a 50/50 combination of brown rice together with another grain to produce an even lighter energetic effect. Be sure to use a sturdy pot with a heavy lid when boiling brown rice so that moisture does not escape.

Preparation time: 65 to 70 minutes
Serves 4 to 5

Ingredients
- 1 cup brown rice
- 2 cups water

Preparation
- Place the soaked rice and soaking water in a pot.
- If you are adding any partially refined or cracked grain, add it at this time along with any additional water needed to keep the 1:2 grain-to-water ratio.

- Bring the water to a boil over a medium-high flame.
- When the water begins to boil add a small pinch of sea salt or kombu sea vegetable.
- Cover, place a flame deflector under the pot, and reduce the heat to the lowest setting.
- Simmer on low for 1 hour.
- Remove the rice using a moistened wooden paddle and place the rice in a serving bowl. Cover the rice with a bamboo mat until serving time.

Favorite Brown Rice and Grain Combinations
- Pearled barley
- Hato mugi barley
- Farro
- Cracked wheat
- Sweet brown rice
- Quinoa
- Rye

⊰◆⊱

VEGETABLE FRIED RICE

Fried rice is a rich and satisfying dish that works best using leftover rice.

Preparation time: 10 to 15 minutes
Serves 4

Ingredients
- 1½ cups leftover rice
- ⅓ cup carrot, diced
- ½ cup onion, diced
- ⅓ cup scallion, diced into ¼-inch-thick pieces
- 1⁄16 to ⅛ teaspoon sea salt
- ¾ to 1 teaspoon shoyu

- Fresh ginger juice, to taste
- 1 tablespoon light sesame oil or olive oil
- ½ cup water

Preparation

- Pour the oil in a cast-iron wok or stainless steel skillet and gently heat over a low flame.
- Add the onion and begin sautéing. When the onions begin to glisten, add a tiny pinch of sea salt and continue to sauté.
- Add a little water to moisten the skillet, then add the carrots.
- Continue to sauté for 2 to 3 minutes for an al dente texture. For a softer texture, cover and simmer the vegetables for another 2 to 3 minutes.
- Add the scallions and combine with the other vegetables.
- Season lightly with 3 or 4 drops of the shoyu and gently fold the vegetable mixture over to blend the seasoning.
- Reduce the flame, add a little more water to the bottom of the pan, then add the rice.
- Place a cover on the pot and simmer for 1 to 2 minutes to allow the rice to soften.
- Lightly season with the remainder of the shoyu and blend well with the rice and vegetables. At the very end of cooking, add the fresh grated ginger juice or pepper.
- Place the rice in a serving bowl and cover with a bamboo mat.

Variations

- Use thin slices of snow peas or edamame in place of the scallion.
- Use only one vegetable, such as spring onions or scallions.
- Add sliced mushrooms for a rich, earthy taste.
- Black or red pepper may be used for additional seasoning.

FRIED RICE WITH FRESH HERBS AND VEGETABLES

This is a lighter, more refreshing version of my traditional vegetable fried rice.

Preparation time: 10 minutes
Serves 4

Ingredients
- 1½ cups cooked medium- or long-grain rice
- 1 cup red onion, sliced in ⅛-inch-thick half-moons
- ½ cup thinly sliced leeks
- 1 to 2 tablespoons light sesame or olive oil
- ¼ to ⅓ cup chopped cilantro or fresh parsley, stems removed
- ⅛ to ¼ teaspoon sea salt
- Dash umeboshi vinegar
- Fresh-squeezed lemon or lime juice
- Water
- Toasted sunflower seeds, optional garnish

Preparation
- Pour the oil in a cast-iron wok or stainless steel skillet and gently heat over a low flame.
- Add the onions to the skillet and sauté. If the pan becomes dry, add a small amount of water to the skillet to moisten the onions.
- When the onions are evenly coated with oil, add a pinch of salt and a splash of umeboshi vinegar.
- Add the leeks and continue to sauté the vegetables until they reach the desired texture. I prefer to keep them on the crunchier side for this dish.
- Add a little more water to moisten the pan and the leftover rice.
- Gently fold the vegetables into the rice using a wooden spatula.

- Lightly season the rice with a few drops of umeboshi vinegar.
- Turn off the flame and add the chopped fresh herbs and fresh-squeezed lime juice to taste.
- Use the spatula to gently blend all the ingredients.
- Place the rice in a serving bowl and cover with a bamboo mat until serving time.

❖

MILLET WITH SWEET VEGETABLES

Millet is a whole grain that is helpful for upper-body problems. It is very balancing for the central organs and good for stabilizing the blood sugar.

Preparation time: 1 hour
Serves 4 to 5

Ingredients
- 1 cup millet
- ½ cup diced onions
- ⅔ cup diced sweet vegetables, such as cabbage, carrots, or squash
- 3¼ to 4 cups water
- ¹⁄₁₆ teaspoon sea salt

Preparation
- Place the millet in a bowl and check for any small pebbles or unwanted debris, then rinse until the water is clear and set aside.
- Place the onions on the bottom of the pot with just enough water to cover and bring to a boil. Add a tiny pinch of sea salt (just a few grains) and cook 5 minutes or until the water begins to evaporate.
- Layer any round vegetables (such as cabbage) you are using on top of the onions, followed by any root vegetables, then the millet.

- Add the remaining water and a tiny pinch of sea salt.
- Cover and bring to a boil on a medium flame.
- Place a flame deflector underneath the pot and simmer on low for 40 minutes.
- Remove the grain from the pot, place in a serving dish, and cover with a bamboo mat until serving.

Favorite Vegetable Combinations
- Onion, cabbage, carrots
- Onion, cauliflower
- Onion, leeks, parsnips
- Onion, sweet potatoes
- Onion, cabbage, parsnips
- Onion, leeks, carrots

BARLEY BEAN STEW

Preparation time: 1½ hours
Serves 4 to 6

Ingredients
- 1 cup pearled barley, washed
- 1 cup precooked white beans with ⅓ cup of their cooking liquid. Organic canned beans work well too, as does fried tempeh.
- 1½ cups diced onions
- 1 cup diced root vegetables. Choose one or a combination of carrots and/or parsnips.
- 1 cup diced leeks or celery
- ½ to ¾ teaspoon sea salt
- 2¼ cups water
- 1 to 2 tablespoons olive oil or light sesame oil

Preparation

- Place the onion in a pot with ¼ cup of water.
- Turn on the flame and begin to cook the onions. When the onions begin to glisten, add a small pinch of sea salt (about ¹⁄₁₆ teaspoon).
- Allow the onions to cook on their own for 3 to 5 minutes.
- Layer the leeks and celery on top of the onions, followed by the root vegetables and pearled barley.
- Add additional water and bring to a boil.
- Add another ⅛ teaspoon sea salt, cover, and place a flame deflector under the pot.
- Lower the flame and simmer on low for 30 minutes.
- Add the white beans and the remaining salt. Gently fold the beans into the stew to blend the ingredients and the seasoning. Cook for another 20 minutes.
- For a richer flavor, sauté ½ cup diced onions and/or leeks together with the white beans, then mix to combine with the barley and vegetables.

♦

MUSHROOM BARLEY BEAN STEW

Preparation time: 1½ hours
Serves 4 to 6

Ingredients

- 1 cup pearled barley, washed
- ¼ cup rolled or steel-cut oats, optional
- 1½ cups diced onions
- 1 cup diced leeks
- ½ cup diced carrots or rutabagas
- 1 cup precooked white beans with their cooking liquid; canned beans may also be used

- 3 medium-sized dried shiitake mushrooms, soaked in ½ cup water then diced
- ⅓ cup dried maitake mushrooms, soaked in ½ cup water, then strained. Keep the soaking water to use in cooking.
- ½ cup cleaned and sliced cremini mushrooms
- ½ cup fresh shiitake mushrooms, sliced
- ½ cup maitake (hen of the woods) and/or chanterelle mushrooms
- ½ to ¾ cup chopped parsley
- 1½ to 1¾ teaspoons sea salt
- 4 cups water
- 4 tablespoons olive oil
- ¼ teaspoon toasted sesame oil
- 2 teaspoons white wine

Preparation

- Gently heat a small amount of olive oil (2 tablespoons), add the onions and begin to sauté.
- Add a splash of water and a pinch of sea salt (about ⅟₁₆ teaspoon).
- Add the dried shiitake, dried maitake, and the soaking water.
- Add the leeks, followed by the root vegetables.
- Layer the oats then the barley on top of the vegetables.
- Add 3 cups of water and ¼ teaspoon of sea salt.
- Place a lid on the pot leaving a small crack and bring to a boil.
- Place a flame deflector under the pot, lower the flame and simmer on low for 30 minutes.
- While the barley and vegetables are cooking prepare the mushrooms.
- Using a cast-iron pan, gently heat ¼ teaspoon toasted sesame oil and 2 tablespoons olive oil.
- Add the mushrooms in order of thickness, adding the more delicate ones last and sauté.
- Add ½ cup water, a splash of white wine, and ¼ teaspoon sea salt.
- Continue sautéing for another 3 to 5 minutes.

- Add the sautéed mushrooms, the white beans, and additional salt to the stew.
- Fold to blend the ingredients and the seasoning.
- If you like a creamier consistency add ½ to 1 cup of water.
- Cover and cook for another 15 to 20 minutes.
- Remove the lid and add most of the parsley, then fold to blend the herbs.
- Place in a serving bowl and garnish with the remaining parsley.

⤏◈⤎

KASHA

This is a traditional Ukrainian style recipe using a two-part cooking method that takes only one half hour to prepare. You can serve the kasha as a grain dish or add it to bow tie pasta for a delicious "kasha and bow tie" dish.

Preparation time: 30 minutes
Serves 4

Ingredients
- 1 cup roasted kasha
- 2 cups water
- 1 pinch sea salt (1/16 to 1/8 teaspoon)
- 1 cup diced onion
- ½ cup water
- ½ to 1 teaspoon olive oil
- 1/8 teaspoon sea salt

Preparation
- Place the roasted kasha in a pot.
- In a separate pot bring 2 cups of water to a boil. Add a small pinch of salt to the water and pour the boiling water over the kasha.

- Cover the pot, reduce the flame, and place a flame deflector under the pot.
- Simmer on low heat for 20 minutes.
- While the kasha is cooking prepare the sautéed onions.
- Add a small amount of water to a skillet and the diced onions. Begin to sauté the onions. When the onions begin to change color add ¹⁄₁₆ teaspoon of salt and continue to sauté until the onions are translucent.
- Add additional water as needed. When the onions are soft allow any water to reduce and add ½ to 1 teaspoon of olive oil and another ¹⁄₁₆ teaspoon of salt. Use your wooden utensil to blend the salt, oil, and onions together and sauté for another 3 to 5 minutes.
- When the kasha is cooked place it in a serving dish. Add the sautéed onions and use a wooden spatula to mix the onions together with the kasha.

FARRO WITH DRIED PORCINI AND GREEN PEAS

Preparation time: 1 hour
Serves 6

Ingredients

- 2 cups farro
- 1½ tablespoons olive oil
- 1 to 2 cloves of garlic, peeled and cut in half lengthwise, optional
- White wine, a splash to 1 tablespoon, optional
- 1 cup chopped onions

- 1½ cups dried porcini mushrooms, soaked and strained to remove debris. Retain the soaking water to use in cooking. Any larger mushrooms may be cut.
- 1 cup green peas, fresh or frozen. If you use fresh peas allow them to cook into the stew for 10 minutes.
- 4½ cups water
- 1 to 1½ teaspoons sea salt
- ½ cup chopped parsley
- Cracked black pepper to taste, optional

Preparation

- Heat the olive oil in a pot over low heat.
- Add onions and begin to sauté add the garlic, a pinch of sea salt and sauté for a minute.
- Add the farro and begin sautéing to evenly coat the grain with the oil and blend with the onions.
- Add white wine and gently fold.
- Add the porcini and the strained soaking liquid.
- Add the water and sea salt.
- Cover leaving a small crack in the lid, turn up the flame, and bring to a boil.
- Cover completely, place a flame deflector under the pot, lower the flame, and simmer for 35 minutes. If using fresh peas, add at this time and cook for another 10 minutes.
- If you like a more creamy texture add ¼ cup of water in the last 5 minutes and cook for an additional 5 minutes.
- Add finely chopped parsley and fold into the stew.
- Add a little finishing splash of olive oil if you like and a little crack of pepper.

FARRO WITH WHITE BEANS AND KALE

Preparation time: 1 hour
Serves 2 to 4

Ingredients
- 1 cup farro
- 2 cups water
- 1 cup diced onions
- 1 cup precooked white beans
- ½ cup finely chopped kale
- ¼ cup extra virgin olive oil
- ¾ to 1 teaspoon sea salt
- sliced or whole garlic cloves, optional
- black or red pepper flakes, optional

Preparation
- Place farro and water in a pot and bring to a boil.
- Add a small pinch of sea salt.
- Cover, place a flame deflector under the pot, and simmer on low heat for 35 to 40 minutes.
- Pour enough olive oil into a separate pan to coat the bottom. Turn on the flame and begin to heat the oil.
- Add the onions and begin to sauté.
- Add a few tablespoons water, ⅛ teaspoon sea salt, and continue to sauté. Add the garlic and/or red pepper flakes if you are using them.
- Add the white beans and a little of the bean juice.
- Add additional sea salt and continue to simmer over a medium-low flame for 10 minutes.
- Add the chopped kale, fold to blend all the ingredients together. Simmer for another 7 to 10 minutes.
- Use a wooden utensil and add the farro to the vegetables and beans. Gently fold to blend the ingredients.

- For additional richness and flavor, drizzle a little olive oil over the grain and add another small pinch of sea salt, about ⅛ teaspoon. Add black pepper if using.
- Fold to blend all the ingredients.
- Place the farro in a serving bowl and cover with a bamboo mat until ready to serve.

⊸✦⊷

PORCINI FARRO RISOTTO

Preparation time: 50 minutes
Serves 4 to 6

Ingredients
- 2 cups pearled farro
- 2 to 2½ tablespoons olive oil
- 1 to 2 cloves of garlic, peeled and cut in half lengthwise
- White wine, approximately ⅛ cup
- 1 cup chopped shallots
- 1½ cups dried porcini mushrooms, soaked in 1 cup water and strained to remove debris. Retain the soaking water to use in cooking.
- 4½ cups water
- ¾ to 1 teaspoon sea salt
- Cracked black pepper to taste, optional

Preparation
- Heat the olive oil in a pot over low heat.
- Add shallots and begin to sauté. Add the garlic, and a pinch of sea salt, and sauté for a minute.
- Add the farro and begin sautéing to evenly coat the grain with the oil and blend with the shallots.
- Add white wine and gently fold.

- Add the porcini and the strained soaking liquid.
- Add the water and sea salt.
- Cover leaving a small crack in the lid, turn up the flame, and bring to a boil.
- Cover completely, place a flame deflector under the pot, lower the flame, and simmer for 40 minutes. Remove the lid and check the consistency. If you like a more creamy texture add ¼ cup of water and cook for another 5 to 7 minutes.
- Add a little finishing splash of olive oil if you like and a crack of pepper.

⊰◈⊱

GRILLED SWEET CORN

Preparation time: 20 to 25 minutes
Serves 6

Ingredients

- 6 cobs organic non-GMO sweet corn
- 3 to 4 tablespoons organic brown rice syrup
- ½ teaspoon umeboshi paste
- 3 tablespoons extra virgin olive oil
- ⅛ teaspoon sea salt
- ½ teaspoon umeboshi vinegar

Preparation

- Pour the brown rice syrup in prep bowl.
- Add the umeboshi paste and mix together using a small whisk or wooden utensil.
- Add the olive oil and continue to mix.
- Add the sea salt and the umeboshi vinegar.
- Mix all ingredients thoroughly.

- Brush the sauce on raw or partially cooked corn. Make sure to coat it evenly.
- Place the corn directly on the grill and cook to the desired texture. As the corn cooks, you can add extra sauce.
- You can also make this dish using your oven with a setting of 350 degrees.

The "sauce" will stay fresh in the refrigerator in a sealed glass jar. If the ingredients begin to separate just stir well before the next use.

⊸◇⊷

POLENTA

Preparation time: 50 minutes to 1 hour
Serves 4

Ingredients
- 1 cup corn grits or polenta
- 5 cups water
- ¼ to ½ teaspoon sea salt
- 1 to 1½ tablespoons extra virgin olive oil, optional

Preparation
- Pour 4 cups water in a pot and begin to heat over a medium-high flame.
- Just before the water comes to a full boil, add the sea salt and begin to sift the cornmeal into the pot. This was traditionally done by using one hand as a funnel, while constantly stirring with the other hand. Stirring is very important to prevent clumping!
- Gradually add the remaining water, a little at a time.
- Continue this method until all the grain is used.

- Add the olive oil, if using, and continue stirring to blend the oil with the grain.
- Continue stirring until the polenta is thick and creamy.
- Lower the flame and place a flame deflector under the pot, cover and simmer on the lowest setting for 30 minutes.
- Serve immediately, or pour the hot polenta into a flat Pyrex pan. As the polenta cools, it will firm up and set. You can serve firm polenta at room temperature, or you can steam, pan-fry, or grill it.

⊲◇⊳

PERUVIAN QUINOA WITH BLACK BEANS AND AVOCADO

Preparation time: 45 minutes to 1 hour
Serves 4

Ingredients

- 1 cup white quinoa, or a mixture of white and red quinoa
- 1¾ cups water
- 1/16 teaspoon sea salt for cooking the quinoa
- 1 cup diced red onion
- 2½ to 3 tablespoons olive oil
- 1½ cups precooked black or red beans
- ½ to ¾ teaspoon sea salt
- 2¼ teaspoons umeboshi vinegar
- ⅓ to ½ cup chopped cilantro
- 1 avocado, diced
- Fresh-squeezed lime juice, to taste
- Red chili or jalapeño pepper, seeds removed and finely sliced, optional

Preparation

- Place the quinoa and 1¾ cups water in a pot and bring to a boil.
- Add a small pinch of sea salt, cover, and place a flame deflector under the pot.
- Lower the flame and simmer on low for 15 minutes.
- Remove the quinoa from the pot, place in a bowl, and set aside.
- Heat the olive oil in a separate pan.
- Add the red onions and begin to sauté.
- When the onions begin to glisten, add a small pinch of sea salt, ¼ cup water, and continue to sauté.
- Add the black beans and a small amount of bean cooking liquid, to keep the mixture moist.
- Add the remaining sea salt and fold to blend the seasoning.
- Lower the flame and let simmer 6 to 7 minutes.
- Turn off the flame, then add the cooked quinoa.
- Drizzle 1 tablespoon olive oil over the grain.
- Add half the chopped cilantro, the avocado, and a little fresh-squeezed lime juice.
- Gently fold to mix all the ingredients together.
- Place in a serving dish and garnish with a little freshly made guacamole if desired.

BULGUR WHEAT SALAD

Preparation time: 45 minutes
Serves 2 to 4

Ingredients

- ½ cup bulgur wheat or quinoa for a gluten-free version
- 1 cup water
- Pinch sea salt

- ½ cup diced red onion (raw or lightly blanched)
- ½ cup chopped cucumber
- ½ to ⅓ cup finely chopped parsley
- 2 to 2½ tablespoons olive oil
- ¼ to ½ teaspoon sea salt
- ¼ to ½ teaspoon umeboshi vinegar
- 1½ to 2 tablespoons fresh-squeezed lemon juice
- ⅓ cup chopped tomatoes, optional

Preparation

- Place the onion and cucumber in a bowl.
- Add a small pinch of sea salt and use your hands to gently mix the salt with the vegetables.
- Put a small plate over the vegetables to lightly press them. Set vegetables aside while you cook the bulgur.
- Place bulgur and water in a pan, turn on the flame, and bring to a boil.
- Add ¼ teaspoon sea salt. Cover, reduce heat to low, place a flame deflector under the pot, and cook for 20 minutes.
- Immediately remove the bulgur from the pot and place in a serving dish. Use a wooden utensil moistened with olive oil to gently fluff the grain and get rid of any clumps.
- Remove the plate from the diced vegetables, and pour off any liquid.
- Add the parsley to the vegetables, then the olive oil and umeboshi vinegar, and combine.
- Add the vegetables to the warm bulgur, together with a squeeze of fresh lemon.
- Gently mix with a wooden utensil to thoroughly blend all the ingredients.

BULGUR WHEAT WITH SAUTÉED RED ONION AND PEAS

Preparation time: 25 minutes
Serves 4

Ingredients

- 1 cup medium-grind bulgur wheat or quinoa for a gluten-free version
- 2¼ cups water
- ¾ cup diced red onion
- 1 cup green peas, fresh or frozen
- ½ to ¾ cup finely chopped parsley or fresh mint
- 2 to 2½ tablespoons olive oil
- ½ to ¾ teaspoon sea salt
- ¼ to ½ teaspoon umeboshi vinegar

Preparation

- Place 1 cup bulgur and 2 cups water in a pot, turn on the flame and bring to a boil.
- Add ¼ teaspoon sea salt. Cover and reduce heat to low setting.
- Place a flame deflector under the pot, and cook for 15 minutes.
- Turn off the flame, remove from the stove, and let sit covered for 5 minutes.
- While the bulgur is cooking prepare the vegetables.
- Gently heat 1½ tablespoons of olive oil in a skillet.
- Add the red onion, add ⅛ teaspoon of sea salt, and begin to sauté.
- Add a dash of umeboshi vinegar and continue sautéing.
- Add the green peas. If fresh, cover the pot and give them about 3 to 10 minutes to soften.
- Add ½ tablespoon olive oil and additional salt.
- Add ¼ cup water and continue sautéing for 2 minutes.

- Turn off the flame.
- When the bulgur is cooked add to the cooked onions and peas and use a wooden utensil coated with olive to toss.
- Add the chopped herbs and gently fold to blend with the grain.
- Serve warm or at room temperature.

—◈—

FINE BULGUR

Fine bulgur is a lighter option to the medium grind. It works great for bulgur salads served chilled or at room temperature.

Preparation time: 30 minutes
Serves 4

Ingredients
- 1 cup fine bulgur
- 1½ cups water
- ⅛ teaspoon sea salt

Preparation
- Place the bulgur in a bowl.
- Bring salted water to a boil.
- Pour boiling water over the bulgur, cover, and let stand for 30 minutes.
- Remove the cover and fluff with a fork or wooden utensil.

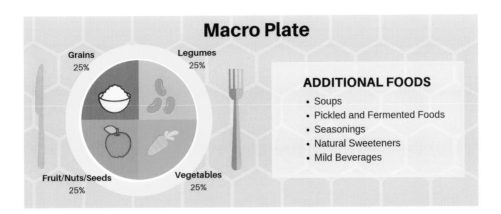

ABOVE: The macrobiotic diet is inspired by the eating habits and lifestyles of the world's longest standing civilizations. However, this chart has been updated to fit the modern lifestyle. BELOW: The macrobiotic food pyramid represents the importance of finding structure, daily habits, and harmony to improve stress management, mental health, and physical health.

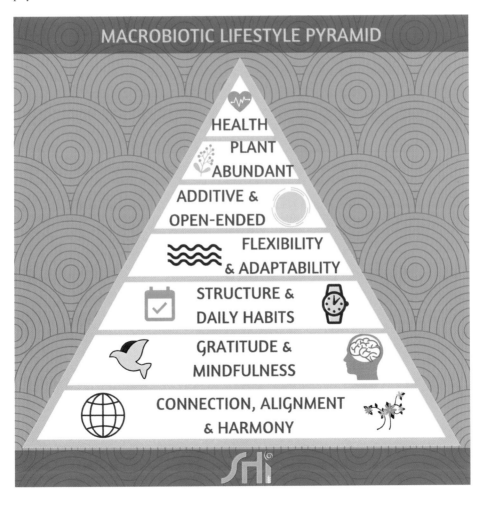

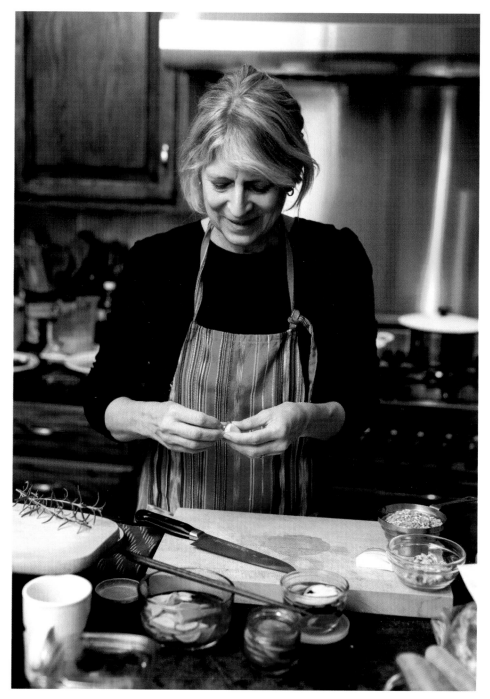

Preparing quick umeboshi vinegar pickles. Red, black, daikon, and watermelon radishes are all nice additions to salads, as a garnish or as a digestive at the end of a meal.

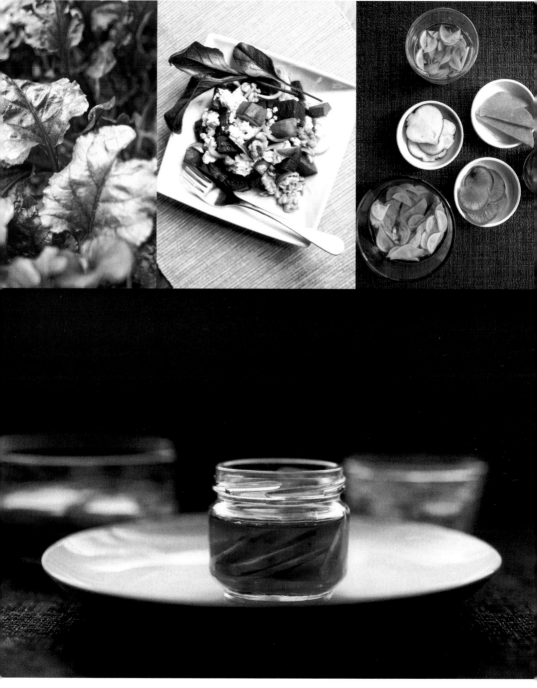

The fermentation process and final dish; beet salad with
pickled red onions, raw walnuts, and tofu cheese.

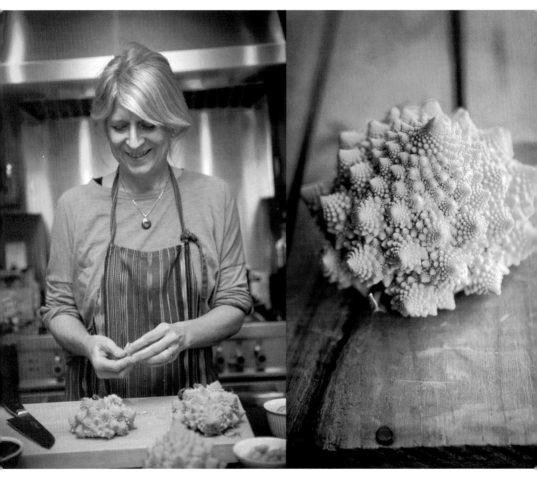

Uniquely shaped and versatile, romanesco works well with pasta,
cracked grains, or on its own, sautéed Mediterranean style.

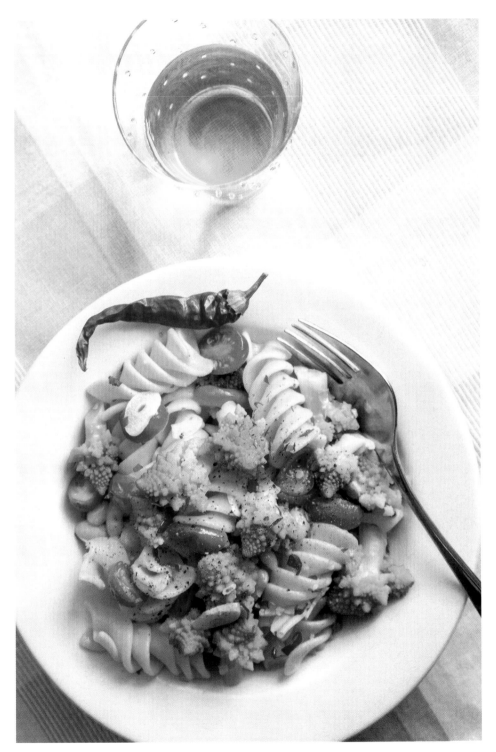

Fusilloni pasta with olive oil, garlic, romanesco, grape tomatoes, cannelloni beans, and dried cayenne pepper served with a slightly chilled Roero Arneis.

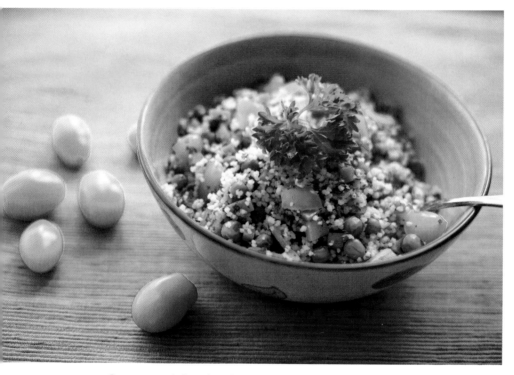

Couscous salad with red onions, carrots, orange cherry tomatoes, green peas, and finely chopped parsley.

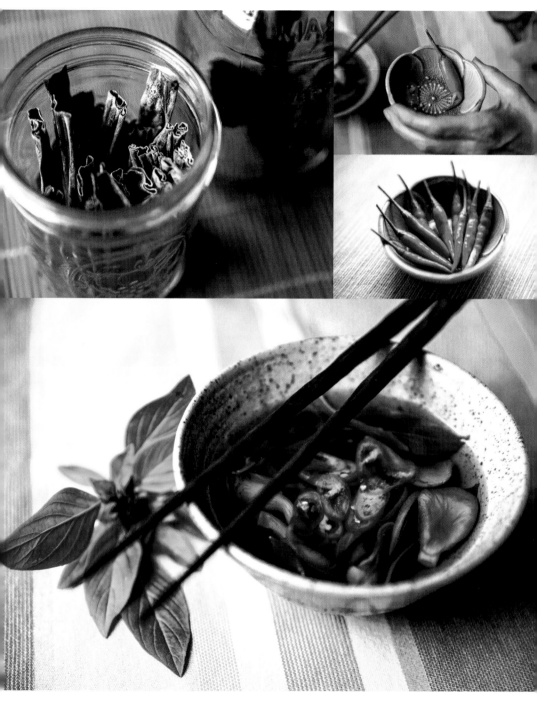

Spicy clear soup with Thai basil and chilies.

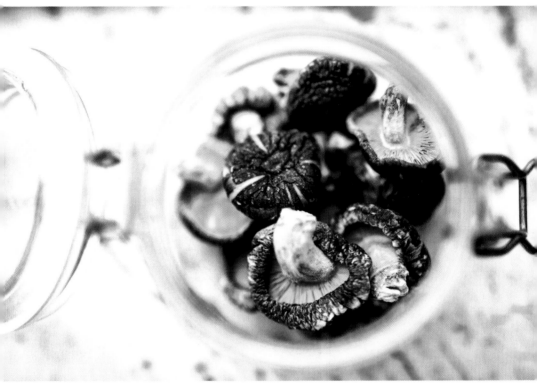

Sun-dried Donko Shiitake mushrooms.

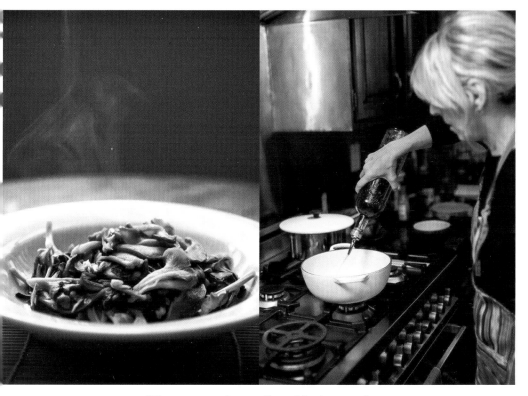

Watercress with a medley of fresh sautéed oyster,
shiitake, and maitake mushrooms

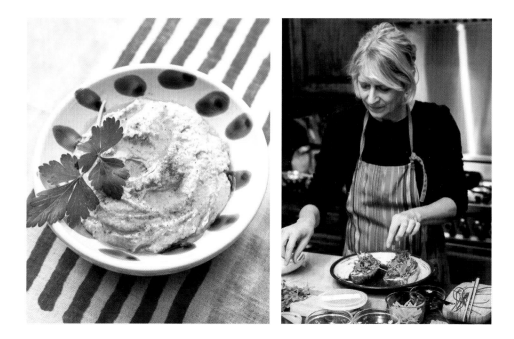

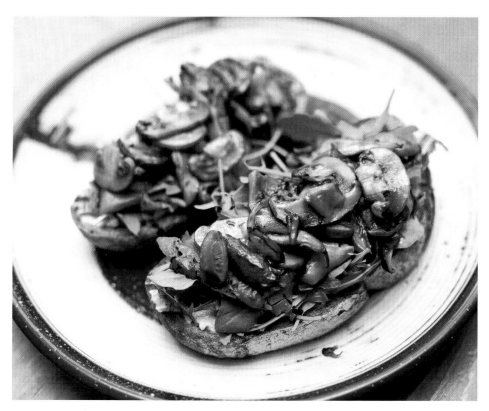

Open-face sandwich with steamed sourdough bread, hummus, arugula, roasted red peppers, and sautéed mushrooms.

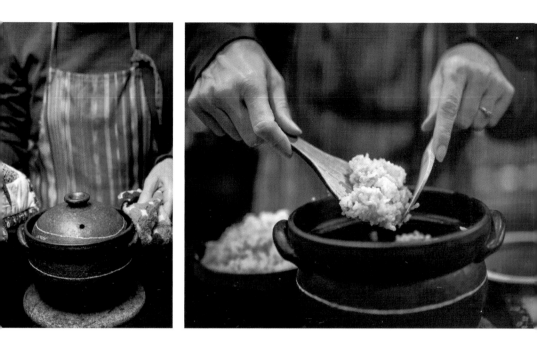

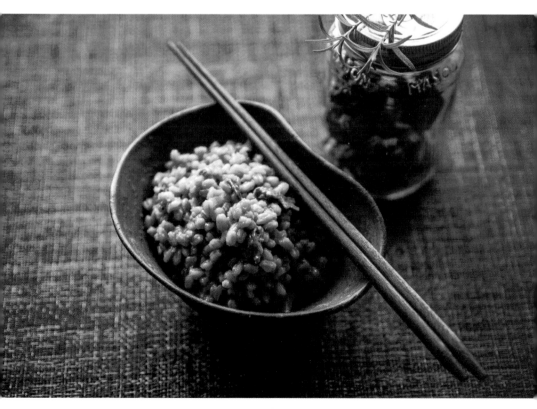

TOP LEFT AND RIGHT: Japanese Donabe pot—best way to cook rice!
BOTTOM: Porcini farro risotto.

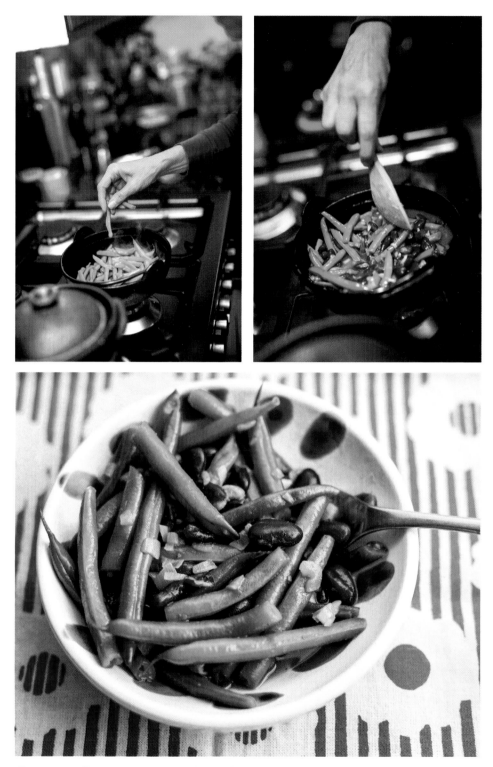

Preparing a Pennsylvania Dutch family favorite, green beans with kidney beans.

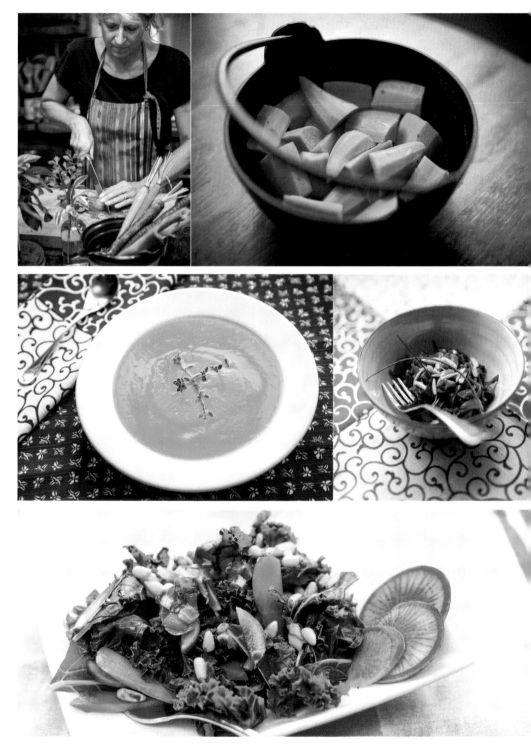

TOP AND CENTER LEFT: Rainbow carrots, steamed sweet potatoes, and creamy butternut squash soup. CENTER RIGHT: Sweet and sour red cabbage with shaved almonds. BOTTOM: Blanched vegetable salad with kale, red onions, red radishes, and carrots, garnished with lightly toasted pine nuts and pickled watermelon radishes.

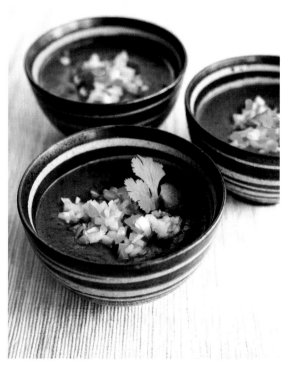

Creamy black bean soup topped with pico de gallo, served with Susan's guacamole and organic blue corn chips.

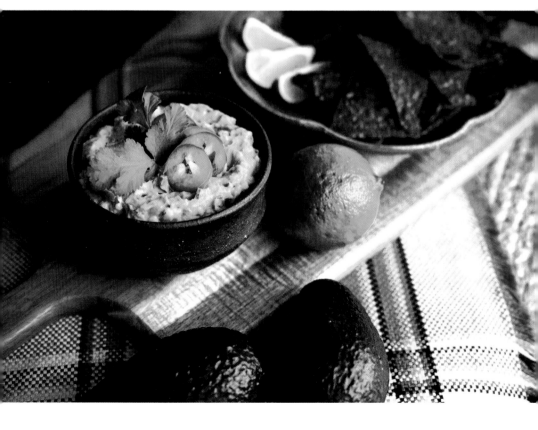

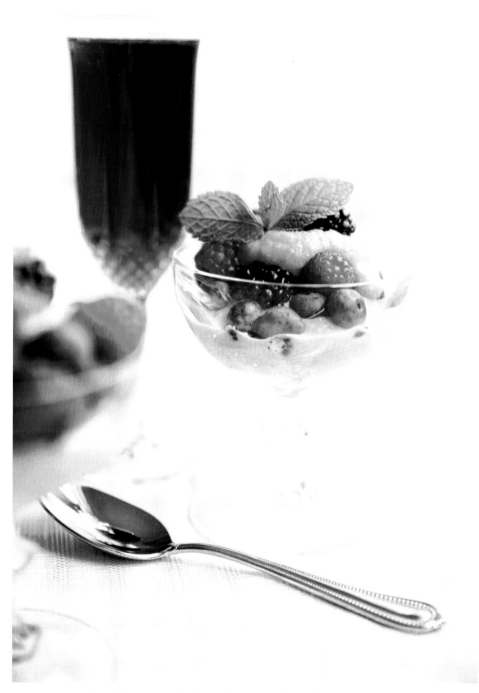

Fresh berries with almond crème and sparkling grape juice.

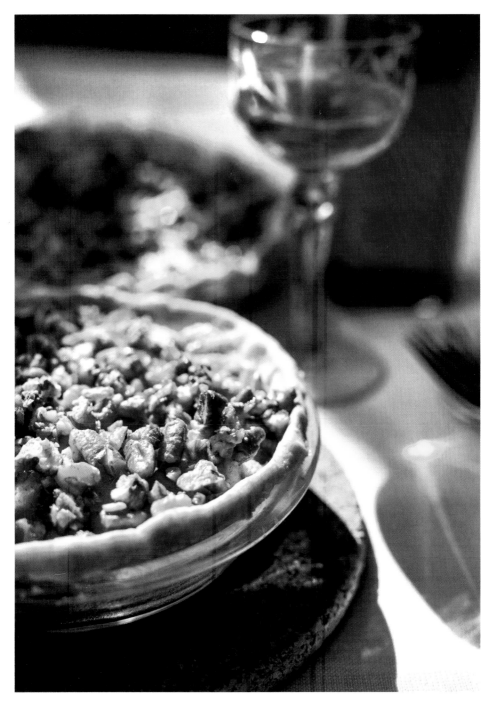

Apple pecan tart with dessert wine.

COUSCOUS VEGETABLE SALAD WITH RED ONION, CARROT, AND PEAS

Preparation time: 45 minutes

Serves 2 to 4

Ingredients

- 1 cup couscous
- 2 cups water
- ⅓ cup carrots, diced
- ⅓ cup green peas
- ½ cup red onion, diced
- ⅓ cup finely chopped parsley
- 1½ tablespoons extra virgin olive oil
- ¼ teaspoon toasted sesame oil
- ⅛ teaspoon sea salt
- 1½ to 2 teaspoons shoyu
- 2 to 2½ teaspoons umeboshi vinegar
- black pepper (optional)

Preparation

- Place the water and sea salt in a pot and bring to a boil.
- Place couscous in a bowl.
- Pour the boiling water over the couscous.
- Cover the bowl and let sit for 5 minutes, or 8 minutes when using whole-wheat couscous.
- Rub a little olive oil on your hands or use an oiled wooden spatula to break up any lumps and fluff the couscous.
- Cover couscous with a mat and set aside while you cook the vegetables.
- Gently heat a few drops of oil in a skillet, then add the onion and sauté.
- When the onion begins to glisten, add a pinch of salt and a little water.

- Add the carrots and continue to sauté. Cover and simmer for 2 to 3 minutes.
- Season the vegetables with shoyu.
- Add the green peas, turn off the flame, and gently fold to mix all of the vegetables.
- Add the couscous, a drizzle of olive oil, and the chopped parsley.
- Gently fold to mix all ingredients.
- Add the umeboshi vinegar and a little black pepper if using, and fold to blend the seasonings.
- Place in a bowl and cover with a mat until you are ready to serve.

Variations
- Substitute cooked chickpeas for the green peas.
- Add seitan or fried tempeh for a heartier dish.

TRADITIONAL HAND ROLLED COUSCOUS WITH SAFFRON AND PEAS

Preparation time: 20 minutes
Serves 4

Ingredients
- 1½ cups of hand rolled couscous
- ½ to 1 packet saffron, freshly ground
- 2¼ cups water
- ¼ cup extra virgin olive oil
- Fresh English peas or hulled green peas removed from their pods and blanched
- 1 small pinch sea salt (approximately ¹⁄₁₆ teaspoon)

- Fresh chopped mint or basil, ⅓ to ½ cup
- Black pepper to taste

Preparation

- Pour the water in a pot.
- Gently begin to heat then add the saffron just before the water begins to boil.
- Add the couscous to the boiling water.
- Cover and allow the water to return to a boil.
- Turn off the flame and let sit for 7 to 10 minutes.
- Remove the cover and place in a bowl.
- Drizzle oil over the couscous and lightly season with a pinch of sea salt.
- If you are using fresh minced herbs add them at this time.
- Add the cooked peas and additional olive oil if you like.
- Gently fold to blend the seasonings.
- Add a little fresh cracked pepper if you like.
- Place in a serving dish and serve warm or at room temperature.

❖

SAFFRON RISOTTO

Preparation time: 1 hour
Serves 4

Ingredients

- 2 cups risotto rice
- 1½ tablespoons olive oil
- 1 to 2 cloves of garlic, peeled and cut in half lengthwise
- A splash of white wine, approximately ⅛ cup
- 1 cup diced onions
- 1 cup diced carrots

- ½ cup green peas
- 2 quarts vegetable stock
- ¾ to 1 teaspoon sea salt
- A few strands of saffron (⅛ to ¼ teaspoon)
- Cracked black pepper to taste, optional

Variations
- Use chopped asparagus or green beans in place of the peas.
- Add additional summer vegetables, such as yellow squash or zucchini.

Preparation
- Heat the olive oil in a pot over low heat.
- Add onions and begin to sauté until the onions begin to glisten, then add the garlic and a pinch of sea salt. Continue to sauté.
- Add the rice and sauté until the rice is evenly coated with the oil-and-onions mixture.
- Add white wine to just cover the rice. When the wine is absorbed, add ¼ cup stock. Gently stir after adding the stock to prevent the rice from sticking. Once the rice has absorbed the stock, add the saffron and carrots and additional sea salt at this time. Gently fold all ingredients together.
- Continue adding the stock in small increments, about ¼ to ½ cup at a time, and folding until you are close to reaching the texture you desire. This takes approximately 25 to 35 minutes.
- Add the peas near the end of cooking and mix throughout the risotto.
- Add black pepper and a drizzle of olive oil to finish off the dish.

MUSHROOM SAFFRON RISOTTO

Preparation time: 1 hour
Serves 4

Ingredients
- 2 cups risotto rice (Carnaroli or Vialone Nano risotto rice)
- 1½ tablespoons olive oil
- 1 to 2 cloves of garlic, peeled and cut in half lengthwise (optional)
- White wine, approximately ⅛ cup
- ½ cup diced onions or shallots
- 2 quarts mushroom stock made with dried porcini and dried shiitake
- 3 to 5 dried shiitake
- ½ cup dried porcini; soaked and strained to remove debris. Retain the soaking water to use in cooking.
- 2 cups combination of sliced fresh shiitake, chanterelles, and royal trumpets mushrooms.
- 1 to 1½ teaspoon sea salt
- 1 packet saffron (⅛ to ¼ teaspoon)
- Cracked black pepper to taste, optional

Stock Preparation
- Fill a stock pot with 9 cups of water.
- Soak the dried shiitake directly in the water.
- Soak the dried porcini an a separate bowl with 1 cup of water.
- Allow the porcini to soak for 20 to 30 minutes, while you are preparing your other ingredients.
- Turn on the flame and begin to heat the stock.
- Add ½ teaspoon of sea salt
- Strain the liquid off of the porcini and add it to the stock pot with a genrous pinch of sea salt.
- Chop the porcini to use in the risotto.

Preparation

- Gently heat the olive oil in a pot.
- Add the onions and begin to sauté.
- Add the garlic, a small pinch of sea salt.
- Add the rice and sauté until the rice is evenly coated with the oil-and-onion mixture.
- Add white wine to just cover the rice.
- When the wine is absorbed, add ¼ cup stock and the saffron.
- Gently stir after adding the stock to prevent the rice from sticking.
- When the rice has absorbed the stock, add the chopped mushrooms and remaining salt and fold to blend all ingredients and seasoning.
- Continue adding stock in small increments, about ¼ to ½ cup at a time and folding until you are close to reaching the texture you desire. This takes approximately 25 to 35 minutes.
- Add black pepper and a drizzle of olive oil to finish the dish.

NOODLES

Noodle Cooking Tips

Preparation time: 2 to 10 minutes

Serves 3

Ingredients

- 1 package of noodles such as udon, soba, or somen

Preparation

- Bring 1 to 2 quarts of water to a boil. When the water is boiling add the noodles.
- Cook the noodles until they are tender.
- Drain the noodles in a colander while running cold water over the noodles.
- Place the noodles back in the pot, fill the pot with cold water, and drain again.
- Repeat this process 3 times.
- Asian-style noodles are made with salt so they do not require salt when cooking but do require draining and rinsing several times.
- Rinsing the noodles in the pot helps eliminate excess salt.

UDON NOODLES WITH SAUTÉED VEGETABLES

Preparation time: 30 minutes
Serves 3 to 4

Ingredients

- 1½ cups water
- ½ teaspoon toasted sesame oil
- 1 tablespoon light sesame oil or 2 tablespoons olive oil
- 1 pack precooked udon noodles
- 1½ cup onions, sliced into ¼-inch half-moons
- ½ cup carrots, cut into thin matchsticks
- 3 to 4 stalks of bok choy, cut on the angle, stems removed from the leaves
- ¾ teaspoon sea salt
- ¼ to ½ teaspoon shoyu
- Fresh grated ginger juice and/or shichimi, optional

Preparation

- Gently heat the oil in a deep pan or wok.
- Add the onions and begin to sauté.
- Add a little water and ¼ teaspoon sea salt and continue to sauté.
- Add the carrots and additional water and the rest of the salt. Cover and simmer for 3 to 5 minutes.
- Add the bok choy bottoms and sauté for a minute, then add the bok choy leaves.
- Add the udon and the shoyu.
- Add the spice, if using.
- Gently fold to blend all the ingredients and seasonings together.

FRIED SOBA

Soba or buckwheat noodles are great for physical activity and endurance. Because of its strengthening qualities it is considered to be "good luck" in Japan and is often served on New Years as the first food of the year.

Preparation time: 20 minutes
Serves 2 to 3

Ingredients

- 1 package precooked soba noodles
- ½ to 1 teaspoon toasted sesame oil
- ½ to ¾ cups water
- ½ to 1 teaspoon shoyu
- ¼ teaspoon mirin
- A dash shichimi
- ½ teaspoon green nori flakes
- 1 scallion finely sliced

⊰◈⊱

HOT AND SPICY HERBED NOODLE BROTH

Ingredients

- 1 pack of precooked udon or somen noodles
- 1 medium to large dried shiitake mushroom
- 2- to 3-inch piece kombu
- 6 cups water
- ¾ teaspoon sea salt
- ½ cup onions, cut into thin half-moons
- ¼ cup of mung bean sprouts or cabbage

- Oyster and enoki mushrooms
- 5 drops shoyu, about ⅛ teaspoon
- 2 to 3 drops umeboshi vinegar
- 3 to 4 drops spicy sesame oil
- Cilantro or pea shoots to garnish each bowl
- Shichimi, optional
- When serving, add a little fresh lemon to each bowl.

Broth Preparation

- Place the water in a pot together with the kombu and dried shiitake.
- Bring the water to a boil, then lower the flame to a rolling boil and continue cooking for 2 to 3 minutes.
- Remove the kombu and shiitake.
- Add a small pinch of salt and the onions.
- Slice the dried shiitake and return it to the pot.
- Add 2 to 3 drops of spicy sesame oil.
- Add the mung bean sprouts and oyster mushrooms.
- Add the remaining ¼ teaspoon sea salt, reduce the flame, and simmer for another 5 minutes.
- Add the shoyu and simmer another 4 to 5 minutes.
- Add the umeboshi vinegar.
- Add the garnish.
- Place noodles in individual serving bowls and ladle hot broth over the noodles.
- Add a squeeze of fresh lemon.
- Garnish each bowl with fresh pea shoots or additional cilantro; add shichimi for a mildly spicy taste, if desired.

Pasta Cooking Tips

Preparation time: Dry pasta 8 to 15 minutes; fresh pasta 2 to 3 minutes

Serves 4

Ingredients

- 1 lb. package of pasta
- 100 percent durum semolina or a gluten-free option
- 6 quarts water
- 1 to 1½ tablespoons sea salt

Cookware

- Deep stock pot or pasta pot

Preparation

- Bring water to a rolling boil.
- Add a generous amount of salt.
- Add the pasta to the boiling water.
- Stir frequently in the first few minutes to prevent sticking.
- Stir intermittently throughout the cooking.
- Follow the suggested cooking time on the package, checking the texture.
- For best results, cook pasta al dente, since it will continue to cook with the sauce.
- Use a colander to strain the pasta. Do not rinse.
- Save the cooking water to use in the sauce. The starch in the water thickens the sauce and helps the sauce adhere to the pasta.

- If you are cooking a small amount use a large wire vegetable skimmer (aka spider) to pull the pasta from the pot then add it directly to the sauce.
- The cooking time will depend on what type of pasta you use. If you are mixing the pasta directly with a sauce, undercook the pasta slightly to prevent overcooking.

PASTA SAUCES

Note: Heat the water for the pasta so it is ready to go while you make the sauce. The cooking time will depend on what type of pasta you use. Try to time it so that the pasta will be done at the same time that you finish the sauce. If you are mixing the pasta directly in with the sauce, undercook the pasta slightly, as it will continue to cook when it is mixed with the sauce.

ONIONS, KALE, AND SUN-DRIED TOMATO SAUCE

Preparation time: 30 to 40 minutes
Sauce makes approximately 4 servings; ½ package of pasta serves 2

Ingredients
- 2 cups diced onions
- ½ cup sun-dried tomatoes, reconstituted in 1 cup of water
- 3 to 5 leaves kale, chopped. Use more kale if desired.
- 1 to 2 cloves garlic
- A dash of white wine, approximately 2 ounces
- 3 to 4 tablespoons extra virgin olive oil
- 1 to 1½ teaspoons sea salt
- 1½ to 2 cups water

- Black pepper or red chili pepper to taste
- Toasted sourdough bread crumbs

Preparation

- Heat 3 tablespoons of olive oil in a saucepan.
- Add the onions and begin to sauté. Add a little bit of water to prevent the oil from getting too hot. Add ⅛ teaspoon sea salt and continue to sauté.
- Add the garlic and a splash of white wine and continue to sauté.
- Add the sun-dried tomatoes, including their soaking liquid.
- Add the kale, additional water, and more salt. Cover the pot, lower the flame, and allow to simmer for few minutes.
- Add a little black pepper and a drizzle of olive oil.
- Cook pasta al dente and toss the pasta with the vegetables and sauce.
- Add a little fried bread crumbs to each individual dish.

Variations

- Add black olives to the sauce.

⊰◈⊱

CAULIFLOWER AND BABY ARUGULA SAUCE

Preparation time: 30 to 40 minutes
Sauce makes approximately 4 servings; ½ package of pasta serves 2

Ingredients

- 2 cups diced onions
- ½ head of cauliflower, cut into bite-size florets, approximately 2½ to 3 cups
- ½ to 1 cup finely grated carrots

- 2 cups baby arugula
- 2 to 3 tablespoons extra virgin olive oil
- 3 to 4 cups water
- 1½ to 2 teaspoons sea salt
- Black pepper and or red pepper
- 1 to 2 cloves of garlic, optional

Preparation

- Gently heat a small amount of olive oil in a pan.
- Add the onions and begin to sauté.
- Add a small amount of water, garlic, and a nice pinch of sea salt.
- Add the cauliflower florets, cover, and simmer for 5 to 8 minutes.
- Add some of the pasta cooking liquid and a little more salt.
- Add the grated carrots.
- Add the baby arugula.
- Add additional olive oil and a little pepper.
- Add a little fresh-squeezed lemon.
- Serve hot over pasta.

⋙◈⋘

BROCCOLI AND WHITE BEANS

Preparation time: 30 to 40 minutes
Sauce makes approximately 4 to 6 servings
1 package of pasta serves 4

Ingredients

- 1½ cups diced onions
- 1 bunch of broccoli, florets separated and stems peeled
- ½ to 1 cup cooked cannellini beans
- 1 cup cherry tomatoes, cut in half, optional
- 1 to 2 cloves garlic, thinly sliced or left whole

- 5 to 6 tablespoons extra virgin olive oil
- 3 to 4 cups of liquid; use a combination of fresh water and the liquid from the cooked pasta
- 2 to 3 teaspoons sea salt
- White wine
- Red and/or black pepper, optional

Preparation

- Gently heat the olive oil in a pan.
- Add the onions and begin to sauté.
- Add a small amount of white wine and garlic. Continue to sauté.
- Add a little bit of water and the broccoli stems, cover, and simmer for 1 minute.
- Add the white beans and sea salt. Cover and simmer on low heat for another 3 minutes.
- Add the broccoli florets and additional water from the pasta cooking liquid. If you like a brothier sauce, add more liquid. Add a little more salt, cover, and simmer for 2 to 3 minutes.
- Add the cherry tomatoes, a drizzle of olive oil, additional salt if needed, and a crack of black pepper.
- Simmer uncovered for a few minutes so that the salt blends in with the other ingredients.
- Serve over pasta or add pasta directly to the sauce.

KASHA VARNISHKES

Preparation time: 30 minutes
Serves 2 to 4

Ingredients

- ½ package of farfalle pasta
- Precooked kasha

- 2½ cups carrots cut into thin matchsticks
- 5 tablespoons olive oil
- ¼ teaspoon sea salt
- ½ bunch finely chopped parsley
- ½ cup pasta cooking liquid

Cookware

- Stainless steel skillet
- Stock pot to cook pasta

Preparation

- Heat the olive oil in a skillet, add the carrots, and begin to sauté.
- Add a small pinch of sea salt (⅟₁₆ teaspoon) and continue to sauté.
- Add half of the reserved pasta liquid and continue to sauté the carrots until they are tender.
- Add the rest of the cooking liquid and the remaining sea salt.
- Add the cooked pasta, the kasha, and parsley and use a wooden spatula to blend all the ingredients.
- Place in a serving dish and enjoy.

PESTO

Preparation time: 15 to 20 minutes
Serves 8

Ingredients

- ⅔ cup high-quality extra virgin olive oil
- 2 teaspoons fresh lemon juice
- ½ cup lightly toasted pine nuts
- 2 cups packed fresh basil leaves
- 2 to 3 cloves garlic
- ¼ to ½ teaspoon sea salt

- ½ teaspoon umeboshi vinegar
- ½ cup pitted Castelvetrano olives
- ⅓ cup juice from the olives

Preparation

- Gently toast the pine nuts over a low flame.
- Turn constantly to keep them from burning.
- Place in a bowl and allow to cool for 5 minutes.
- Add the olive oil and lemon juice to the food processor.
- Add the pine nuts and blend for 2 minutes using a pulse setting.
- Add the garlic and seasoning and pulse for a minute.
- Add the fresh basil, pulse for 2 minutes, then blend until the leaves are chopped.
- Add the olives and olive juice, pulse for 2 minutes then blend to a smooth consistency. For a creamy texture, add a little of the pasta cooking liquid before blending.
- Add pesto to cooked pasta.

⤚◇⤙

ROMANESCO FRESH TOMATO

Preparation time: 30 to 40 minutes
Serves 4 to 6

Ingredients

- 1 package Italian-style pasta
- 1 cup diced onions
- 4 cups romanesco florets
- 1 cup heirloom tomato, peeled and diced; I like to use the yellow or orange tomatoes.
- ½ cup oil-packed sun-dried tomatoes, diced
- 2 to 3 cloves garlic, thinly sliced or left whole
- 5 to 6 tablespoons extra virgin olive oil

- 3 to 4 cups of liquid; use a combination of fresh water and the liquid from the cooked pasta
- 2 to 3 teaspoons sea salt
- A splash of white wine; about 1 to 2 tablespoons
- Red and/or black pepper, optional
- Micro basil, optional

Preparation

- Gently heat the olive oil in a pan.
- Add the onions and begin to sauté.
- As the color of the onions changes add a pinch of sea salt and fold to blend.
- Add a small amount of white wine and garlic. Continue to sauté.
- Add the diced tomatoes and 1 to 2 ladles of pasta cooking liquid. Simmer 2 to 3 minutes.
- Add the romanesco, additional liquid, and a pinch of sea salt.
- Cover and simmer for 3 to 4 minutes.
- Add the sun-dried tomatoes, a drizzle of olive oil, and ½ to 1 cup pasta liquid.
- Simmer uncovered for 3 more minutes so that the salt blends in with the other ingredients.
- Add pasta directly to the sauce. Drizzle olive oil over the pasta and add another pinch of salt.
- Gently toss the pasta with the sauce and serve immediately.

<hr>

SPICY CAULIFLOWER SAUCE

Preparation time: 30 minutes
Begin preparing the pasta water while you are preparing the sauce.

Ingredients

- 1 package of pasta

- 1 head cauliflower separated into medium-sized florets
- 2½ cups onions, diced
- 2 to 3 cloves of garlic, peeled and sliced thin or left whole
- ½ to ¾ cup grated carrots
- 2 cups of whole peeled tomatoes
- Hot pepper flakes, a dash of harissa (¼ teaspoon), or both
- ¼ cup extra virgin olive oil
- ¼ to ⅓ cup oil-cured Moroccan olives, diced
- 2 tablespoons capers
- 1 tablespoon barley miso
- 3 to 4 cups of liquid; use a combination of fresh water and the liquid from the cooked pasta
- Salt and pepper to taste
- 1½ to 2 teaspoons sea salt

Preparation

- Gently heat olive oil in a pan, add the onions, and begin to sauté.
- Add a little water and the garlic and continue to sauté.
- Add salt, pepper flakes, and harissa.
- Add a small ladle of pasta cooking liquid.
- Add the grated carrots.
- Add the tomatoes and liquid.
- Add the miso and a little more olive oil, cover, and let simmer for 8 minutes.
- Add the cauliflower florets and cover, let simmer for 4 to 5 minutes.
- Remove the lid and add a little more pasta cooking water.
- Add additional olive oil if needed.
- Add the black olives and capers and cook for 2 minutes.
- Add the pasta, a drizzle of olive oil, and additional salt to taste.
- Toss the pasta with the sauce and serve immediately.

ZUCCHINI, ONION, AND CARROT SAUCE

Preparation time: 30 to 40 minutes
Serves 4

Ingredients

- 1 package Italian-style pasta
- 1½ cups onions sliced into ⅛-inch half-moons
- 3 cups zucchini cut into half rounds
- 1½ cups carrots cut into fine matchsticks
- 1 to 2 cloves garlic, thinly sliced or left whole
- 5 to 6 tablespoons extra virgin olive oil
- 3 to 4 cups of liquid; use a combination of fresh water and the liquid from the cooked pasta
- 2 to 3 teaspoons sea salt
- Red and/or black pepper, optional

Preparation

- Gently heat the olive oil in a pan.
- Add the onions and begin to sauté.
- Add the garlic, ½ cup water, and a pinch of sea salt. Continue to sauté.
- Add a cup of the pasta cooking liquid and the zucchini. Cover and simmer for 1 to 2 minutes.
- Add the carrots, another 1 to ½ cup of liquid and sea salt.
- Cover and simmer on low heat for another 3 minutes.
- Add additional olive oil, additional pasta cooking liquid, salt, then fold.
- Simmer uncovered for a few minutes so that the salt blends in with the other ingredients.
- Add pasta directly to the sauce and fold to mix the ingredients. Serve immediately.

SOUPS

Soups are an important part of a healthful diet. Both strengthening and balancing, aim to have one serving of vegetable soup per day. There are two main categories of soup: savory and sweet. Both savory soups and sweet soups are delicious and healthful, although the health benefits are different for each.

Savory soups activate the digestive system and build healthy intestinal flora, helping clean out our intestines. Savory soups are seasoned with miso, sea salt, or a combination of salt and shoyu. Miso soup is the most commonly consumed savory soup in the macrobiotic diet. In addition to its delicious taste, miso is also a wonderful probiotic. Miso soup can be enjoyed 5 to 7 times per week.

Sweet soups are mildly sweet, and are often creamy in texture. The sweetness and consistency are derived by using a combination of cooked sweet vegetables. Sweet vegetables relax the central organs, which has a stabilizing effect on our blood sugar. Sweet vegetable soups are also very soothing, with their satisfying, nourishing texture. We recommend using only sea salt for seasoning sweet vegetable soups. Enjoy sweet vegetable soup about two times per week.

BASIC MISO SOUP

Miso soup strengthens and activates our digestive systems. Miso helps clean the intestinal villi and creates healthy bacteria and enzymes in the digestive tract. Enjoying miso soup regularly strengthens our digestion and alkalizes our overall condition. Note that miso soup is meant to be brothy, so be conservative when deciding how many vegetables to add!

Preparation time: 10 minutes

Ingredients

- Wakame sea vegetable, 1 to 2 inches wakame per cup of water
- 2 to 4 thin slices of root or round vegetables per cup of water
- ⅛ to ¼ cup leafy greens, finely chopped
- Miso, use ½ to 1 level teaspoon miso per 1 cup water. Be sure to buy your miso from a reputable health food store. Barley miso, brown rice miso, and sweet-tasting brown rice miso are all excellent options.
- 1 cup water per serving, plus an additional ⅛ cup (for two servings, measure out 2⅛ cups water)
- Scallion, finely chopped for garnish

Preparation

- Soak the wakame in water for one to two minutes, or until it is soft enough to cut. Discard the soaking water and cut the wakame into even pieces.
- Measure the water and pour into a stainless steel pot. Place the wakame in the pot, turn on the flame, and bring to a boil.
- Add the root and/or round vegetables and cook for 4 to 5 minutes.
- While the vegetables are cooking, measure out the miso into a small bowl. Take a small ladle of the stock and use a wooden utensil to dilute the miso with the ladleful of stock. The resulting consistency should be thin enough that it will easily dissolve when added back to the pot.

- Add the leafy greens to the pot, then add the diluted miso to the boiling water.
- Turn your flame on its lowest setting and simmer for 3 to 4 minutes.
- Place a ladle full of soup in a small bowl, garnish with finely chopped scallions, and serve.

⊸◆⊷

DAIKON AND DRIED SHIITAKE MISO SOUP

Daikon and dried shiitake miso soup dissolves fat and softens hardness in the intestines. It is also good for lowering cholesterol and losing weight.

Preparation time: 10 to 15 minutes

Ingredients

- Wakame sea vegetable, use 1 to 2 inches per cup of water
- 2 to 3 pieces thinly sliced daikon radish per cup of water
- 1 to 2 dried shiitake mushrooms, soaked and thinly sliced
- ⅛ to ¼ cup leafy greens, finely chopped
- ½ to 1 level teaspoon miso per cup of water
- 1 cup water per serving, plus an additional ⅛ cup (for two servings, measure out 2⅛ cups water)
- Scallions, finely chopped for garnish

Preparation

- Soak the wakame in water for one to two minutes or until it is soft. Discard the soaking water and cut the wakame into equal pieces.
- Measure the water for the total number of servings you want, including the shiitake soaking water. Pour the liquid into a

pot, add the wakame and the shiitake, and bring to a boil over a medium flame.

- Add the daikon and cook for 4 to 5 minutes.
- Measure the miso and place in a small bowl. Add a little stock and use a wooden utensil to dissolve the miso.
- Add the leafy greens to the pot, then add the diluted miso to the boiling broth. Immediately lower the flame and simmer for 3 to 4 minutes. Garnish with finely chopped scallions and serve.

⊰◈⊱

SUSAN'S MINESTRONE MISO SOUP

Serves 5 to 7

Ingredients

- Wakame sea vegetable, 2 to 3 inches wakame per cup of water
- ½ medium-sized onion sliced in ¼-inch half-moons
- ½ cup sliced green cabbage
- ½ cup broccoli florets
- 3 plum tomatoes, skin removed or small yellow, orange, and red heirloom tomatoes. Fresh tomatoes offer a better taste and are less acidic!
- Miso, use ½ to ¾ level teaspoon miso per 1 cup water.
- 1 cup water per serving, plus an additional ⅛ cup (for two servings, measure out 2⅛ cups water)
- Italian parsley or fresh basil
- Organic extra virgin olive oil
- Optional ingredient: fresh sliced garlic. Add after the onions.
- For a heartier soup add pasta and/or precooked beans

Preparation

- Soak the wakame in water for one to two minutes, or until it is soft enough to cut. Discard the soaking water and cut the wakame into even pieces.
- Measure the water and pour into a stainless steel pot. Place the wakame in the pot, turn on the flame, and bring to a boil.
- Add the onions and cook for 4 to 5 minutes.
- Add the cabbage and cook another 5 minutes.
- While the vegetables are cooking, measure out the miso into a small bowl. Take a small ladle of the stock and use a wooden utensil to dilute the miso with the ladleful of stock. The resulting consistency should be thin enough that it will easily dissolve when added back to the pot.
- Add the tomatoes and a drizzle of olive oil.
- Add the diluted miso to the boiling water.
- Cover then turn your flame on its lowest setting and simmer for 3 minutes.
- Remove the lid and add the broccoli, cover, and simmer an additional 3 to 4 minutes.
- Add a little chopped Italian parsley or fresh basil just before serving.

⊸◈⊷

BUTTERNUT SQUASH SOUP

Preparation time: 35 to 40 minutes
Serves 5 to 6

Ingredients

- 3 cups diced onions
- 6 cups butternut squash, peeled and cut into 3-inch cubes
- 5 to 6 cups water
- ¾ to 1 teaspoon sea salt

- Garnish options: fried tarragon, minced parsley, green nori flakes

Preparation
- Place the onions in a pot with 1½ cups of the water.
- Bring to a boil, then add ⅛ teaspoon sea salt, reduce the flame to medium-low, and simmer uncovered for 5 minutes.
- Add the squash.
- Add the rest of the water and ¾ teaspoon salt. Cover and bring to a boil.
- Reduce the flame and simmer on low for 25 to 30 minutes or until the vegetables are soft.
- Remove from the stove and purée with an immersion blender until smooth and velvety.
- Place in individual serving bowls and garnish as desired.

⊰◇⊱

CAULIFLOWER CORN CHOWDER

Preparation time: 30 to 35 minutes
Serves 4 to 6

Ingredients
- 3 cups onions, diced
- ½ to 1 head cauliflower, about 5 to 6 cups chopped florets
- ½ cup leeks, cut into ⅛-inch slices
- 1 to 2 ears of non-GMO corn removed from the cob. Use a fine grater to extract the remaining juice and pulp from the cobs.
- 1 tablespoon of organic extra virgin olive oil
- 5 to 6 cups water
- ¾ teaspoon sea salt
- Garnish with fresh herbs such as dill, mint, or green shiso.

Preparation

- Place diced onions in a pot with 1 cup water, just enough to cover the onions by an inch.
- Turn on the flame and bring to a boil.
- Add a pinch of sea salt and continue to cook onions for several minutes or until they become translucent.
- Add cauliflower and enough additional water to cover the vegetables by an inch.
- Add a generous pinch of sea salt, cover, and bring to a boil on a medium-high flame.
- When water begins to boil, cover, and simmer on medium-low heat for approximately 15 minutes.
- Add the grated corn pulp.
- Use an immersion blender to purée until smooth and creamy in texture.
- Pour a small amount of olive oil in a saucepan and turn on the flame.
- Add the corn and begin to sauté.
- Add a small pinch of sea salt ($\frac{1}{16}$ to $\frac{1}{8}$ teaspoon) and gently mix with the corn.
- Add the sliced leeks and continue to sauté until the corn is tender.
- Add the sautéed corn and leeks to the soup and gently stir to blend all ingredients.
- Place in a serving bowl and garnish with chopped fresh herbs.

Note: You can adjust the consistency by increasing or decreasing the amount of vegetables and water. If soup becomes too thick, add additional water until desired consistency is reached.

CREAM OF BROCCOLI SOUP

Preparation time: 45 minutes
Serves 6 to 7

Ingredients

- 2½ cups onions, diced
- ½ cup leeks, diced
- 3 heads broccoli, stems peeled and diced, flower-cut into florets and placed in a separate bowl
- 1 cup cauliflower, cut into florets
- 7 cups water
- 1 teaspoon sea salt
- Herbs (parsley, cilantro, thyme, etc.), finely chopped for garnish

Preparation

- Place the onions and 2 cups of the water in a stock pot and bring to a boil.
- Add ⅛ teaspoon of sea salt and boil the onions for 3 to 4 minutes.
- Add the leeks, then the cauliflower and the broccoli stems.
- Add the remaining 5 cups water and the rest of the salt. Cover and bring to a boil.
- Lower the flame and simmer for 15 minutes.
- Add the broccoli florets, cover, and simmer another 5 to 7 minutes.
- Remove the pot from the stove and use an immersion blender to purée the soup.
- Garnish with your favorite fresh herbs.

Variations

- For a richer taste, sauté thin slices of leek and add them to the soup. The leeks add a new dimension of flavor and are also pleasing to the eye.

CAULIFLOWER AND LEEK SOUP

Preparation time: 45 minutes
Serves 4 to 6

Ingredients

- 3 cups onions, diced
- ½ cup leeks, diced
- ½ to 1 head cauliflower, about 5–6 cups chopped florets
- 5 to 6 cups water
- ¾ teaspoon sea salt
- Parsley, finely chopped for garnish

Preparation

- Place diced onions in a pot with 1 cup water, just enough to cover the onions by an inch.
- Turn on the flame and bring to a boil.
- Add a pinch of sea salt and continue to cook the onions for several minutes or until they become translucent.
- Add the leeks, cauliflower, and enough additional water to cover the vegetables by an inch.
- Add a generous pinch of sea salt, cover, and bring to a boil on a medium-high flame.
- When water begins to boil, cover, and simmer on medium-low heat for approximately 20 minutes or until the vegetables are tender.
- Use a hand food mill or an immersion blender to purée until smooth and creamy in texture.
- Place in a serving bowl and garnish with finely chopped parsley.

Note: Adjust the consistency by increasing or decreasing the amount of vegetables and water. If soup becomes too thick, add additional water until desired consistency is reached.

COOL CUCUMBER SOUP

Preparation time: 20 minutes
Serves 4 to 6

Ingredients

- 3 cups onions, diced
- ½ cup leeks, diced
- 3 to 4 cups chopped cauliflower florets
- 3 to 4 cucumbers, de-seeded then cut into thick half rounds making 4 to 5 cups
- 5 to 6 cups water
- ¾ teaspoon sea salt
- Fresh mint and fresh dill, for garnish or as part of the seasoning

Preparation

- Place diced onions in a pot with 1 cup water, just enough to cover the onions by an inch.
- Turn on the flame and bring to a boil.
- Add a pinch of sea salt and continue to cook the onions for several minutes or until they become translucent.
- Add the leeks, cauliflower, and enough additional water to cover the vegetables by 2 inches.
- Add a generous pinch of sea salt, cover, bring to a boil on a medium-high flame; reduce flame and simmer on medium-low heat for approximately 7 to 10 minutes or until the vegetables are tender.
- Add the cucumber.
- For an herbal flavor add a little mint or fresh dill before you purée the soup.
- Use a hand food mill or an immersion blender to purée until smooth and creamy in texture.
- Place in a serving bowl and garnish with fresh herbs.

Note: Adjust the consistency by increasing or decreasing the amount of vegetables and water. If soup becomes too thick, add additional water until desired consistency is reached.

⊰◈⊱

SWEET POTATO SOUP WITH CARROTS AND GINGER

Preparation time: 40 minutes
Serves 5 to 6

Ingredients

- 3 cups diced onions
- 4 cups sweet potatoes, peeled and cut into 1-inch cubes
- 2 cups diced carrots
- 5 to 6 cups water
- ¾ to 1 teaspoon sea salt
- 1-inch knob fresh ginger, grated with juice reserved
- Garnish options: fried tarragon, minced parsley, fried parsley

Preparation

- Place the onions in a pot with 1½ cups of the water. Bring to a boil, then add ⅛ teaspoon sea salt, reduce the flame to medium low, and simmer uncovered for 5 minutes.
- Add the sweet potatoes and the carrots.
- Add the rest of the water and ¾ teaspoon salt. Cover and bring to a boil.
- Reduce the flame and simmer on low for 20 minutes or until the vegetables are soft.
- Remove from the stove and purée with an immersion blender until smooth and velvety. Grate the ginger using a fine

ginger grater, then squeeze the juice into the soup, stirring to incorporate.

- Place in individual serving bowls and garnish with your favorite choice of fresh herbs.

<hr />

CLEAR SOUP

Preparation time: 30 minutes
Serves 4 to 6

Ingredients
- 1 medium to large dried shiitake mushroom
- 2- to 4-inch strip kombu
- 6 cups water
- ¾ teaspoon sea salt
- ½ cup onions, cut into thin half-moons
- 5 drops shoyu, about ⅛ teaspoon
- 2 pieces fried mochi or fresh tofu per bowl of soup
- A small amount of baby kale to garnish each bowl

Soup Preparation
- Place the water in a pot together with the kombu and dried shiitake.
- Bring the water to a boil, then lower the flame to a rolling boil and continue cooking for 2 to 3 minutes.
- Remove the kombu and shiitake.
- Add the onions and a small pinch of salt.
- Slice the shiitake and return it to the pot.
- Add the remaining ¼ teaspoon sea salt, reduce the flame, and simmer for another 5 minutes.
- Add the shoyu and simmer another 4 to 5 minutes.

Mochi Preparation

- Leave this step until right before you are ready to serve the soup!
- Cut the mochi into 1-inch-square pieces.
- Place a small amount of light sesame oil in the bottom of a skillet and turn on the flame.
- Add the mochi and begin frying on a low temperature.
- After 1 to 2 minutes, turn the mochi over and fry on the other side until soft.

To Serve

- Place 1 or 2 pieces of fried mochi in each bowl.
- Garnish with some baby greens.
- Ladle the hot clear soup over top of the ingredients and serve hot.

SPICY CLEAR SOUP

Preparation time: 15 minutes
Serves 4 to 6

Ingredients

- 1 medium to large dried shiitake mushroom
- 5 or 6 fresh or dried oyster mushrooms
- 2- to 4-inch strip kombu
- 6 cups water
- ¾ teaspoon sea salt
- ½ cup onions, cut into ¼-inch half-moons
- Baby bok choy
- Fresh herbs such as cilantro or Thai lemon basil
- 2 to 3 drops of toasted spicy sesame oil, optional and a delicious touch!
- 5 drops shoyu, about ⅛ teaspoon

Soup Preparation

- Place the water in a pot together with the kombu and dried mushrooms.
- Bring the water to a boil, then lower the flame to a rolling boil and continue cooking for 2 to 3 minutes.
- Remove the kombu and shiitake.
- Add the onions and a small pinch of salt.
- Slice the dried mushrooms and return it to the pot.
- If you are using any fresh mushrooms add them at this time.
- Add the remaining ¼ teaspoon sea salt, reduce the flame, and simmer for another 5 minutes.
- If you desire a hot taste add the spicy sesame oil.
- Add the baby bok choy bottoms and shoyu, then simmer about 2 minutes.
- Add the leafy greens.
- Serve hot and garnish each bowl with a little fresh Thai basil and or cilantro.

⟨◊⟩

CREAMY BLACK BEAN SOUP

Preparation time: 90 minutes
Serves 5 to 6

Ingredients

- 1½ cups black beans, soaked 6 to 8 hours
- 4 cups diced onions
- 6 cups water
- 1-inch piece kombu sea vegetable, rinsed
- 1½ teaspoons sea salt
- Fresh cilantro or basil
- ¼-inch-thick slices or medium-sized diced pieces avocado
- Umeboshi vinegar

- Fresh lime juice; 1-inch thick wedge or slightly more
- Cayenne, jalapeño, or other hot pepper to taste (seeds and vein removed)
- 1 to 2 cloves fresh garlic
- 1 to 1½ teaspoons extra virgin olive oil
- ⅛ teaspoon cumin, optional
- ⅛ teaspoon smoked paprika, optional

Preparation
- Rinse and soak the dry beans 6 to 8 hours or overnight.
- Discard the bean soaking water, add some fresh water, and rinse the beans.
- Place the diced onions in a pressure cooker and add enough water to cover (2 cups).
- Bring the water to a boil, then add the kombu.
- Lower the flame and cook the onions for 4 to 5 minutes.
- Add the garlic and hot peppers.

RED BEAN SOUP

Preparation time: 45 minutes
Serves 4 to 6

Ingredients
- 3 to 4 cups cooked red beans or kidney beans, reserving the cooking liquid
- 3 cups diced onions
- ¾ cup diced celery
- 1 cup diced carrots
- ½ cup leeks or scallion, thinly sliced
- 6 to 7 cups water
- 2½ teaspoons sea salt

- For sautéed vegetables:
- 1 cup diced onions
- ½ cup leeks and/or scallions, thinly sliced
- 1 teaspoon olive oil
- 1 teaspoon toasted sesame oil
- Fresh cilantro or Italian parsley, finely chopped
- Optional: black and/or red pepper, thinly sliced fresh garlic

Preparation

- Place the onions and 3 cups of the water in a stock pot and bring to a boil.
- Add ⅛ teaspoon sea salt, lower the flame, and simmer the onions for 3 minutes.
- Add the celery and simmer another minute. If using the garlic, add it at this time.
- Add the carrots, beans, additional water, and sea salt.
- Cover and bring to a boil. Lower the flame, place a flame deflector under the pot, and simmer 15 minutes.
- While the soup is simmering, prepare the sautéed vegetables.
- Gently heat the toasted sesame and olive oils in a skillet.
- Add the onions and begin to sauté. When the onions begin to sweat, add a small pinch of sea salt and a scant ¼ cup water. Cook until the onions are translucent.
- Add the leeks and/or the scallions, and continue to sauté. Add more water as needed to keep the pan moist. When the vegetables are soft, add them to the soup pot.
- Add another ½ teaspoon of sea salt, cover, and simmer for another 10 minutes.
- Add the pepper and the fresh herbs. Simmer uncovered for another 5 minutes.
- Serve hot and garnish with the finely chopped fresh herbs.

SPLIT PEA SOUP

This soup is so popular that I always have to make extra, so this recipe makes a large quantity of soup. You can always make half of the amount or freeze some for a later day.

Preparation time: 3 hours
Serves 8 to 10

Ingredients
- 4 cups split peas
- 4½ cups diced onions
- 1 cup diced leeks
- ½ cup finely diced burdock
- 10 to 12 cups water
- 2½-inch strip kombu sea vegetable, rinsed
- 1½ to 2 tablespoons sea salt
- 1 teaspoon shoyu
- Black and/or red pepper, to taste
- Fresh herbs (I like parsley or sweet basil), finely chopped
- Optional: a splash of red wine and a drizzle of olive oil and/or deep-fried sourdough croutons

Preparation
- Place the onions and 4 cups of the water in a deep stock pot. Split peas foam during the initial cooking, so using a deeper pot will prevent a huge mess on your stove.
- Bring the water to a boil and cook the onions for 4 minutes.
- Add the leeks, then the burdock.
- Layer the peas on top of the vegetables.
- Add 6 cups of water and bring to a boil, uncovered.
- Skim off any excess foam, lower the flame to a relaxed rolling boil, and continue to cook uncovered until the foaming diminishes.
- Place a flame deflector under the pot, cover, and lower the flame.

- Simmer on low for 1½ hours. Check the peas and use a wooden spoon to stir the soup.
- Cover and continue to cook until the peas are completely soft, about 2 hours.
- Add the salt and stir with a wooden spoon. Cover and simmer for 15 minutes.
- Add any additional water to reach the desired consistency.
- Add the shoyu, pepper, and any of the optional ingredients.
- Simmer for another 5 minutes, then garnish with the fresh herbs and serve.

⊰◈⊱

PURÉED CHICKPEA SOUP

Preparation time: 2 hours
Serves 5 to 6

Ingredients
- 1½ cups chickpeas or white beans, soaked 6 to 8 hours
- 4 cups diced onions
- 6 cups water
- 1-inch piece kombu sea vegetable, rinsed
- 1½ teaspoons sea salt
- Fresh herbs such as sweet basil, thyme, or oregano; choose one fresh herb or a combination of herbs
- Fresh lemon juice; 1-inch-thick wedge or slightly more
- Black pepper to taste

Preparation
- Rinse and soak the dry beans 6 to 8 hours or overnight.
- Discard the bean soaking water, add some fresh water, and rinse the beans.

- Place the diced onions in a pressure cooker, then add enough water to cover (2 cups).
- Bring the water to a boil, then add the kombu.
- Lower the flame and cook the onions for 4 to 5 minutes.
- Add the soaked beans and the remaining water.
- Bring the water to a boil. Skim off any foam that rises.
- Place the lid on the pressure cooker and bring to full pressure.
- Place a flame deflector under the pot, reduce the flame, and pressure cook for 50 to 60 minutes (if using cannellini beans, cook for 30 minutes).
- Remove the pot from the stove, take the pressure down, and remove lid.
- Return the pot to the stove and turn the flame on low.
- Add the sea salt, bring to a light boil, and simmer for 10 minutes.
- Turn off the flame and use a hand immersion blender to purée the soup.
- Return the pot to the stove, then add the fresh herbs.
- Garnish with a drizzle of olive oil, fresh herbs, and black pepper to taste.

BEANS

Soaking and Preparing Beans

- Soak beans for 6 to 8 hours or overnight. Discard the soaking water and use fresh water to cook the beans.
- Cook the beans with a 1-inch-long strip of kombu sea vegetable. Kombu makes the beans soft and more digestible.
- Use just enough water to cover the top of the beans. For beans that do not require soaking, such as lentils and split peas, cover the beans with 2 inches of water. Be sure to cook the beans until they are soft before adding any salt. A common mistake is to leave the beans undercooked; undercooked beans are slightly crunchy, not very digestible, and cause gas and bloating.
- Reduce the liquid in the pot before salting the beans. When you add salt, the beans release more liquid. Allow 15 minutes for the salt to blend with the beans.
- When cooking beans on their own, I recommend using a pressure cooker, which drastically reduces cooking time. I prefer boiling my beans when making bean stews.

Cooking Times

- Boiled beans take approximately 3 hours, from start to finish.
- Pressure-cooked beans: timing begins when the beans reach full pressure.
- 15 to 20 minutes for quick-cooking varieties, such as black turtle beans, cannellini beans, navy beans, lima beans, black-eyed peas, and pinto beans.

- 50 to 60 minutes for longer-cooking varieties, such as chick-peas, yellow soybeans, black soybeans, and kidney beans.
- Canned beans: it is completely acceptable to use canned beans in place of cooking dry beans to save yourself some time. I like using the Eden brand, readily available in many grocery stores. This brand is organic and unseasoned, and the can contains no BPAs.

⸺◈⸺

AZUKI BEANS WITH SEASONAL SWEET VEGETABLES

You may be familiar with the classic version of this dish made with kombu and squash. When squash is not in season, use other seasonal sweet vegetables. Both are delicious, nutritious, and strengthening.

Preparation time: approximately 3 hours
Serves 6 to 8

Ingredients

- 1½ cups azuki beans, washed and soaked 6 to 8 hours. Keep the soaking water and use when cooking the beans.
- 1 medium-sized winter squash such as kabocha, buttercup, or butternut, cut into 2-square-inch pieces. Keep the skin on or leave it off, whatever you prefer.

-or-

- 2 medium-sized onions, diced
- 2 carrots, diced
- 1 to 2 parsnips, diced
- 1 square inch of kombu sea vegetable, rinsed
- Water
- ½ to ¾ teaspoon sea salt
- ¼ to ½ teaspoon shoyu

Preparation

- If you are using onions, cook them on their own for a few minutes before adding the rest of the vegetables and beans. Otherwise, place the kombu and vegetables in the pot.
- Layer the beans on top of the vegetables and add water just to cover the top of the beans.
- Place a lid on the pot, leaving it partially uncovered.
- Bring to a boil, then cover completely. Place a flame deflector under the pot, lower the flame, and simmer 50 minutes to 1 hour.
- Check the liquid level to ensure that the beans are still covered by liquid. Add additional water if needed or use a wooden utensil to immerse the beans in the liquid.
- Replace the cover and continue to simmer on low until the beans are soft, approximately 1½ hours.
- Lightly season with the sea salt and gently fold the ingredients over to blend the salt.
- Continue to simmer for another 10 minutes.
- Add the shoyu and fold to blend. Continue to simmer for another 7 minutes, then serve.

⊰◇⊱

LENTIL SWEET POTATO STEW

This stew is a riff on Azuki Beans with Sweet Vegetables. This is a slightly lighter version, perfect for warmer weather or relaxing your overall condition. This dish is so naturally sweet that it requires very little seasoning.

Preparation time: approximately 3 hours
Serves 6 to 8

Ingredients

- 2 cups green or brown lentils, sorted and washed
- 3 cups sweet potatoes, peeled and diced

- 2½ cups diced onions
- 1½ cups diced carrots
- Water
- 1-inch strip kombu
- ¾ teaspoon sea salt

Preparation

- Place the onions in a pot with 2 cups water and bring to a boil.
- Add the kombu, lower the flame, and simmer the onions for 3 to 4 minutes.
- Layer the sweet potatoes on top of the onions, then add the carrots, then add the lentils.
- Add enough water to cover the lentils by 2 inches.
- Bring the water to a boil. Skim off any excess foam.
- Cover the pot, lower the flame, place a flame deflector under the pot, and simmer for 55 to 60 minutes.
- Remove the cover and check the water level. Add more water to just cover the lentils if necessary. Otherwise, use a wooden spoon to immerse the lentils under the liquid. Re-cover and simmer on low until the lentils are soft, about 1 to 1½ hours.
- Remove the cover and use a wooden utensil to fold the top into the bottom. If the stew is creamy, add the sea salt. If the dish is still a little watery, let simmer uncovered until the liquid is reduced and the lentils are creamy in texture, then add the salt. Fold the top into the bottom to blend all of the ingredients.
- Partially cover the pot and simmer for another 15 to 20 minutes.

CHICKPEA STEW

Preparation time: approximately 2 hours
Serves 4 to 6

Ingredients
- 1 cup chickpeas, washed and soaked
- 1-inch-square piece of kombu
- 2 onions, diced
- 2 stalks celery, sliced thin
- 2 to 3 carrots, diced
- Water
- ½ to ¾ teaspoon sea salt
- ¼ teaspoon shoyu
- Finely chopped fresh herbs, optional

Preparation
- Pour the soaking liquid off of the beans and rinse them several times.
- Place onions in a pressure cooker with a small amount of water to cover, then bring to a boil.
- Add the kombu and allow the onions to cook for another 4 to 5 minutes.
- Layer the celery on top of the onions, then the carrots, and then the chickpeas.
- Add enough water just to cover the top of the beans.
- Bring to a boil and skim off any foam.
- Place the lid on the pressure cooker and bring to full pressure.
- Place a flame deflector under the pot, lower the flame, and cook for 50 minutes.
- Allow the pressure to come down naturally or run cold water over the bottom of the pot until the pressure releases.
- Remove the lid and test one of the beans to see if it is thoroughly cooked. If the beans are tender, season with sea salt

and cook for another 15 to 20 minutes, partially covered. Let any excess liquid cook off before adding the shoyu.

- Add the shoyu and cook for another 5 minutes, then the fresh herbs, if using.

⊸◈⊶

SAVORY LENTIL STEW WITH SAUTÉED ONIONS AND LEEKS

Preparation time: approximately 3 hours
Serves 8

Ingredients
- 3 cups brown or French lentils, sorted and rinsed
- 3 medium-sized onions, diced, approximately 4 cups
- 1-inch piece kombu
- 6 cups water
- 1 cup thinly sliced leeks
- 2 tablespoons olive oil
- 1¾ teaspoons sea salt, total
- 1¼ teaspoons shoyu
- Splash of white wine
- Red and/or black pepper, optional
- 1 to 2 cloves of garlic, finely chopped, optional
- Finely chopped fresh herbs, such as basil, optional

Preparation
- Place the onions in a pot together with the kombu and 1 cup of water.
- Bring the mixture to a boil and cook for 4 to 5 minutes.
- Add the lentils and enough water to cover by two inches. Bring to a boil and skim off any foam that rises to the top.

- Cover the pot. Place a flame deflector under the pot, lower the flame, and simmer on low for 45 to 50 minutes.
- Lift the lid and check the water level. If most of the water is absorbed, add additional water to cover the top of the lentils. You can also use a wooden spoon to immerse the lentils under the cooking liquid.
- Cover and continue to cook until the beans are soft, approximately 1 to 1½ hours. When the beans are tender, add 1¼ teaspoons sea salt. Fold the top into the bottom to blend the salt throughout the dish.
- In a separate skillet, heat 2 tablespoons of olive oil on a low flame.
- Add the onions and begin sautéing. When the onions begin to change color add ⅛ teaspoon sea salt, and ¼ cup water, and continue to sauté for 5 minutes.
- Add the leeks and another ¼ cup of water, and sauté for another 5 minutes.
- Add the shoyu and mix with the sautéed vegetables.
- Add the sautéed vegetables to the lentil pot and add the remaining ¼ teaspoon salt.
- Add a splash of white wine and a drizzle of olive oil.
- Gently fold the bottom layer to the top to blend all the seasonings with the lentils. Simmer for another 5 minutes to blend all the ingredients thoroughly, and serve.

HEARTY LENTIL STEW WITH FRIED BREAD

This recipe is a hit with everyone. The fried bread adds a whole other dimension of satisfaction.

Preparation time: approximately 3 hours
Serves 8

Ingredients
- 2 cups lentils, sorted and washed
- 2 medium-size onions, diced
- 1 cup diced carrots
- ½ cup diced celery
- 1-inch strip kombu, rinsed
- ½ to ¾ teaspoons sea salt
- Water
- ½ teaspoon shoyu
- Good-quality sake or red wine, optional
- 2 or 3 slices un-yeasted sourdough bread
- Safflower oil

Preparation
- Place onions in the heavy pot and add water to just cover the onions. Bring to a gentle boil and add the kombu. Cook for 2 to 3 minutes or until you notice a slight change in the color of the onions.
- Add the remaining ingredients in the following order: celery, carrots, and lentils.
- Add enough water to cover the lentils by 2 inches and bring to a boil.
- Place a lid on the pot, lower the flame, place a flame deflector under the pot, and simmer on low for approximately 45 minutes.

- Check the water level to assure there is enough water for the lentils to continue to cook. If the lentils appear dry, add just enough water to cover. The lentils should be a little juicy before adding the bread, since the bread will absorb a good amount of liquid and thicken the stew.
- If the water level is slightly lower than the lentils, take a wooden spoon and immerse the lentils in the liquid.
- Continue to cook the beans until they are soft, then add the sea salt.
- Gently fold the mixture over to blend the salt, and simmer on low for 15 minutes.
- Season with shoyu, fold again, and simmer for 7 minutes.
- Add the deep-fried bread and simmer another 5 minutes, then add the red wine or sake and simmer another 5 minutes.

Deep-Fried Bread
- Fill the pot with 3 inches of oil and heat to 350 degrees.
- Place the bread in the hot oil and fry on each side until golden brown.
- Place fried bread on an unbleached paper towel to drain off excess oil.
- Cut into squares or break into pieces.

⊰◈⊱

BLACK SOYBEAN STEW

Preparation time: 2 hours
Serves 6 to 8

Ingredients
- 1½ cups black soybeans, soaked 6 to 8 hours. Using the soaking liquid is optional. Some people find it to cause gas.
- 1 to 2 dried shiitake soaked and diced, the soaking water saved

- 1½ cups onions, diced
- 1 cup leeks, diced
- 1 cup carrots, diced
- 1½-inch strip of kombu seaweed
- 1 teaspoon sea salt
- ¼ to ½ teaspoon shoyu
- 1 to 1½ tablespoons barley malt
- ¼ to ½ teaspoon fresh grated ginger and/or ginger juice
- Water to cover the beans

Preparation

- Place the onions in a pressure cooker, add ¼ cup of water, bring to a boil, then simmer for 3 minutes.
- Add the kombu, dried shiitake, and shiitake soaking water.
- Add the leeks, then the carrots. Layer the black soybeans on top of the vegetables.
- Add the soaking liquid or water to cover the beans by ½ inch and bring to a boil.
- Black soybeans produce a lot of foam. Use a fine mesh skimmer to remove the foam.
- When the foaming slows, place the lid on the pressure cooker and bring to full pressure.
- Place a flame deflector under the pot, lower the flame, and cook for 60 minutes.
- Remove the pot from the stove. Run cool water over the pot to lower the pressure.
- When the pressure drops open the lid.
- Test one of the beans to see if it is soft. If it is tender, then place the pot back on the stove.
- Add a small pinch of sea salt and simmer, uncovered, to reduce the liquid until it is even with the beans.
- Add the shoyu, cook for 4 minutes.
- Add the barley malt and continue to simmer for 2 to 3 minutes.
- Turn off the flame, allow to cool for a couple minutes before adding the ginger.
- Serve in a small bowl along with the cooking juice.

WHITE BEAN BURDOCK VITALITY STEW

This dish is particularly strengthening to the kidneys, immune system, and nervous system. It is helpful for people trying to strengthen their sexual vitality.

> Preparation time: 2 to 3 hours
> Serves 6

Ingredients

- 2 cups yellow soybeans or great northern beans, washed and soaked 8 hours
- 2 cups onions, diced
- 1 cup leeks, diced
- ½ cup carrots, diced
- ½ cup burdock, diced
- 1-inch strip kombu
- ½ to ¾ teaspoon sea salt
- ¼ to ¾ teaspoon shoyu
- Water to cover the beans

Preparation

- Place kombu on the bottom of the pot together with the onions.
- Add a little water and bring to a boil. Lower flame and simmer onions for a few minutes.
- As onions begin to change color, layer the leeks, carrots, burdock, and beans on top of the onions.
- Add water along the sides of the pot, just enough to cover the beans.
- Cover the pot and bring to a boil on a medium flame.
- Place a flame deflector under the pot, lower the flame, and cook for 50 minutes.
- Remove the lid to check the water level. As beans soften the water absorbs.

- The water level needs to remain just above the beans, add additional water if needed.
- Continue to simmer until beans are tender.
- When the beans are soft add the sea salt and allow to cook for 15 minutes.
- Add the shoyu and fold the bottom into the top, cook for 5 minutes.
- Serve while hot!

⊰◈⊱

SWEET AND SOUR BAKED BEANS

Preparation time: 3 hours
Serves 6

Ingredients
- 1½ to 2 cups navy or great northern beans, washed and soaked 8 hours
- 2 to 2½ cups onions, diced (Using more onions makes a sweeter dish.)
- 1 cup celery, diced
- 1½ cups carrots, diced
- 1-inch strip kombu
- ½ to ¾ teaspoon sea salt
- ¼ to ¾ teaspoon shoyu
- ¾ to 1 teaspoon umeboshi paste
- 1 to 1½ teaspoons prepared mustard
- 1 to 1½ tablespoons barley malt
- Water to cover the beans

Preparation
- Place kombu on the bottom of the pot together with the onions.

- Add a little water and bring to a boil. Lower the flame and simmer onions for a few minutes.
- As onions begin to change color add the celery. Layer carrots and beans on top of the onions.
- Add water along the sides of the pot, just enough to cover the beans.
- Cover the pot and bring to a boil on a medium flame.
- Place a flame deflector under the pot and lower the flame and cook for 50 minutes.
- Remove the lid to check the water level. As beans soften the water absorbs.
- The water level needs to remain just above the beans, add additional water if needed.
- Continue to simmer until beans are tender.
- When the beans are soft add the sea salt and allow to cook for 10 minutes.
- Add the shoyu and fold the bottom into the top, cook for 5 minutes.
- Add the umeboshi paste and fold.
- Add the barley malt and fold.
- Add the mustard and fold to mix all ingredients.
- Simmer on low for another 4 minutes to allow the flavors to blend together.
- Serve while hot!

Optional variations for a richer flavor

- Preheat your oven to 350 degrees.
- Dice 1 to 2 medium onions, sauté in 1 teaspoon toasted sesame oil blended with a little water.
- Season the onions with ¼ to ½ teaspoon smoked paprika and ¹⁄₁₆ teaspoon sea salt.
- Add the onions to the beans and bake in the oven for 5 to 7 minutes.

SWEET BLACK SOYBEANS

Preparation time: 1½ to 2 hours
Serves 6 to 8

Ingredients
- 1½ cups of black soybeans; sorted, washed and soaked for 6 to 8 hours
- 1 square inch of kombu
- ½ cup of dried chestnuts, soaked
- 1 teaspoon of sea salt
- ¼ to ½ teaspoon of shoyu
- 1 tablespoon of barley malt
- Water

Preparation
- Place the black soybeans, chestnuts, and the soaking water in a pressure cooker together with a piece of kombu.
- Turn on the flame and bring the water to a boil.
- Black soybeans produce a lot of foam. Use a fine mesh skimmer to remove the foam.
- When the foaming slows place the lid on the pressure cooker and bring to full pressure.
- Place a flame deflector under the pot, lower the flame, and cook for 60 minutes.
- Remove the pot from the stove. Run cool water over the pot to lower the pressure.
- When the pressure drops open the lid.
- Test one of the beans to see if it is soft. If it is tender then place the pot back on the stove.
- Add a small pinch of sea salt and simmer, uncovered, on medium-low heat to allow some of the liquid to reduce.
- Add the shoyu, cook for 4 minutes.

- Add the barley malt and continue to simmer for 2 to 3 minutes.
- Serve in small individual serving bowl.

⊸◈⊷

WHITE BEANS WITH SAUTÉED ONIONS AND KALE

Preparation time: 15 to 20 minutes
Serves 4

Ingredients
- 1½ to 2 cups precooked white beans
- 2 tablespoons olive oil
- 1½ cups diced onions
- 3 to 4 leaves kale, stems separated from the leaves and sliced thin and leaves chopped. You can also substitute broccoli or escarole for the kale.
- 1 cup water
- ¾ to 1 teaspoon sea salt

Preparation
- Pour the olive oil into a skillet and gently heat on medium-low heat. Add the onions and begin to sauté.
- When the onions are evenly coated with oil, add a small pinch of sea salt. Add a little more water to keep the pan moist and continue to sauté the onions.
- Add the kale stems and cover. Lower the flame and simmer for 2 minutes.
- Add the leaves and the additional water. Cover and simmer for another 2 minutes.
- Add the precooked beans and the sea salt. Gently fold the top into the bottom to blend all of the ingredients together.

- Cover and simmer for 7 minutes.
- Remove the cover, add a drizzle of olive oil, and season to taste with pepper.
- Gently fold to blend the seasoning with the beans and greens.

⟨◆⟩

WHITE BEANS WITH SAUTÉED CABBAGE, ONIONS, AND CARAWAY

My father, Jared Schwalm, came up with this creation.

Preparation time: 15 minutes
Serves 4

Ingredients
- 1 cup onions, diced or cut into ¼-inch half-moons
- 2 cups green head cabbage, sliced thin
- 2 cups precooked white beans
- 2 tablespoons extra virgin olive oil
- ½ to ¾ teaspoon sea salt
- ½ teaspoon umeboshi vinegar
- 1 to 2 tablespoons caraway seeds
- A dash of celery seed, about 1/16 teaspoon

Preparation
- Gently heat 2 tablespoons of olive oil in a cast-iron pot.
- Add the onions and begin to sauté.
- When the onions begin to sweat, add a pinch of sea salt and a little water to the pan. Add the cabbage and continue to sauté.
- Add a sprinkle of caraway and a dash of celery seed.
- Add the white beans, a generous pinch of salt, a dash of pepper, and blend to combine.

- Reduce flame and continue to sauté slowly for another 2 to 3 minutes.
- Add a dash of umeboshi vinegar at the end of cooking, and mix well.
- Place in a serving dish and cover with a bamboo mat.

⋘◈⋙

ITALIAN-STYLE WHITE BEANS AND GREENS

Preparation time: 10 to 15 minutes
Serves 4 to 5

Ingredients
- 1½ to 2 cups precooked cannellini beans
- 4 cups chopped broccoli rabe, stems separated from the flowers and leaves
- 2 to 3 tablespoons olive oil
- ¾ teaspoon sea salt
- ¾ cup water or bean cooking liquid
- 1 to 2 cloves of garlic, sliced thin or left whole
- Red pepper flakes, to taste

Preparation
- Gently heat 2 tablespoons of olive oil in a cast-iron or sauté pan.
- Add the stems of the greens and begin to sauté.
- Add a little liquid, the garlic, and a good pinch of pepper flakes.
- Add the flowers, the leaves, and a pinch of salt.
- Cover the pot and simmer for a minute.
- Add the beans and the additional salt. Gently fold to blend all the ingredients and simmer for 5 minutes.

- Add a drizzle of olive oil and continue to simmer for another 2 to 3 minutes.

Variation
- Use broccoli or escarole in place of the broccoli rabe.

⬥

M'PANATA, OR WHITE BEANS WITH GREENS AND FRIED BREAD

I first tried this recipe at one of our favorite South Philadelphia restaurants, Ristorante Tre Scalini. My version of this recipe is inspired by Chef Francesca DiRenzo's traditional recipe from her hometown, Monteroduni, Isernia in the Molise region of Italy. I think you will find this dish to be one of the most delicious and satisfying bean dishes of all time.

Preparation time: 10 to 15 minutes
Serves 4

Ingredients
- 1½ to 2 cups precooked cannellini beans
- 4 cups chopped broccoli rabe, stems separated from the leaves and the flowers
- 2 to 4 pieces broken bread crumbs, sautéed in olive oil
- ¾ teaspoon sea salt
- 2 to 3 tablespoons extra virgin olive oil
- A dash red pepper flakes
- 1 to 2 cloves of garlic, sliced thin or left whole
- ½ cup water

Preparation
- Gently heat the olive oil in a sauté pan.
- Add the stems and begin to sauté.

- Add a little water and the garlic and pepper flakes.
- Add the flowers, the leaves, and a pinch of salt.
- Cover the pot and simmer for a minute, then add the bread crumbs.
- Add the beans and the remainder of the salt. Gently fold to blend all of the ingredients.
- Simmer for 5 minutes, or until the bread softens.
- Add a drizzle of olive oil and continue to simmer for another 2 to 3 minutes.
- Variation: I have used kale in place of broccoli rabe, also very yummy!

REFRIED BEANS

Preparation time: 15 minutes
Serves 4 to 6

Ingredients
- 4 cups precooked pinto or turtle beans
- 2 medium onions, diced
- 2 tablespoons extra virgin olive oil
- Water and/or bean cooking liquid
- 1½ to 2 teaspoons sea salt
- 1 to 2 scallions, sliced thin
- Chopped cilantro, sliced jalapeño, or cayenne pepper, optional

Preparation
- Heat the olive oil in a deeper skillet or saucepan.
- Add the onions and begin to sauté.
- When the onions begin to sweat, add a pinch of sea salt and 2 or 3 tablespoon of water or bean cooking liquid. If you are using fresh peppers, add them at this time.

- Continue sautéing until the onions become translucent.
- Add the beans and the rest of the sea salt.
- Fold to blend the seasoning,
- Place a flame deflector under the pot, lower the flame, and simmer for 10 minutes.
- Use the back of a wooden spoon to mash the beans to your desired texture.
- Garnish with chopped cilantro and scallions.

⊰◈⊱

GREEN BEANS AND KIDNEY BEANS

This is an old family recipe common to the Pennsylvania Dutch region where I grew up. It is light, nourishing, and particularly good during the seasonal harvest.

Preparation time: 20 to 30 minutes
Serves 4 to 6

Ingredients
- 3 to 4 cups green and/or yellow beans, wash and snip the ends to remove the string, and cut them in half if they are long.
- 2 cups of precooked kidney beans with their juice
- ¾ cup finely diced onions
- ½ cup finely sliced celery
- ⅛ teaspoon toasted sesame oil
- 1 to 1½ tablespoons extra virgin olive oil
- 3 to 4 cups water
- ¾ to 2 teaspoons sea salt
- 1 clove sliced garlic, optional
- ⅛ to ¼ teaspoon spiced paprika for a smoky flavor, optional

Preparation

- Pour toasted sesame oil followed by a tablespoon of olive oil into a heavier pot.
- Turn on the flame and heat for a minute. Add the onions in the pot and begin to sauté.
- When the color changes on the onions add the garlic and a pinch of sea salt and sauté for 5 minutes.
- Add the celery and continue to sauté for another 3 minutes.
- Layer the green beans on top of the onions, add 2 cups water, and a pinch of sea salt.
- Cover and bring to a gentle boil on a medium-high flame.
- Lower the flame and simmer on low for 7 minutes.
- Add the kidney beans with the juice, additional oil, and salt, then fold to blend ingredients.
- Add additional water if you like more juice.
- Cover and cook for 3 minutes.
- Remove the cover and add the smoked paprika, fold to blend seasoning.
- Simmer uncovered for another couple minutes to reduce some of the liquid and allow the seasoning to fully blend.

⊰◇⊱

QUICK FIX WHITE BEAN BURDOCK STEW

Preparation time: 20 minutes
Serves 4

Ingredients

- 2 cups precooked great northern or navy beans, save the juice to use in cooking
- 1 cup onions, diced

- 1 cup thinly sliced leeks
- ½ cup burdock, diced
- ½ cup carrots, diced
- 2 tablespoons extra virgin olive oil
- ½ to ¾ teaspoon sea salt
- Optional: Chopped fresh herbs such as parsley, lemon thyme, and sage, or a combination

Cookware
- A deeper cast-iron pot with a tight-fitting lid.

Preparation
- Gently heat 2 tablespoons of olive oil in a deeper cast-iron pot.
- Add the onions and begin to sauté.
- When the onions begin to sweat, add a pinch of sea salt and a little water to the pan.
- Add the burdock and continue to sauté.
- Add the carrots and ½ cup of cooked bean juice, cover, reduce the flame.
- Simmer on low for 7 minutes.
- Add the leeks and fold to blend the vegetables.
- Layer the beans on top of the vegetable and season with the remaining sea salt.
- Fold several times to blend the seasoning, cover, and simmer for another 7 minutes.
- Add the fresh herbs before you are ready to plate.
- Place in a serving dish and cover with a bamboo mat.

BAKED BEANS

Preparation time: 2 hours
Serves 6

Ingredients
- 2 cups great northern beans, washed and soaked 8 hours
- 2 to 2½ cups onions, diced (Using more onions makes a sweeter dish.)
- 1 cup celery, diced
- 1½ cups carrots, diced
- 1-inch strip kombu
- ¾ to 1 teaspoon sea salt
- 1½ to 2 tablespoons tomato paste
- ½ to ¾ teaspoon smoked paprika
- ¼ to ½ teaspoon cumin
- ⅛ teaspoon dry mustard
- 1 to 1½ tablespoons barley malt
- Water to cover the beans
- 1 teaspoon toasted sesame oil
- 1½ to 2 tablespoons olive oil
- Cayenne pepper or chili pepper flakes, optional

Preparation
- Discard the soaking liquid and rinse the beans.
- Place the rinsed beans and the kombu in a pressure cooker.
- Add enough water to cover the beans by an inch and bring to a boil.
- Use a fine mesh skimmer to remove the foam that rises to the top of the pot.
- Place the lid on the pressure cooker and bring to full pressure.
- Place a flame deflector under the pot, lower the flame, and cook for 20 minutes.
- As the beans cook begin to prepare the vegetables. After 20 minutes turn off the flame and allow the pressure to release.

- In the second pot gently heat a little toasted sesame oil combined with olive oil.
- Add the diced onions and begin to sauté.
- Add a little water and the celery and continue to sauté.
- Add the carrots and additional water if needed.
- Add the tomato paste.
- Remove the beans from the pressure cooker and pour them over the vegetables.
- Place a flame deflector under the pot, lower the flame, and simmer until the beans are soft.
- Add the sea salt and the spices and cook for another 10 minutes.
- Add the barley malt and additional sea salt if needed.
- Simmer on low for another 4 minutes to allow the flavors to blend together.

Optional variations for a richer flavor:
- Preheat your oven to 350 degrees
- Bake in the oven for 5 to 7 minutes.

⟨◆⟩

SUMMER CHICKPEA VEGETABLE STEW

Preparation time: 20 to 30 minutes
Serves 4 to 6

Ingredients
- 2 cups of precooked chickpeas with their juice
- 1 medium-size onion cut into ¼-inch half-moons
- 1½ cups of carrots cut into a partial roll cut
- 1½ cups zucchini cut into ½-inch half rounds
- 1½ cups summer yellow squash cut into ½-inch half rounds
- 3 tablespoons of extra virgin olive oil

- 4 to 5 cups water
- 1½ to 2 teaspoons sea salt
- 1 to 3 cloves garlic sliced thin
- Fresh herbs such as lemon basil, lemon thyme or use a combination.

Preparation

- Pour enough olive oil in the bottom of the pot and turn on the flame.
- Place onions in the pot and begin to sauté.
- Add a small pinch of sea salt and allow the onions to cook for another 4 to 5 minutes.
- Layer the carrot on top of the onions, and add the bean juice and additional water to cover the vegetables.
- Cover and bring to a gentle boil on a medium-high flame.
- Lower the flame and simmer for 15 minutes.
- Add the summer vegetables, and additional salt, cover and cook for 7 minutes.
- When the vegetables reach the texture you desire add the fresh herbs and turn off the flame, then place in a serving bowl.

HUMMUS

A traditional dish that both kids and adults enjoy. It makes a delicious snack or use it in a sandwich together with vegetables. Hummus will keep in the refrigerator for 1 week.

Preparation time: 15 to 20 minutes
Serves 4 to 6

Ingredients
- 2 cups of precooked organic chickpeas
- ½ cup bean juice
- ¼ cup roasted tahini
- 1 to 2 cloves minced garlic (optional)
- ⅛ to ¼ teaspoon sea salt
- ⅛ teaspoon pepper
- ½ teaspoon umeboshi paste
- 1 tablespoon umeboshi vinegar
- ½ cup extra virgin olive oil
- Fresh-squeezed organic lemon juice, to taste

Preparation
- Place beans and salt in a blender together with a little of the bean juice. Add other ingredients and blend until desired consistency.
- Hummus is great with fresh vegetables, pita, or with chips.

TOFU, TEMPEH, AND NATTO

TOFU

MARINATED TOFU

Marinated tofu can be used in sandwiches, wraps, salads, or sushi.

Preparation time: 5 to 7 minutes
Marinate time: minimum 3 hours or overnight or longer
Half a block of tofu will make 3 sandwiches or approximately 6 sushi rolls.

Ingredients
- Half a block of organic tofu, firm or extra firm
- 1 part umeboshi vinegar (¼ cup umeboshi vinegar)
- 3 to 4 parts water (¾ to 1 cup water). Use more water for a milder flavor.

Preparation
- Rinse the tofu and cut into half-inch-thick slices or strips.
- Place the tofu on a clean cotton towel or paper towel. Place another towel on top and gently press out excess water.

- Place the cut tofu in a flat Pyrex dish.
- Mix the umeboshi vinegar and water in a measuring cup, then pour over the tofu. The tofu should be fully immersed in the liquid. You can place a bamboo mat on top of the tofu to keep it immersed.
- Allow the tofu to marinate at least 3 hours. I like to make this and let it sit overnight in the refigerator.

⊰◈⊱

SIMMERED TOFU

Preparation time: 10 minutes
Half a block of tofu will make 3 sandwiches or 6 sushi rolls

Ingredients
- ½ block organic tofu, extra firm
- 2 teaspoons shoyu
- 2 teaspoons umeboshi vinegar
- ½ teaspoon mirin
- 6 teaspoons water

Preparation
- Rinse the tofu and cut into ½-inch-thick slices.
- Measure the liquid ingredients and pour into a stainless steel sauce or frying pan.
- Place the tofu in the pan and turn on the flame to medium.
- Bring the liquid to a very gentle boil, lower the flame, and simmer for 2 to 3 minutes on each side.
- Remove the tofu from the pot and place on a plate or dish, and allow it to cool before serving.

TOFU CHEESE

Use tofu cheese in salads, in lightly cooked vegetable dishes, or in pasta.

Preparation time: 5 minutes
½ block tofu makes approximately 2 cups tofu cheese

Ingredients
- ½ block organic tofu, extra firm
- ⅛ cup umeboshi vinegar

Preparation
- Rinse the tofu, then place in a bowl. Use one hand to begin crumbling the tofu while also pouring the umeboshi vinegar into the bowl with the other hand. The texture should remain firm.

⊰◈⊱

HIYAYAKKO ("COLD TOFU")

This recipe was created and adapted from my personal experience of eating "cold tofu" in a number of Japanese restaurants. I order it without the bonito.

Tofu is a traditional food of Asian cuisine and may be prepared in a variety of ways. Chilled tofu is a light and fresh dish which is so simple and perfect for summer. There are many different toppings you can try and this is the way I like to prepare it.

Preparation time: 7 to 10 minutes
Serves 3 to 4

Ingredients
- One block fresh tofu
- 2 to 3 inches freshly grated ginger
- 2 to 3 finely chopped scallions

SUSAN'S PONZU SAUCE

Ingredients
- 2 tablespoons shoyu
- 1 teaspoon mirin
- ½ teaspoon umeboshi vinegar
- ¼ teaspoon brown rice vinegar
- Hot chili peppers or shichimi, optional

Preparation
- Rinse and dry 1 block of tofu.
- Cut into equal size pieces approximately 2 inches long and 1 inch thick.
- Use a dry clean cloth or paper towel and lightly press to tofu to remove excess water.
- Place the tofu on a serving dish.
- In a separate bowl mix your sauce.
- Garnish each piece of tofu with fresh grated ginger followed by scallion.
- If you are using bonito put a little on each piece of tofu.
- Pour the sauce over top of the tofu and serve or dip individual pieces of tofu in the sauce.

TEMPEH

Tempeh is a fermented bean product with a dense consistency and texture. It is a delicious source of protein with a hearty bite and is extremely versatile. Tempeh needs to be boiled in order to make it digestible.

Boiled Tempeh
- Boil the tempeh in a mixture of 9 parts water to 1 part shoyu, a small piece of kombu, and a few slices of ginger. The tempeh will keep in the cooking liquid for up to 1 week.

Fried Tempeh
- Place about ⅛ to ¼ inch of safflower oil in a cast-iron frying pan. Cut tempeh into desired-size pieces. Fry on each side until the tempeh reaches a golden brown color.
- Place the fried tempeh on unbleached paper to drain off excess oil.

Serving Suggestions
- Cut into cubes and add to light vegetable dishes or salads.
- Cut into strips and use in wraps, fajitas, or nori rolls.
- Use in sandwiches.

⊰◇⊱

NATTO

Natto is a fermented soybean product that is said to have an acquired taste.

Natto has numerous health benefits including strengthening digestion, cardiovascular function, and clarifies thinking. It is high in calcium, so it is great for the bones, skin, and hair. It is also said that eating natto helps make us brilliant and beautiful.

Preparation time: 10 minutes

3 ounces of natto serves two

Ingredients

- 3 ounce pakage of natto
- 1 finely chopped scallion
- ½ sheet of toasted nori, torn finely
- ¹⁄₁₆ to ⅛ teaspoon shoyu (begin by adding ¼ teaspoon and add additional if desired)
- ¼ teaspoon stone ground mustard or Dijon style

Preparation

- Place natto, toasted nori, scallions, and shoyu in a bowl. Whip together with chopsticks. You will know the ingredients are mixed well when the consistency becomes sticky and stringy. Natto may be eaten together with rice, toasted nori, with noodles or in miso soup. Natto is also delicious with fried mochi and toasted nori.

NATTO WITH SAUERKRAUT

Prepartion time: 5 to 7 minutes

3 ounces of natto serves 2

Ingredients

- 3 ounce package of natto
- 2 to 3 tablespoons sauerkraut
- ¹⁄₁₆ to ⅛ teaspoon shoyu
- ⅛ to ¼ teaspoon mustard, optional
- Spicy variation: use kimchi in place of sauerkraut

SUBSTANTIAL LONG-COOKED VEGETABLE DISHES

These long-cooked vegetable dishes are considered to be substantial because of their strengthening qualities and their ability to provide us with health benefits for up to 3 days.

NISHIME VEGETABLES

Nishime is a style of cooking that creates a settling energetic effect. Vegetables are cut into medium to large chunks and steamed until they become meltingly soft and tender. In nishime-style cooking, a small piece of kombu seaweed is cooked with the vegetables. The use of kombu, together with the longer cooking time, brings out the protein and carbohydrate qualities in the dish. Nishime is also a layered dish: lighter vegetables are layered on the bottom, followed by round vegetables in the middle, and root vegetables on top. From an energetic perspective, layering this dish enhances its settling qualities. This dynamic cooking method provides us with lasting energy, harmonizes our central organs, and keeps our blood sugar stable.

Preparation time: about 45 minutes
A 1-quart pot yields approximately 4 to 5 servings

Ingredients
- 1-square-inch piece of kombu, rinsed and/or soaked
- $\frac{1}{16}$ to $\frac{1}{8}$ teaspoon sea salt

- ⅛ to ¼ teaspoon shoyu
- Water to cover the bottom of the pot by ¼ to ½ inch
- A variety of vegetables cut into 1- to 2-inch chunks. I recommend using sweet vegetables with this dish (refer to vegetable list, p. 193).
- Round vegetables, cut into wedges or half-rounds.
- Root vegetables, cut using a partial or full roll cut about 1 to 2 inches in length
- Hearty-style leafy greens (such as celery or leeks)
- On occasion you can also use dried shiitake mushrooms in nishime cooking.

Cookware

- This dish works best using a heavy pot with a tight-fitting lid. The dish will also turn out much better if the vegetables fit tightly into the pot, leaving very little space. As mentioned above, a 1-quart pot will yield 4 to 5 servings.

Preparation

- Place kombu on the bottom of the pot.
- Add the first layer of vegetables.
- Add ¼ to ½ inch water to cover the bottom of the pot.
- Continue layering the vegetables.
- Add a tiny pinch of sea salt, cover, and bring to a boil over a medium flame. When the water begins to boil, steam will begin to build inside the pot. You may see the steam or notice a little condensation on the side of the pot. You may even hear the water begin to boil. All these signs are an indication that the water inside the pot is boiling.
- Turn the flame down and simmer on low for an average of 25 to 30 minutes, or until the vegetables are tender. The cooking times will vary, depending on the vegetables you use and the size of the pieces.
- Remove the lid and lightly season with a few drops of shoyu.
- Place the lid back on the pot, then pick up the pot and give it a gentle shake to blend the shoyu with any liquid remaining

in the pot. Return the pot to the stove and cook for another 4 minutes.
- Remove the pot from the stove and let it stand for a few minutes before placing the vegetables in a serving dish.

⋙◈⋘

ARAME WITH SWEET VEGETABLES

Preparation time: 30 to 40 minutes
Serves 6

Ingredients
- ½ package arame, about 25 grams, soaked until soft, soaking water discarded
- 4 cups onions, sliced into ¼-inch half-moons
- 2½ cups carrots, cut into thin matchsticks
- Approximately ½ cup water
- ¹⁄₁₆ teaspoon sea salt
- ¾ to 1 teaspoon shoyu
- ¼ teaspoon mirin
- ⅛ to ¼ teaspoon sesame oil, optional

Preparation
- Place the onions in a pot with enough water to cover, and turn flame to medium-low.
- When you notice the onions begin to "sweat," add a pinch of sea salt.
- Continue to cook the onions for 3 minutes.
- Layer the carrots on top of the onions and the arame on top of the carrots.
- Add enough water to reach the bottom portion of the arame.
- Cover and bring to a boil on a medium-high flame.
- Reduce the heat to medium-low and simmer for 15 minutes.

- Remove the lid and check the level of the liquid in the pot. There should be about 1½ inches of liquid left in the bottom of the pot. If there is still too much liquid in the pot, crack the lid and allow some of the liquid to reduce before seasoning.
- Add the sesame oil if using, followed by the shoyu.
- Add the mirin.
- Gently fold to blend the seasoning with the ingredients.
- Replace the cover, reduce the heat, and simmer on low for another 5 minutes.

Variations

- For a richer taste, layer crumbled tofu under the arame.
- For a lighter dish, add green peas, snow peas, or edamame at the end of cooking.

⊷◈⊷

ROOTS AND GREENS

Preparation time: 10 to 20 minutes
Serves 3 to 8, depending on the size of the vegetable. One bunch of radishes or turnips will serve 3 to 4, while a daikon radish will serve 6 to 8.

Ingredients

- Choose one of the following: daikon, red radishes, turnips, or carrots.
- Separate the roots from the stems and leaves, making sure to leave the small connection between the root and stems intact on the root. Cut root portion into matchsticks or half-rounds, or dice them. Finely chop the stems and leaves, separating the leafy parts from the thicker portions of the stems.
- ¹⁄₁₆ teaspoon sea salt
- ⅛ to ¼ teaspoon shoyu
- ¼ to ½ cup water

Preparation

- Gently heat enough water to cover the bottom of the pan.
- Add the roots and begin sautéing. If you are using carrots, add ½ teaspoon sesame oil to the pan when sautéing.
- When the roots begin to "sweat," add a tiny pinch of salt and continue to sauté.
- Add about ¼ cup water, cover, and simmer a few minutes until the roots are about halfway cooked.
- Pull the roots to one side of the pot and add the stems. Fold the roots over the stems, cover, and continue to simmer for 2 to 3 minutes.
- Once again, move the roots and stems to one side, add the leaves, and fold the roots on top of the greens. Allow to simmer another minute before lightly seasoning with the shoyu. Fold the top into the bottom to blend everything together.

⊰◈⊱

CLASSIC KINPIRA

This dish is delicious and hearty. It it is helpful for strengthening blood quality, the bones, and the central nervous system.

Preparation time: 30 to 40 minutes
Serves 6

Ingredients

- 2 cups burdock, cut into thin matchsticks or shaved
- 2 cups carrots, cut into thin matchsticks or shaved slightly thicker than the burdock
- 2 cups lotus root, cut into half-rounds
- ¼ teaspoon light or toasted sesame oil
- 1/16 teaspoon sea salt
- ½ cup water
- Shoyu, approximately ½ teaspoon

- Mirin, approximately ⅛ teaspoon
- Fresh ginger juice, to taste, or shichimi

Preparation
- Add several drops of sesame oil to the skillet and gently heat on a medium-low flame.
- Add the burdock to the pan and begin to sauté.
- When the burdock is coated evenly with oil, add a pinch of sea salt and continue to sauté until the color begins to deepen, approximately 4 minutes.
- Add the lotus root and sauté until it begins to sweat, then add the carrot.
- Add a little water to the bottom of the skillet, then cover and simmer until vegetables are tender, about 7 to 9 minutes.
- Lightly season with the shoyu and mirin, cover, and cook another 4 to 5 minutes.
- At the very end of cooking, add a squeeze of fresh-grated ginger juice or a dash of shichimi.

⊸◈⊸

SWEET VEGETABLE KINPIRA

This is a lighter version of the "classic" sauté and simmer style using sweet vegetables.

Preparation time: 30 to 40 minutes
Serves 4

Ingredients
- 2 cups onions, cut into ¼-inch-thick half-moons
- 2 cups root and/or round vegetables, cut into thin matchsticks or slices
- ¼ to ½ teaspoon light sesame oil
- ¹⁄₁₆ to ⅛ teaspoon sea salt

- ½ cup water
- ¼ teaspoon shoyu
- Optional: fresh-grated ginger juice

Preparation

- Pour the sesame oil into a skillet, turn on the flame to medium-low to gently heat the oil.
- Add the onions and begin to sauté. When you notice a slight change in color, add a small pinch of sea salt.
- Add approximately ¼ cup water and continue sautéing until the onions become translucent.
- Add the harder, more fibrous vegetables to the pan and let cook 1 minute. Then add the rest of the vegetables and continue to sauté.
- Add just enough water to keep the pan moist, then cover and simmer until the vegetables are tender.
- Lightly season with a few drops of shoyu.
- Fold to blend the seasoning, cover, and simmer for another 4 to 5 minutes.
- Turn off the flame, then add a squeeze of fresh-grated ginger juice.
- Gently fold to blend with the vegetables.
- Place in a serving dish and cover with a bamboo mat.

⊸◈⊶

CANDIED SWEET POTATOES

Preparation time: 30 minutes
Serves 2, using 1 medium sweet potato per person

Ingredients

- 2 sweet potatoes, peeled and cut lengthwise into 2-inch-thick slices

- 2 tablespoons brown rice syrup
- 1 tablespoon barley malt
- ½ to 1 teaspoon pure maple syrup
- 1 teaspoon extra virgin olive oil
- Water
- Small pinch sea salt, between ¹⁄₁₆ and ⅛ teaspoon

Preparation

- Place the sweet potatoes in the pan with just enough water to cover the bottom of the pan. Cover and bring to a boil.
- Lower the flame and steam on low heat for 5 minutes.
- Remove the lid and drizzle a little olive oil over the sweet potatoes, then add a pinch of salt, cover, and continue to steam for 10 minutes.
- In a separate bowl, mix the rice syrup, barley malt, and maple syrup together. Pour over top of the sweet potatoes, replace lid, and continue to cook until the potatoes are tender. As the potatoes cook, the sauce will reduce, forming a sweet glaze.

❧

MEDITERRANEAN SAUTÉED VEGETABLES

This is one of my "go-to" dishes when I want something quick with a little more substance. It is simple to prepare, yet offers a nourishing and satisfying quality. As an added bonus, everyone who tries it seems to love it!

Preparation time: 10 to 15 minutes
Serves 4 to 6

Ingredients

- 1 bunch of broccoli or a small head of cauliflower, or round green cabbage

- ⅛ to ¼ teaspoon sea salt
- 2 to 3 tablespoons extra virgin olive oil
- ¼ to ½ cup of water

Cookware
- Deep stainless steel or cast-iron sauté pan with lid

Preparation
- Cut vegetables into medium to larger florets, or into 2-inch pieces if using cabbage.
- Peel and slice the stems into matchsticks proportionate to the size of the florets.
- Add enough water to cover the bottom of the pan, then turn on the flame to medium-low.
- Place the stems and florets in the pan, cover, turn the flame to medium, and steam for 2 minutes.
- Remove the lid and drizzle olive oil over the vegetables, then add a pinch of sea salt.
- Cover and continue to steam for another minute.
- Remove the lid and gently fold to blend the seasonings.
- Return the cover and continue cooking about 7 minutes, or until the vegetables reach the desired texture. The longer you cook the vegetables, the sweeter they will be. Remove vegetables from the pot, place in a serving dish, and cover with a bamboo mat.

⊂◈⊃

SAUTÉED BROCCOLI RABE

Preparation time: 7 to 10 minutes
Serves 2

Ingredients
- 1 bunch broccoli rabe, stems, leaves, and florets separated

- 2 to 3 tablespoons extra virgin olive oil
- ⅛ to ¼ teaspoon sea salt
- Water
- Dried red pepper flakes, optional

Preparation
- Cut the stems on an angle into 2-inch-long pieces.
- Add enough water to cover the bottom of the pan, then turn the flame to medium-low and place the stems in the pan.
- Cover and steam for 1 to 2 minutes.
- Add the leaves, cover, and steam for another minute.
- Add the florets, a drizzle of olive oil, and a pinch of salt.
- Gently fold the ingredients to blend the seasoning and continue to sauté until tender but still slightly crunchy.
- Place in a serving bowl and cover with a bamboo mat.

BOILED DAIKON WITH SWEET MISO-TAHINI SAUCE

Preparation time: 35 to 45 minutes
Serves 2 to 4

Ingredients
- 1 tablespoon sweet brown rice miso or barley miso
- 2 tablespoons roasted tahini
- 2 tablespoons brown rice syrup
- 1 large daikon or 2 medium-size daikon radishes, peeled and cut ¼- to ½-inch thick on the diagonal
- 1 pinch of sea salt, about ⅛ teaspoon

Preparation

- Place cut daikon in a pot with water to cover and a small pinch of sea salt.
- Bring to a boil on a medium-high flame then cover. It is okay to leave the lid slightly cracked as to not make a mess on your stove.
- Lower the flame and simmer until the daikon is tender, approximately 30 to 40 minutes depending on the thickness and texture of the daikon.
- While the daikon is cooking prepare the sauce.
- Place 1 slightly rounded tablespoon of miso in a bowl then dilute with a tablespoon of the daikon cooking water; mix well to a smooth consistency.
- Add 2 tablespoons of tahini and blend together with the miso to form a thick paste.
- Add 2 tablespoons of brown rice syrup, stir well until all ingredients are blended into a thick, smooth paste.
- When the daikon is thoroughly cooked place each piece on a flat serving platter and allow to cool for a minute before adding the sauce. A wire spider utensil works best to allow the excess liquid to drain. It works best if you only take a few pieces of daikon at a time. This helps to prevent the sauce from running and making your dish look messy.
- Place a small amount of sauce on each piece of daikon and serve immediately, while hot.

Note: If you have extra sauce it will easily keep in the refrigerator for about a month.

SAUTÉED ONIONS, CABBAGE, AND TOMATOES WITH MISO

Preparation time: 20 minutes
Serves 4 to 6

Ingredients

- 1 medium onion, sliced into ¼-inch half-moons
- 5 to 6 cups green cabbage, cut into 1-inch pieces
- 3 cups plum tomatoes (peeled and diced)
- 1 to 2 tablespoons extra virgin olive oil
- ¹⁄₁₆ to ⅛ teaspoon sea salt
- ¾ to 1 cup water. If using canned tomatoes use less water.
- ½ teaspoon aged barley miso per cup of liquid

Preparation

- Gently heat a few drops of olive oil.
- Add the onions and begin to sauté.
- As you are sautéing add a small amount of water to the sides of the pot.
- When the onions begin to show a slight change in color add a small pinch of sea salt.
- Gently fold to blend the ingredients. Continue sautéing for another couple minutes.
- Add a small amount of water to the sides of the pot then layer the cabbage on top of the onions. Add additional water, enough to half cover the cabbage.
- Lower the flame and simmer for 5 minutes.
- Add the diced tomatoes to the cabbage and fold to blend all the ingredients.
- Measure the amount of miso and use a little of the cooking water to dilute the miso.
- Make a well in the middle of the vegetables and add the miso.

- Cover and simmer for 5 minutes.
- Remove the cover and add a drizzle of olive oil.
- Fold the bottom into the top to allow the seasonings to blend evenly with the vegetables. Simmer for another 2 to 3 minutes.
- This dish may be served as a side dish, over rice, noodles, or pasta.

⊸◈⊶

SAVORY SESAME BURDOCK

For strength and vitality.

Preparation time: 25 to 30 minutes
Serves 2 to 4

Ingredients
- 1 cup of cut burdock. I recommend using a partial roll cut.
- ¾ cup of water or water to cover
- A small pinch sea salt
- ½ teaspoon toasted sesame oil
- ¾ teaspoon shoyu
- ¼ teaspoon mirin
- ½ teaspoon umeboshi vinegar

Preparation
- Place the cut burdock in a pot with enough water to cover the burdock.
- Turn on the flame and bring the water to a boil.
- Add a tiny pinch of sea salt (¹⁄₁₆ of a teaspoon).
- Cover the pot, lower the flame, and simmer for 10 minutes.
- Crack the lid and continue to simmer, allowing most of half the liquid to reduce, leaving about ⅛ inch to cover the bottom of the pot.
- Add the toasted sesame oil.

- Add the shoyu, mirin, and umeboshi vinegar.
- Gently fold the bottom into the top to allow the ingredients to mix.
- Continue to simmer on low until almost all of the remaining liquid reduces.
- Place in a small serving dish and cover with a bamboo mat until you are ready to eat.

Variations
- Garnish with some plain toasted sesame seeds
- For a spicy effect, add a little hot spice, like shichimi during the seasoning, or use spicy toasted sesame oil in place of the regular sesame oil.

⊰◇⊱

SWEET AND SOUR BEETS

Preparation time: 30 to 35 minutes
Serves 4 to 5

Ingredients
- 4 to 5 beets, peeled and sliced into ½ inch thick half-rounds
- 1½ cups red onions cut into ¼-inch-thick half-moons
- ¼ teaspoon toasted sesame oil
- ¾ cup water
- 1/16 to ⅛ teaspoon sea salt
- ½ teaspoon olive oil
- 1 to 2 tablespoons brown rice syrup
- 1 to 1½ teaspoons brown rice vinegar or fresh-squeezed lemon juice (⅓ wedge of lemon)

Preparation
- Gently heat a small amount of toasted sesame oil.

- Add the red onion and begin to sautéing the onions.
- When the onions are evenly coated with oil add a small pinch of sea salt and continue to sauté another 2 to 3 minutes.
- Add enough water to cover the bottom of the pot by 1 to 1½ inches. The more water you use the more juice it will yield.
- Layer the beets on top of the onions.
- Add a pinch of sea salt, cover and cook until you see a little steam emerging from the pot.
- Lower the flame and simmer on low for 20 minutes, until the beets are almost soft.
- You can use a wooden skewer or toothpick to check the tenderness.
- Drizzle a small amount of olive oil over the beets.
- Add the rice syrup.
- Cover and continue to simmer until the beets have reached the perfect texture you desire.
- Carefully remove the beets from the pot and place in a serving dish.
- Add fresh-squeezed lemon juice or brown rice vinegar to the beet juice.
- Pour the juice over the beets before serving.

◇

SWEET AND SOUR LOTUS ROOT

Preparation time: 35 minutes
Serves 4 to 6

Ingredients

- 4 cups fresh lotus root cut into ½-inch rounds (about 2 to 3 small roots). Use loose-packed lotus roots rather than roots that have been vacuum sealed. Lotus root is often packed in straw-filled crates. Choose the more round bulbous roots.

These are better quality and have more vitality, thus offering us more vitality when we eat them!

- ¹⁄₁₆ to ⅛ teaspoon sea salt
- 3 to 4 cups water
- 1 to 2 teaspoons toasted black sesame seeds

Preparation

- Place the lotus root in a pot and cover with water.
- Add a small pinch of sea salt.
- Bring to a boil, cover, and simmer for ½ hour. After the first 15 minutes, begin preparing the sauce.
- Remove the lotus, place in a serving dish, and cover with the hot sauce.
- Garnish with toasted black sesame seeds.

Sauce Ingredients

- ½ cup grated lotus root
- ⅓ cup water
- 1 tablespoon rice syrup
- ¼ to ½ teaspoon brown rice vinegar, to taste
- Toasted black sesame seeds and grated fresh ginger juice, optional

Sauce Preparation

- Measure ⅓ cup of water and pour it into a pot.
- Squeeze the grated lotus root and the juice to the water.
- Add a pinch of sea salt.
- Bring to a boil, lower the flame, and simmer for 3 minutes until the liquid thickens. Add rice syrup and brown rice vinegar.
- Pour the sauce over the lotus root.
- Garnish with toasted black sesame seeds before serving.

SWEET AND SOUR RED CABBAGE

Preparation time: 20 to 25 minutes
Serves 4 to 5

Ingredients

- 5 to 6 cups red cabbage sliced into ½-inch strips
- 1 cup red onions cut into ¼-inch half-moons
- ¼ teaspoon toasted sesame oil
- ½ cup water
- ⅛ to ¼ teaspoon sea salt
- 1 teaspoon olive oil
- ⅛ teaspoon umeboshi vinegar
- 1 to 2 tablespoons brown rice syrup
- 1 to 1½ teaspoons brown rice vinegar
- ½ to 1 teaspoon caraway seeds

Preparation

- Gently heat a small amount of toasted sesame oil in a cast-iron pot.
- Add the red onions and begin to sauté.
- When the onions are evenly coated with oil add a small pinch of sea salt and the umeboshi vinegar.
- Add a little water and continue to sauté another 2 minutes.
- Add the red cabbage and a little more water. Continue sautéing.
- Add enough water to cover the bottom of the pot by 1 to 1½ inches.
- Add the remaining sea salt, cover, and cook until you see a little steam emerging from the pot.
- Lower the flame and simmer on low for 15 minutes.
- Remove the lid and drizzle a small amount of olive oil over the vegetables.
- Add the caraway seeds.

- Add the rice syrup and fold to blend all the ingredients.
- Cook uncovered for another 2 to 5 minutes.
- Add the brown rice vinegar and fold to blend the ingredients.
- Place in a serving dish along with the juice and cover with a bamboo mat.

⟞◇⟝

VEGAN CAULIFLOWER AU GRATIN

Preparation time: 20 minutes
Serves 4 to 6

Ingredients

- 5 cups cauliflower or 1 medium head, cut into larger florets
- $\frac{1}{16}$ to $\frac{1}{8}$ teaspoon sea salt
- 1 to 2 tablespoons extra virgin olive oil
- 1 block extra firm tofu
- ½ cup roasted tahini
- 1 tablespoon green nori flakes or finely chopped parsley
- ¼ to ½ cup of umeboshi vinegar
- ½ to ¾ cup water

Preparation

- Place the tofu in a bowl and use your hands to crumble it while adding the umeboshi vinegar.
- Add the tahini and the nori flakes or parsley and mix all in together.
- Pour the water into a slightly deeper pan. More water makes a slightly creamier dish.
- Place the cauliflower florets in the pot, cover, and begin to steam the cauliflower for 1 minute.
- Add a drizzle of olive oil and the sea salt. Cover and steam for another minute.

- Layer the tofu mixture on top of the cauliflower, cover, and continue steaming for 3 minutes.
- Add a finishing touch of olive oil and cook uncovered until the tofu becomes creamy in consistency. Place in a serving dish and cover with a bamboo mat.

LIGHT VEGETABLE DISHES

Lightly cooked vegetable dishes are important to include with every meal. They provide us with fresh, uplifting energy and keep our internal condition hydrated. When we eat lightly cooked vegetable dishes on a regular basis, we do not need to drink gallons of water every day. Because these dishes are cooked quickly, they sharpen our reflexes, allowing us to think and react more quickly, a wonderful benefit for both work and play!

QUICK SAUTÉED BABY SPINACH

Preparation time: 4 to 5 minutes
Serves 2 to 4

Ingredients

- 1 bunch or box of spinach. Wash the spinach by filling a bowl and dunking it in the water. You may have to pour off the water and dunk several times to remove excess debris. Even when purchasing "triple washed" boxed vegetables I still prefer to wash again.
- ¼ cup water
- 3 to 5 drops toasted sesame oil
- ⅛ teaspoon sea salt

- ¼ teaspoon shoyu
- 3 to 5 drops mirin

Variation combining oils

- 1 drop toasted sesame oil
- ½ teaspoon extra virgin olive oil
- ¼ teaspoon sea salt
- ⅛ teaspoon shoyu
- Fresh-squeezed lemon or mirin
- Red pepper, optional

Preparation

- Use a stainless steel skillet.
- Gently begin to heat just enough water to cover the bottom of the pan.
- Add the toasted sesame oil.
- Add the spinach and begin to sauté for approximately 10 seconds.
- Add the sea salt and gently fold to blend the seasoning. If using olive oil, drizzle a little oil over the top of the vegetables, then add a little sea salt and fold to blend the seasoning.
- Add the shoyu and fold.
- Add either fresh-squeezed lemon juice or mirin and fold to blend all the flavors.
- Place in a serving dish and cover with a bamboo mat.
- Optional: For a light spicy taste add a smidge of red pepper.

QUICK SAUTÉED ROMAINE
WITH TOFU CHEESE

Preparation time: 7 to 8 minutes
Serves 2 to 4

Ingredients
- 1 head romaine lettuce, washed and broken into 2-inch pieces. Separate the lower thick part of the leaf from the thinner, deeper green part. (Baby greens may be kept whole.) When washing lettuce it is preferable to use a dunk method, filling a bowl with water and submerging the lettuce. This helps to remove any debris and grit. You may need to dunk several times.
- ¼ cup water
- ⅛ teaspoon sea salt
- 1 tablespoon extra virgin olive oil
- ½ to ¾ cup tofu cheese
- Black pepper, optional

Variation using sesame oil
- 1 drop toasted sesame oil
- 3 to 4 drops light sesame oil
- A small pinch sea salt
- ¼ teaspoon shoyu
- 3 drops mirin
- ½ to ¾ cup tofu cheese

Preparation
- Add just enough water to cover the bottom of a stainless steel skillet.
- Over a medium-low flame add the lower white part of the lettuce leaf and begin to sauté for approximately 10 seconds.
- Add the thinner green part of the leaves.

- Drizzle a little oil over the top, then add a little sea salt and fold to blend the seasoning. Place in a serving dish then add 1 to 2 tablespoons of tofu cheese.
- Optional: For a light spicy taste add a smidge of black pepper.

⤝◈⤞

QUICK STEAMED GREENS

Quick steamed greens are a lightly cooked vegetable dish with more settling energetic qualities. Steamed greens should be bright, crunchy, and a little deeper in color than blanched greens. Use only one type of leafy green per serving. Broccoli can be considered a leafy green.

Preparation time: 1 to 2 minutes
2 to 3 leaves serves 1 person

Ingredients
- Choose a leafy green from the "regular use" list, p. 191.
- Squeeze of fresh lemon juice, optional

Preparation
- Wash the vegetables well to remove unwanted debris and dirt.
- Separate the leaves from the stems with a sharp knife.
- Cut the stems on an angle.
- More fibrous stems should be sliced thinly, approximately ⅛ to ¼ inch in width. Juicier stems (such as bok choy or napa cabbage) may be cut thicker, approximately ½ to 1 inch in length.
- Cut the leaves on an angle, approximately 1 to 2 inches in length.
- Place ¾ to 1 inch of water in the bottom of a pot and place the steamer basket over the pot.
- Cover and turn the flame to medium-high.
- When the pot is filled with steam, add the stems to the basket.

- Cover and steam for 20 seconds or longer. The more fibrous the stem, the longer you will need to cook them, up to 1 minute in some cases.
- Add the leaves, cover and continue steaming for another 30 seconds or longer. Again, the texture of the greens varies according to the vegetable type, the growing season, and the environment.
- When done, the greens should still be crunchy, but tender enough to chew easily.
- Remove the greens from the basket and place in a serving dish. Cover with a bamboo mat until serving.
- Optional: For an even lighter, more refreshing effect, add a squeeze of fresh lemon on your greens.

⋯◈⋯

BLANCHED VEGETABLE SALAD

This light and colorful dish is a combination of root, round, and leafy green vegetables. The method of preparation and the combination of the different types of vegetables creates a dynamic energetic effect that helps to activate circulation from deep inside our bodies.

Preparation time: 10 to 15 minutes
Serves 2 to 3

Ingredients
- Choose a minimum of 2 different vegetables, from different categories, or use the combination listed below:
- 4 to 5 leafy greens, thinly sliced 1 inch wide by 2 inches in length
- 1 to 2 cups round vegetables, quartered and sliced thinly
- ½ cup root vegetables, cut into matchsticks ideally not thicker than ½ inch
- A small pinch of sea salt
- Enough water to fill the pot halfway up

- Cookware and utensils
- A stainless steel pot
- A "spider" or mesh vegetable skimmer (to remove vegetables from the water)

Preparation

- Fill a pot halfway with water and bring the water to a boil over a medium flame.
- Add a pinch of sea salt.
- In an open pot, blanch one vegetable at a time, starting with the mildest in taste and lightest in color. When you add the vegetables, the water may stop boiling.
- When the color of the vegetables brightens, remove the vegetable from the pot and place on a plate. Cover with a bamboo mat and drain off any excess water.
- After the water returns to a boil, add the next vegetable and repeat the process.
- Repeat the entire process for all of the vegetables.
- Allow the vegetables to cool, then gently mix in a bowl.
- Cover with a bamboo mat until ready to serve.
- Optional: Sprinkle brown rice vinegar or umeboshi vinegar on your blanched salad.

‹◊›

QUICK SAUTÉED VEGETABLES— RED ONION, BOK CHOY, CARROT

Preparation time: 10 to 15 minutes
Serves 4

Ingredients

- 1 medium onion, sliced into thin half-moons

- 1½ cups root vegetables, cut into thin matchsticks
- 4 to 6 leafy greens leaves, stems and leaves separated and cut ½-inch thick on the angle
- 1 to 2 teaspoons light sesame oil or 1 tablespoon extra virgin olive oil
- ⅛ teaspoon sea salt
- ¼ to ½ cup water
- Several drops shoyu

Note: Sautéed vegetables cook quickly. They should be bright, colorful, and crunchy.

Preparation

- Gently heat the oil in a saucepan, skillet, or other sauté pan.
- Tilt the pan so the oil spreads out evenly and lightly coats the bottom.
- Add the onions, turn up the flame, and begin to sauté.
- Add a little water, a pinch of sea salt, and continue to sauté for 2 minutes.
- Add the leafy green stems and more water if needed to keep the pan moist, continue to sauté.
- Add the leaves, followed by the root vegetables, and continue sautéing.
- When the colors begin to deepen, approximately 1 to 2 minutes, you are ready to season. Make sure you have a little juice in the bottom of the pan. If the pan is dry, add a little more water.
- Add a few drops of shoyu to the juice, then continue sautéing to blend the seasoning.
- Remove the vegetables from the skillet, place in a serving dish, and cover with a bamboo mat until ready to serve.
- Optional: Add a little spice, such as red pepper flakes or ginger juice. Chili pepper may be added after the onions at the beginning of cooking. A squeeze of fresh ginger juice may be added at the very end of cooking.

QUICK SAUTÉED LEAFY GREENS

This is a light preparation style where I begin by slightly steaming the greens, then adding oil and seasoning. The greens are juicy but still retain their crunchy texture.

Preparation time: 7 to 8 minutes
Serves 2 to 4

Ingredients
- ½ to 1 bunch leafy greens, washed and cut into larger pieces (approximately 2 to 3 inches in length and width). Baby greens may be kept whole.
- ⅛ teaspoon sea salt
- 1 tablespoon extra virgin olive oil or several drops of light sesame oil
- If using olive oil, season only with sea salt.
- Season with 5 to 6 drops of shoyu if using sesame oil.

Preparation
- Gently heat just enough water to cover the bottom of the pan.
- Add the stems, cover, and steam for 20 to 30 seconds.
- Add the leaves, cover, and steam for another 10 seconds.
- Drizzle a little oil over the top, then add a little sea salt and fold to blend the seasoning.
- Finish cooking the greens using a sauté method, approximately 20 to 30 more seconds. Place in a serving dish and cover with a bamboo mat.
- Optional: Add fresh garlic, red pepper flakes, or fresh ginger juice.

ASIAN-STYLE MUSTARD GREENS

Preparation time: 5 to 7 minutes
Serves 2 to 3

Ingredients

- ½ bunch washed mustard greens, stems and leaves separated
- 2 or 3 drops toasted sesame oil
- 5 or 6 drops shoyu
- 3 drops mirin
- ¼ cup water

Preparation

- Place a small amount of water in a skillet (enough just to cover the bottom of the pan) and turn on the flame.
- Add the stems, cover, and steam for 30 seconds to 1 minute.
- Remove the lid, add the leaves, cover, and steam for an additional 20 to 30 seconds.
- Remove the lid, and then add 2 to 3 drops of toasted sesame oil, 5 drops of shoyu, and 2 to 3 drops of mirin.
- Mix all ingredients together in the pan, using a wooden spatula or chopsticks.
- Place in a serving dish and cover with a bamboo mat.

Variations

- Use spicy toasted sesame oil, cayenne pepper, or shichimi.
- Use watercress, baby kale, or dandelion in place of mustard greens.

SALADS

Raw salads refresh and relax our condition. There are many varieties of lettuces and leafy greens that taste great in salads. Even though it is not usually thought of as a "healthy" choice, I love using iceberg lettuce because it is so refreshing, due to its high water content. You can also mix and match the greens you use in your salads.

SIMPLE ICEBERG SALAD

Preparation time: 10 minutes
Serve 2 to 4

Ingredients
- ½ head iceberg lettuce
- 1 medium cucumber, cut into ½-inch-thick (or thinner) slices
- Optional: Carrots, grated or cut into feathery thin matchsticks
- 1 to 2 red radishes, sliced into thin half-rounds
- Tofu cheese: ⅓ block tofu, crumbled and seasoned with ⅛ cup umeboshi vinegar

Preparation
- Remove the outer leaves and center core of the lettuce.
- Break open the head of lettuce and wash.
- Drain off the excess water. Use a salad spinner or clean cotton dish towels to absorb the excess moisture.
- Break the lettuce up into a bowl.

- Add any additional vegetables you desire and/or tofu cheese.
- Toss together and serve with your favorite dressing.

Dressings:
- A few drops of umeboshi vinegar
- A few drops of brown rice vinegar
- A squeeze of fresh lemon or tangerine
- A few drops of balsamic or red wine vinegar

⊰◈⊱

ARUGULA SALAD

Preparation time: 10 minutes
Serves 2 to 4

Ingredients
- 5 ounces arugula, washed
- Tofu cheese: ⅓ block tofu, crumbled and seasoned with ⅛ cup umeboshi vinegar
- ⅓ cup lightly toasted pine nuts
- ½ to 1 tablespoon olive oil
- Pinch sea salt, about ¹⁄₁₆ teaspoon
- Fresh-squeezed lemon juice to taste
- Fresh-cracked black pepper, if desired

Preparation
- Place arugula in a bowl and add a drizzle of olive oil and a tiny pinch of sea salt, then toss to blend.
- Add the tofu cheese and lemon, and toss to blend.
- Place in a serving dish, and garnish with toasted pine nuts.

Variations
- Add some thin slices of fresh pear or apple.
- Add thin slices of cooked beets.

ARUGULA SALAD WITH SAUTÉED MUSHROOMS

Preparation time: 10 minutes
Serves 4

Ingredients

- 5 ounces arugula, washed
- ½ to 1 lb. fresh mushrooms, such as oyster, beech, or maitake
- ½ red onion, sliced into half-moons
- Tofu cheese: ⅓ block tofu, crumbled and seasoned with ⅛ cup umeboshi vinegar
- Olive oil
- Pinch sea salt, about ¹⁄₁₆ teaspoon
- ¼ teaspoon shoyu
- 3 or 4 drops mirin

Preparation

- Place the washed arugula in a bowl, and add the tofu cheese on top of the arugula.

Mushrooms

- Heat 1 to 2 tablespoons of olive oil in a pan.
- Add the red onion and begin to sauté.
- Add a little water, a pinch of sea salt, and 2 or 3 drops of umeboshi vinegar.
- Add the beech mushrooms, cover the pot, and simmer for 1 minute.
- Add the oyster mushrooms and continue to sauté.
- Add the maitake mushrooms and lightly season with the shoyu and mirin.
- Sauté for another minute to cook the mushrooms and blend the seasonings together.

- Pour the sautéed mushrooms over the arugula and tofu cheese.
- Lightly toss all ingredients together and serve.

⊰◈⊱

VEGAN AVOCADO CAESAR SALAD WITH TEMPEH CROUTONS

Preparation time: 30 to 40 minutes, including the time to cook the tempeh
Serves 4 to 6

Ingredients
- 1 head romaine hearts, washed
- 1 package of tempeh, cooked and cut into 1-inch cubes (see tempeh recipe in the bean section)
- 1 small red onion, cut into ⅛-inch-thick half-moons
- Guacamole or avocado slices (½ to 1 avocado)

Preparation
- Slice the red onion and place in a bowl. Add ¹⁄₁₆ teaspoon of sea salt and 2 or 3 drops of umeboshi vinegar. Use your fingers to gently rub the salt and vinegar into the onion until the color deepens. Set aside until you are ready to assemble your salad.
- Wash the romaine and remove any excess water using a salad spinner or cotton towel.
- Break the lettuce into a bowl.
- Add the red onion and the tempeh and lightly toss with your hands or wooden utensils.
- Add a little freshly made guacamole, toss to coat the lettuce. If you do not have time to make guacamole, add some fresh avocado slices.
- Drizzle a little umeboshi vinegar over the entire salad, then toss to blend the ingredients.

SUSAN'S GUACAMOLE

Preparation time: 15 to 20 minutes
Serves 2 to 4

Ingredients
- 1 avocado
- ½ cup finely diced onions
- Freshly sliced jalapeño pepper, center vein and seeds removed (optional)
- ¼ cup finely chopped cilantro
- Fresh lime juice, to taste
- 1½ to 1¾ teaspoons umeboshi vinegar

Preparation
- Dice the onion and place in a Pyrex bowl. Add ¹⁄₁₆ teaspoon sea salt to the onion and gently mix. Add ½ teaspoon umeboshi vinegar to the onions, mix all ingredients together with your hands, and set aside while you prepare the other ingredients.
- Cut the avocado in half and remove the pit and the rind.
- Place avocado in a bowl together with the marinated onions and the liquid from the onions. Add the cilantro and the jalapeño, if using, and the remaining ¾ to 1 teaspoon umeboshi vinegar to taste. Add the lime juice and gently mix.

This recipe keeps longer than other guacamole recipes because of the umeboshi vinegar. The pickled onions balance the rich vegetable fat of the avocado. You can store the guacamole in a glass or earthenware bowl together with the pit (to maintain freshness). Remove the pit before serving. Serve with good-quality corn chips (made with non-GMO, organic corn and sea salt), lightly blanched or raw carrots or celery sticks, or top off a vegan rice and bean burrito.

BABY ARUGULA GOLDEN BEET AND PEAR SALAD

This easy to prepare salad gives you a gourmet feel using simple ingredients.

Preparation time: 15 minutes
Serves 4

Ingredients
- 5 ounces baby arugula, washed and spun to remove excess water
- 1 medium-size golden beet, peeled, precooked and sliced in ⅛-inch quarter rounds.
- 1 ripened pear sliced length wise, ⅛ inch thick to match the beet. Keep the sliced pear in water with a small pinch of salt to prevent oxidizing.
- ¼ cup tofu cheese
- ¼ cup lightly toasted pine nuts or raw walnuts
- 1 to 2 teaspoons extra virgin olive oil
- ¹⁄₁₆ teaspoon sea salt
- Fresh-squeezed lemon to taste, about ⅓ wedge
- Optional: For a richer and sweeter taste use aged balsamic vinegar in place of lemon.

Preparation
- Place the arugula in a prep bowl, drizzle a small amount of olive oil over the arugula and add a small pinch of sea salt.
- Gently toss the greens using wooden salad utensils to mix the oil and salt evenly.
- Add ¼ to ½ cup of tofu cheese and toss all ingredients together.
- Squeeze fresh lemon juice over the greens and toss again.
- Place the arugula on a serving plate and arrange the beets and pears around the plate in a decorative fashion.
- Garnish the salad with the toasted pine nuts or walnuts.

BEET SALAD

Preparation time: 35 to 40 minutes

Serves 4 to 6

Ingredients

- 4 to 5 medium-size beets, peeled and cut into ½-inch wedges
- 1 cup red onions; sliced into thin half-moons
- Fresh mint
- 2 to 3 teaspoons extra virgin olive oil
- ¼ teaspoon sea salt
- 1 teaspoon umeboshi vinegar
- Fresh-squeezed lemon, ⅓ wedge
- ½ cup tofu cheese
- ⅓ to ½ cup of walnuts
- ¼ to ½ cup water

Preparation

- Place the sliced onions in a small prep bowl.
- Add 2 to 3 drops umeboshi vinegar and a few granules of sea salt.
- Using your fingers, gently massage the onions until they begin to glisten.
- Set the onion to the side and cover with a bamboo mat.

Cooking Beets

Preparation time: 15 to 30 minutes

- Place the beets in a deeper skillet with about an inch of water to cover the bottom of the pan.
- Turn on the flame and bring the water to a boil.
- Add a pinch of sea salt and 3 to 5 drops of umeboshi vinegar.
- Place a lid on the pot, lower the flame, and simmer for 10 minutes.

- Remove the lid, drizzle a teaspoon of olive oil over the beets, then add ⅛ to ¼ teaspoon of sea salt.
- Cover and continue to cook the beets for another 10 to 15 minutes or until the beet reaches the texture you desire. The total cooking time will depend on how firm you like your beets.
- Remove the cooked beets from the skillet and allow them to cool. It is fine to refrigerate them until you are ready to make your salad.
- Place the beets in a prep bowl together with the red onions.
- Drizzle a little olive oil over top followed by a dash of umeboshi vinegar.
- Add a little fresh-squeezed lemon to taste and toss before plating.
- Place the beets and onions in a serving dish.
- Garnish with a little tofu cheese, raw walnuts, and fresh mint.

❖

BIBB LETTUCE WITH SUN-DRIED TOMATOES AND SAUTÉED ONIONS

Bibb lettuce is the perfect combination of tenderness to crunch. For a beautiful presentation I recommend removing the outer leaves, using the inner leaves and leaving them whole. Keep the outer leaves, as they are the perfect size to use on a sandwich.

Preparation time: 7 to 10 minutes
Serves 2 to 4

Ingredients
- 1 head Bibb lettuce, washed and spun
- ½ cup red onions sliced into ¼ inch half-moons
- 3 to 5 sun-dried tomatoes, sliced thin. Choose sun-dried tomatoes that do not have to be reconstituted, pick the softer ones.

- ⅛ cup water
- ⅛ teaspoon sea salt
- 1 to 2 tablespoons extra virgin olive oil
- ½ to ¾ cup tofu cheese
- 1 to 2 tablespoons aged balsamic vinegar
- Optional: A crack of fresh black pepper

Preparation

- Place the lettuce in a prep bowl.
- Add the sliced tomatoes.
- Gently heat 1 tablespoon olive oil in a skillet.
- Add the red onions, a pinch of sea salt and begin to sauté.
- Add a splash of water and continue to sauté for another 1 to 2 minutes.
- Turn off the flame then add the onions to the salad.
- Add the tofu cheese.
- Drizzle additional oil over the top and a few granules of sea salt.
- Using wooden utensils gently toss to blend the ingredients.
- Place in a serving dish then dress with aged balsamic vinegar.
- Optional: For a light spicy taste add a smidge of black pepper.

⊰◈⊱

CABBAGE SLAW

Preparation time: 30 minutes
Serves 2 to 3

Ingredients

- 1 cup finely sliced green cabbage
- ½ cup finely cut carrot matchsticks
- 1/16 to ⅛ teaspoon sea salt
- ⅛ teaspoon umeboshi vinegar

- 1 tablespoon fresh lime juice
- Chopped cilantro and hot sauce, optional

Preparation

- Cut cabbage and the carrots into fine strips and place in a prep bowl.
- Add a small pinch of sea salt.
- Use your hand to gently mix the sea salt with the vegetables.
- The vegetables will begin to give off a little liquid.
- Add a little umeboshi vinegar.
- Move all of the vegetables into the center of a bowl.
- Place a plate on the vegetables and a very light weight on top of the plate.
- Lightly press the vegetables while you are preparing the other ingredients. (About ½ hour, give or take a few minutes!)
- Remove the plate and the weight.
- Pour off any excess liquid, squeeze a little fresh lime on the veg.

⋯◈⋯

MIXED ARUGULA AND BITTER LEAF SALAD

Preparation time: 15 minutes
Serves 4

Ingredients

- 3 ounces baby arugula; washed and spun to remove excess water
- 2 ounces Belgian endive, washed
- 1 ounce radicchio
- ¼ cup tofu cheese
- 1 to 2 teaspoons extra virgin olive oil

- $\frac{1}{16}$ teaspoon sea salt
- Fresh-squeezed lemon to taste, about $\frac{1}{3}$ wedge
- $\frac{1}{8}$ cup toasted pine nuts or walnuts
- Optional: For a richer and sweeter taste use aged balsamic vinegar in place of lemon.

Preparation

- Place the vegetables in a prep bowl, drizzle a small amount of olive oil over top.
- Add a small pinch of sea salt and gently toss using wooden utensils.
- Add $\frac{1}{4}$ to $\frac{1}{2}$ cup of tofu cheese and the rest of the olive oil.
- Squeeze fresh lemon juice over the greens and toss again.
- Place on a serving plate.
- For a rich addition, garnish the salad with the toasted pine nuts or walnuts.

MUSHROOM FENNEL AND BABY ARUGULA

Preparation time: 15 to 20 minutes
Serves 4

Ingredients

- 2 cups of button mushrooms, cleaned and cut into $\frac{1}{4}$-inch slices
- 5 ounces of baby arugula, washed and spun to remove excess water
- 2 cups of fennel, sliced thin
- 2 to 3 teaspoons organic extra virgin olive oil
- $\frac{1}{8}$ teaspoon sea salt

- Fresh-squeezed lemon to taste
- Fresh cracked black pepper, optional

Preparation

- Wash and spin the arugula and place in a large prep bowl.
- Wash and slice the fennel, then place in a separate prep bowl.
- Add a small pinch of sea salt, about $\frac{1}{16}$ teaspoon, and gently begin to massage the fennel for 2 to 3 minutes or until it begins to glisten, then set aside.
- Clean the mushrooms, then cut the stem just below the cap.
- Slice the mushrooms and place in the bowl with the fennel.
- Add 1 drop of olive oil and another pinch of sea salt, then very gently begin to mix the ingredients to blend together. You may want to use wooden spoons to prevent oxidation.
- Add the fennel and mushrooms to the arugula and lightly toss to mix the vegetables.
- Add a drizzle of olive oil and another pinch of sea salt.
- Add a squeeze of fresh lemon juice and a crack of black pepper to taste.

SANDWICHES

Cookware for all sandwiches includes a pot with a steamer basket, preferably the type that sits on top of the pot. After steaming you can keep the bread moist by placing it between bamboo mats. Before assembling sandwiches allow the bread to cool slightly.

Sandwiches are great for packed lunches. Simply wrap the sandwich in parchment paper or purchase little parchment-type sandwich bags. Then place the sandwich in a plastic container to keep it moist and prevent it from smushing. Your sandwich will keep fresh overnight which makes it great travel food. A helpful hint when making food to go is not to overdo the moist spreads and ingredients that can make the bread soggy. I recommend packing any pickles in a separate container.

BURRITOS

Preparation time: 20 to 30 minutes
Serves 4

Ingredients
- 4 cups refried beans (see recipe p. 292)
- 5 to 6 cups shredded lettuce
- Pico de gallo
- Guacamole (see recipe p. 338)
- Hot sauce
- Large flour tortillas
- 1 jalapeño pepper sliced, seeds and capsicum removed

- 1 cup white rice cooked using half water and half tomato juice, optional

Preparation

- Prepare your refried beans following the recipe in the bean section.
- Cut the jalapeño in half lengthwise, then remove the seeds and the vein.
- Use a steamer basket to warm the tortillas, then place them in a bamboo mat and cover with a towel to keep warm.
- Take a tortilla and spread a layer of beans.
- Add the rice, if using.
- Add the lettuce, the pico de gallo, and the guacamole.
- Fold the tortilla over the beans and vegetables.
- Fold the sides into the center then roll the shell to form a tight wrap.

⋘◆⋙

PICO DE GALLO

Preparation time: 10 minutes
Serves 4

Ingredients

- 2 cups fresh diced plum tomatoes, seeds removed. Heirloom tomatoes will make a more delicious sauce, especially if they are the sweeter variety.
- ½ cup chopped onions, diced to match the tomato
- ⅓ to ½ cup chopped cilantro
- ¼ to ½ teaspoon sea salt
- Lime juice to taste, ½ small lime
- ⅛ teaspoon umeboshi vinegar
- Optional: chopped serrano or jalapeño peppers, vein and seeds removed

Preparation

- Place the diced onion in a bowl. Add a pinch of sea salt and umeboshi vinegar. Gently massage the onion until it begins to glisten.
- Set it to the side while you are preparing the other ingredients.
- Remove the top of the tomato, then cut in quarters and remove the seeds.
- Add a pinch of sea salt and use a wooden utensil to blend with the tomatoes.
- If you are using peppers, prepare by removing the seeds and finely chopping.
- Remove the leaves from the sprigs of cilantro and chop coarsely.
- Place all vegetables in a prep bowl together with the cilantro.
- Add the remaining sea salt and toss together to blend the ingredients.
- Add a little fresh-squeezed lime juice and toss.

❖

HUMMUS SANDWICH

Preparation time: 10 minutes
Serves 1

Ingredients

- Steamed un-yeasted sourdough bread or pita
- Lettuce, washed and dried
- 3 to 5 slices seasoned red onion, cut into thin half-moons
- 2 to 3 drops umeboshi vinegar
- Sea salt, a few granules, less than $\frac{1}{16}$ teaspoon
- 3 to 5 slices cucumber
- 1 teaspoon tahini

Preparation

- Place the red onion in a prep bowl. Add a few granules of sea salt and 2 to 3 drops of umeboshi vinegar. Use your fingers to gently mix the seasoning with the red onion, then set to the side.
- Slice the cucumber. I recommend thinner slices.
- Steam the bread until it gives off a freshly baked aroma.
- Place a bamboo mat on a plate.
- Remove the bread from the basket.
- Place the bread on the mat, cover with a second mat and allow the bread to cool a few minutes.
- Use a thin spread of tahini on each slice of bread.
- Use a generous spread of hummus on the bottom half.
- Place the cucumber slices evenly on top of the hummus.
- Strain any liquid and place the red onion evenly on top of the cucumber.
- Cover with lettuce add the top slice of bread.
- For a gooier sandwich add a thin spread of humus to the top slice of bread.
- If packing your sandwich to go, I recommend keeping it whole. If eating at home feel free to cut it in half.

SIMPLE TOFU SANDWICH

This is a great travel sandwich and keeps fresh when wrapped in parchment paper and stored in an airtight baggie. If you are taking it to go, use a little less pickle, or keep your pickled vegetable in a separate container, and add it before eating.

Preparation time: 10 minutes
Serves 1

Ingredients

- Steamed un-yeasted sourdough bread
- Lettuce, washed and dried
- 3 to 5 slices cucumber, sliced thin
- 1 to 2 tablespoons sauerkraut, kimchi, or sliced dill pickle
- Tahini, about 1 to 2 tablespoons
- 2 to 3 teaspoons prepared mustard of your choice
- Marinated or steamed tofu
- Hummus, optional

Preparation

- Prepare the tofu according to my recipe (see p. 300).
- Slice the cucumber.
- Steam the bread until it gives off a freshly baked aroma.
- Place a bamboo mat on a plate.
- Place the bread on the mat, cover with a second mat and allow the bread to cool a few minutes.
- Use a thin spread of tahini on each slice of bread, followed by the mustard.
- Place the cucumber slices across the bottom slice of bread.
- Drain excess liquid from the pickle and add on top of the cucumber.
- Add the tofu. If you like, add a thin spread of mustard on the tofu.
- Cover with lettuce, then add the top slice of bread.
- For a richer sandwich add a thin spread of humus to the top slice of bread.
- If packing your sandwich to go I recommend keeping it whole. If eating at home feel free to cut it in half.

SUSAN'S VEGAN MAYO

Preparation time: 10 minutes
Makes 2 cups

Ingredients
- ½ cup juice from cooked chickpeas.
- 1 to 2 tablespoons cooked chickpeas, optional
- 2 teaspoons lemon juice
- 2 teaspoons apple cider vinegar
- 2 teaspoons Dijon mustard
- 4 teaspoons umeboshi vinegar
- 2 teaspoons brown rice syrup
- ¼ teaspoon caper juice
- ¼ teaspoon sea salt
- ¼ teaspoon dry mustard
- Optional: ⅛ teaspoon wasabi powder or black pepper
- 1½ cups olive oil

Preparation
- Pour all the wet ingredients except the olive oil into a larger glass jar.
- Add the dry ingredients.
- Slowly begin to add the olive oil while blending.
- As you continue to pour, the ingredients will begin to emulsify creating a creamy texture.
- If you like a thicker style mayo, simply add a few chickpeas while blending.

TEMPEH BACON AVOCADO CLUB

Preparation time: 20 minutes
Serves 2

Ingredients

- 4 slices of steamed un-yeasted sourdough bread
- Precooked tempeh using the boiling method (see p. 304)
- ⅛ teaspoon smoked paprika
- ⅛ teaspoon harissa
- ½ teaspoon prepared mustard
- ¼ teaspoon toasted sesame oil
- 2 to 3 tablespoons safflower or sunflower oil for frying
- ½ teaspoon shoyu
- ⅛ teaspoon mirin
- Cabbage slaw, prepared in advance (see p. 342)
- Guacamole, prepared in advance (see p. 338) or Susan's Vegan Mayo (see p. 351) with chopped basil added
- Lettuce and tomato are optional

Preparation

- Place all dry ingredients in a small prep bowl.
- Add the mustard, shoyu, and mirin, then mix to blend well.
- Cut tempeh lengthwise into strips about ⅛- to ¼-inch thick.
- Place about a ⅛ to ¼ inch of safflower oil in a cast-iron frying pan.
- Turn on the flame and begin to heat the oil.
- Fry on one side until the tempeh is golden brown.
- Flip the tempeh, add a spread of the seasoning, while the opposite side is frying.
- Place the fried tempeh on a paper towel to drain off any excess oil.
- Steam the bread until it has a freshly baked aroma.
- Place on a bamboo mat and allow to cool for 2 to 3 minutes.
- Spread guacamole on each slice of the bread.

- Place the tempeh bacon on top, followed by the cabbage slaw.
- Add lettuce and/or tomato.
- Add the top slice of bread.

❖

TEMPEH REUBEN

Preparation time: 5 to 7 minutes
Vegetables make 2 to 3 sandwiches

Ingredients
- 2 to 3 squares of precooked tempeh
- 1 cup sliced cremni mushrooms
- 1 cup onions cut into ¼-inch half-moons
- ½ cup sauerkraut
- ½ teaspoon sesame oil or 1½ tablespoon olive oil
- ½ cup water
- ¹⁄₁₆ to ⅛ teaspoon sea salt
- Whole-wheat or multigrain buns, steamed
- Tomato mayo relish
- Lettuce and pickles, optional

Tomato Mayo Relish Preparation
- Place 2 to 4 tablespoons of Susan's Vegan Mayo (see p. 351) in a prep bowl.
- Add 1 to 1½ teaspoons tomato paste.
- Use a wooden utensil or fork to blend.
- Add ½ teaspoon finely chopped dill pickles.
- Mix well and you are ready to use on your sandwich.

Preparation
- Steam the bun on low heat until it gives off a fresh baked aroma.

- Remove the bun from the steaming basket and wrap it in a bamboo mat to keep it moist. Cut the tempeh in half so you have two ⅛-inch-thick squares.
- Heat a little oil in a skillet, add the tempeh, and cook on each side for 2 to 3 minutes.
- Remove from the pan and place on a plate.
- Add a little more oil to the skillet.
- Add the onions and begin to sauté.
- Add a little water, and when the onions begin to change color add a pinch of sea salt.
- Add the mushrooms and continue to sauté for 3 to 5 more minutes.
- Add the sauerkraut and sauté for another 2 minutes.
- Turn off the flame.
- Spread the relish on each side of the bun. I say be generous!
- Place one half of the tempeh on the bottom part of the bun.
- Spread a little more sauce on the tempeh.
- Add the vegetables.
- Place the other half of the tempeh on top of the vegetables.
- Add the pickles, then the lettuce.
- Add the top of the bun and serve warm.

⊸◈⊶

TOFU BANH MI

Preparation time: 15 to 20 minutes
Serves 2 to 3

Ingredients
- 6 thicker cut slices steamed un-yeasted sourdough bread
- 12 leaves lettuce washed and dried
- ¼ to ⅓ cup kimchi
- 5 cucumber slices per sandwich

- ½ block tofu, pan-fried
- ½ teaspoon yellow mustard or ⅛ teaspoon dry mustard
- ¼ to ½ teaspoon harissa
- 1 teaspoon shoyu
- ½ teaspoon mirin
- 2 teaspoons umeboshi vinegar
- ⅛ teaspoon toasted sesame oil
- 2 to 4 tablespoons extra virgin olive oil
- ¼ to ⅓ cup water for steaming bread
- "Curried Mayo"; 6 to 8 tablespoons of Susan's Vegan Mayo (see p. 351) seasoned with ⅛ teaspoon curry powder or make your own curry using ⅛ teaspoon cumin, ¹⁄₁₆ teaspoon yellow mustard, and ¹⁄₁₆ teaspoon harissa.

PAN-FRIED TOFU

Preparation time: 5 to 7 minutes

- Rinse the tofu and cut into ½-inch-thick slices.
- Press the tofu slices between a clean cloth to remove excess water.
- Add the toasted sesame oil then the olive oil to a pan and gently heat.
- Add the tofu and begin to fry on one side.
- Measure the liquid ingredients and reserve in a prep bowl.
- Add half of the harissa to the liquid, then add the mustard and mix.
- Spread a little of the seasoning mix on the tofu, then turn the tofu over to lightly fry.
- Spread additional seasoning on the fried side.
- Allow the tofu to fry for 3 minutes then turn it over and add more of the sauce mixture.

- Remove the tofu from the pan and allow to cool a bit before assembling your sandwich.
- Spread a little curried mayo on each slice of bread. My advice is to be generous.
- Place sliced cucumbers on one half of the bread.
- Next add the kimchi.
- Layer the fried tofu on top of the kimchi.
- Add the lettuce and the other slice of bread.

PICKLES

Pickles are an important part of creating healthy digestion. Ideally you should try to include a small 1- or 2-tablespoon serving of pickles almost daily. Because pickles are salty, it is important to stick to just one small serving. We recommend having pickles with meals about five times per week.

You can purchase naturally fermented pickles at the local health-food shop or at the farmers' market. When shopping for pickles, such as sauerkraut, look for organic ingredients and sea salt. There should be no preservatives listed on the label.

You can also try making your own pickles at home. It's quite easy, and you can control what vegetables and how much salt go into your homemade pickles. Homemade pickles are also delicious!

QUICK UMEBOSHI VINEGAR PICKLES

Preparation time: 15 minutes; minimum fermentation time: 3 hours
Serving size is approximately 2 tablespoons

Ingredients
- Choose one vegetable or a combination of vegetables. Here are some of my favorites:
- Daikon radishes or red radishes, sliced into half-rounds on the angle
- Cauliflower florets
- Turnips, sliced into thin half-rounds
- Red onions, sliced into ¼- to ½-inch-thick half-moons

- Lotus root, cut into half-rounds
- Red or green cabbage, cut into 1-inch squares or thin slices
- 3 to 3½ parts water per 1 part vegetable
- 1 part umeboshi vinegar per 1 part vegetable

Preparation

- Cut the vegetables and place them in a deep Pyrex bowl.
- Use a liquid measuring cup to measure the liquid ingredients.
- Pour enough liquid to cover the vegetables. Place the small bowl or dish over the vegetables to keep them submerged under the brine.
- Cover the bowl with a bamboo mat or cheesecloth and place in a cool, dark area to ferment.
- The thicker-cut vegetables and the heartier vegetables (such as the turnips) will need to be fermented longer than thinly sliced or softer vegetables. I usually let my pickles ferment overnight.
- Umeboshi pickles will keep in the fridge for up to one week.

⊸◈⊶

QUICK CUCUMBER PICKLES

Preparation time: 10 minutes; fermentation time: 3 hours
Serving size is approximately 1 to 2 tablespoons

Ingredients

- 1 to 2 cucumbers, washed, cut in half lengthwise, seeds removed
- 1 part umeboshi vinegar
- 4 parts water

Preparation

- Slice the cucumber on the angle in ½-inch- to 1-inch-thick slices.

- Place the cucumber slices in a bowl.
- Use a liquid measuring cup to measure the liquid ingredients and pour liquid over the cucumbers to cover.
- Cover the bowl with a bamboo mat or cheesecloth and place in a cool, dark area to ferment for 3 hours.
- Use within 24 hours so that the pickles stay crispy and fresh.

⊲◈⊳

QUICK PRESSED CUCUMBER AND RED ONION FOR SALADS

Preparation time: 30 minutes
Makes enough for a large salad

Ingredients
- ½ cucumber, seeds removed and sliced thinly on the angle
- ½ red onion, sliced into ¼-inch-thick half-moons
- ¹⁄₁₆ teaspoon sea salt
- ¼ teaspoon umeboshi vinegar

Preparation
- Place the sliced onion in a prep bowl.
- Add a small pinch of sea salt and use your hands to mix the salt with the onion. Massage the onion for 2 minutes.
- Add the cucumber to the bowl, then continue to massage the vegetables for another 2 to 3 minutes.
- Add the umeboshi vinegar, then use your hands to gently blend the seasonings.
- Cover with a bamboo mat and allow the vegetables to sit while you assemble the rest of your salad.
- Add the pressed vegetables to your favorite salad base and enjoy.

DESSERTS

APPLE GRAPE KANTEN DESSERT

Fresh fruit kanten is a clean, refreshing dessert that is the perfect ending to a big meal.

Preparation time: 20 minutes to make, and approximately 1 hour to set

Serves 3 to 4

Ingredients
- 2 cups apple juice
- 1 to 2 cups spring or filtered water
- 1 tablespoon agar-agar (also called kanten flakes) per cup of liquid. For three cups of total liquid (apple juice and water), use 3 tablespoons agar-agar.
- 1½ to 2 cups fresh grapes, cut in half and seeds removed

Preparation
- Place the apple juice and water in a pot.
- Add the agar-agar and bring to a slight boil on a medium flame.
- Lower flame and simmer until the kanten dissolves.
- Place the grapes in the serving dish of choice. Use either a large serving dish or individual ramekins. Pour the hot liquid over the fruit and allow the kanten to set, either at room temperature or in the refrigerator.

Variations

- Try using different fruit juices such as grape, white grape, peach, berry, and pear juice. Use different fruit combinations. I like fresh tangerines or cherries.

Serving Suggestions

- Make your kanten look extra-special by using champagne flutes or crystal and garnishing with fresh mint leaves. You can also top your kanten with almond crème or make a fruit mousse, by blending a little of the kanten with amasake.

POACHED PEARS

Preparation time: 15 minutes
Serves 2 to 4

Ingredients

- 2 pears, washed, cored, and quartered
- Water
- 1/16 teaspoon sea salt
- 1 to 2 tablespoons barley malt
- lemon wedge or balsamic vinegar

Preparation

- Place a small amount of water in a deep sauté pan, just enough to cover the bottom.
- Place pears in the pan and add a tiny pinch of sea salt, cover, and bring to a boil on a medium flame.
- Lower the flame and steam for 5 minutes, then drizzle 1 tablespoon of barley malt over top. Note that the cooking time will vary according to the ripeness, variety, and texture

of the pear. The pear should still be slightly crunchy when you add the barley malt.

- Replace the cover and give the pot a gentle shake to mix the sweetener with the cooking liquid.
- Cook pears until they reach the desired texture.
- Squeeze a little fresh lemon or add a little aged balsamic vinegar over top of the pears and gently fold to blend the flavors.
- When the pears reach a desired texture, place in a serving dish. Continue heating the remaining sweet mixture to allow it to reduce, then pour over the plated pears.
- Place in a serving dish.

⊰◇⊱

APPLE SAUCE

Recipe by Barbara Schwalm

Preparation time: 30 minutes
Serves 10

Ingredients

- 3 Granny Smith apples
- 3 Winesap apples
- 3 Rome apples
- 3 McIntosh apples
- 3 Red Delicious apples
- $\frac{1}{16}$ to $\frac{1}{8}$ teaspoon sea salt
- 1 to 2 tablespoons olive oil
- $\frac{1}{2}$ to $\frac{3}{4}$ cup apple juice or cider
- Cinnamon, optional

Preparation

- Wash, core, and quarter the apples, then place them in a bowl with a pinch of salt to prevent oxidation.

- Place apples in a stock pot with liquid to cover the bottom of the pot by 2 to 3 inches.
- Add a small pinch of sea salt.
- Cover and bring to a boil, lower the flame, and simmer until the apples are soft. The cooking time will vary according to the firmness of the apples. Cook about 10 minutes, then check the texture.
- When the apples are soft pour into a hand food mill or food processor. For a chunkier style sauce use a potato masher.
- Add a little olive oil and another pinch of sea salt.

❖

STEAMED SEASONAL FRUITS WITH SWEET KUZU SAUCE

Seasonal fruit is the fruit that is obtained locally within a season.

Preparation time: 15 minutes
1 piece of fruit yields 1 to 2 servings

Ingredients
- Fresh peaches, apples, or pears, washed, cored, and cut into quarters, 2 to 3 pieces of fruit
- 1 to 2 tablespoons rice syrup
- A pinch of sea salt, about 1/16 teaspoon
- 1 slightly rounded teaspoon kuzu per 1 cup liquid
- 1/2 to 1 teaspoon fresh lemon juice
- Water

Preparation
- Fill a deep, wide skillet with about 1/2 inch to 1 inch of water. Use more water for harder fruits such as apples or pears and

less water for softer fruits like peaches. Place fruit in the pot, cut side down.

- Add a tiny pinch of sea salt, turn on the flame to a medium setting, and cover.
- Bring the water to a boil, then lower the flame and gently steam the fruit to the desired texture. The type of fruit you use and the firmness you desire will determine the cooking time. You want the fruit to be tender enough to cut it easily with a spoon but not mushy. Harder fruits take approximately 2 to 5 minutes or longer to cook. Softer fruits may take only 2 to 3 minutes to cook. Check the texture while the fruit is cooking.
- When the fruit is almost tender, add the rice syrup and cook uncovered for another minute.
- Turn off the flame, remove the fruit from the pan, and place it in a serving dish.
- Leave the juice in the pan to make the sauce.
- Measure the kuzu in a separate Pyrex bowl.
- Add ¼ to ⅓ cup water and dissolve the kuzu, using your fingers to break up any clumps.
- Turn the flame on low and add the dissolved kuzu to the juice in the pan while stirring constantly.
- Continue to stir until the liquid comes to a boil and thickens. Turn off the flame and allow the sauce to sit for a minute.
- Drizzle sauce over the fruits and garnish with fresh mint sprig or shiso leaves, lightly toasted walnuts, or pecans.

SAUTÉED APPLES

Recipe by my father, Jared Schwalm

Makes a great topping for pancakes or simply to eat as a dessert.

Preparation time: 15 minutes
Serves 4

Ingredients
- 3 hard, crisp apples: feel free to use a combination which may include Granny Smith if you like a sweet and tart taste.
- 1 tablespoon extra virgin olive oil
- ¼ to ⅓ cup apple cider
- 1 tablespoon vanilla
- 1 teaspoon cinnamon
- ¼ teaspoon nutmeg
- 1 teaspoon kuzu or 1 to 2 tablespoon other flour
- 1/16 teaspoon sea salt

Preparation
- Wash and peel apples, cut into ¼-inch-thick slices. Place cut apples in a bowl of water with a pinch of salt to prevent oxidation.
- Gently heat the oil in a pan.
- Add the apples and a pinch of sea salt, then gently fold to coat with oil.
- Add a splash of apple cider. Turn gently to keep the apples intact.
- Cover and let simmer for 2 to 3 minutes.
- Add the rest of the cider and the seasonings to the liquid.
- Turn to blend all the ingredients.
- In a small Pyrex bowl, dissolve kuzu in 1 to 2 tablespoons apple cider.

- Add the kuzu to the apples and continue to fold. As the liquid comes to a gentle boil the juice will thicken. If you like a thicker sauce use less cider.

Variation
- Use pears in place of apples or mix apples with pears.

⊸◈⊷

ALMOND CRÈME

Sweet, delicious, and rich, almond crème is great with fresh fruit. You can make fancy fruit cocktails or simply serve it as a dip. Either way this is a winner. Almond crème also makes a delicious cake frosting.

Preparation time: 15 minutes
Makes 1½ to 2 cups

Ingredients
- 1 cup raw almonds
- ½ cup amazake, a fermented rice beverage, and ¼ cup rice syrup OR ½ cup brown rice syrup and ¼ to ⅓ cup almond, soy, or rice milk

Preparation
- Blanch the almonds 5 to 7 minutes and remove the skins.
- Place the almonds, rice syrup, and half the amount of liquid ingredients in a blender or food processor. Begin to blend, while adding additional liquid. Feel free to adjust the liquid ratio to achieve the desired consistency.
- This recipe makes 1½ to 2 cups of crème and will keep in the refrigerator for at least 5 days.

PANNA COTTA WITH FRESH FRUIT SAUCE

Preparation time: 1½ hours
Serves 4 to 5

Ingredients

- 2 cups amasake
- 1 cup organic non-GMO soy milk or almond milk
- 2 teaspoons agar-agar flakes (also called kanten flakes)
- 1 to 3 teaspoons maple syrup or 1 tablespoon rice syrup
- ½ teaspoon vanilla extract

Preparation

- Pour liquid ingredients into a pot and gently begin to heat on a low flame.
- Add the kanten flakes and bring the liquid to a very gentle boil.
- Lower the flame and simmer until all of the agar-agar is completely dissolved.
- Turn off the flame.
- Add the maple syrup and stir with a wooden spoon to mix well.
- Add the vanilla and stir.
- Pour the liquid into a bowl or mold and allow it to cool.
- When your dessert sets, gently remove it from the mold and place it on a serving dish together with the sauce.

FRESH FRUIT SAUCE

Ingredients
- Apple or grape juice to cover the bottom of the pan, about ⅛ cup
- 1 cup fresh berries
- Maple syrup or rice syrup, to taste

Preparation
- Add the apple or grape juice to a saucepan with some fresh berries and a few grains of sea salt. Turn on the flame and simmer on low. The liquid will begin to reduce and thicken into a sauce as the berries begin to cook. When the sauce reaches the desired consistency turn off the flame. If the berries are a little tart, you may want to add a little maple syrup or rice syrup to make the sauce sweeter. To serve, place some sauce on a dish, then place the panna cotta on top of the sauce. Garnish with a few fresh berries and a nice fresh sprig of mint.

⟨◈⟩

CARAMEL RICE PUDDING

Preparation time: approximately 1 hour
Serves 2 to 4

Ingredients
- 1 cup organic carnaroli risotto rice
- 5 cups water
- 1 cup apple juice
- ⅛ teaspoon sea salt
- ¼ to ½ teaspoon organic olive oil
- 1 teaspoon vanilla extract
- 2 teaspoons fresh-squeezed orange juice

Preparation

- Heat the apple juice and water together in a pot.
- In a separate, heavier pot, warm the olive oil over a low flame. Add the risotto rice and sauté for 1 to 2 minutes.
- Ladle the warm liquid over the rice, then add the sea salt and stir. Allow the liquid to begin to absorb into the rice almost completely before adding any additional liquid.
- Continue to ladle the liquid into the rice and fold rice after each ladle of liquid is added. When you reach the desired consistency and texture, turn off the flame. If you want a creamier texture, use the entire amount of liquid. If you like the rice to have more texture, use less liquid.
- Add the fresh orange juice and blend with the rice.

Caramel Topping

- ½ cup brown rice syrup
- ½ cup barley malt
- 1 tablespoon water
- 2 to 3 drops umeboshi vinegar
- 1 teaspoon fresh-squeezed orange juice

Preparation

- Put the water, rice syrup, and barley malt in a saucepan.
- Add the umeboshi vinegar and mix well with a wooden spoon.
- Gently heat the mixture until it begins to boil around the edges of the pan.
- Turn the flame off. Add the fresh orange juice and mix well.

Serving Suggestions

- Use individual serving dishes. Ladle a little sauce on the bottom, followed by the rice.
- Pour additional sauce on top, and garnish with roasted pecans and fresh berries.
- You can also create a parfait by layering fresh berries between layers of pudding.

AMASAKE ALMOND KANTEN

Preparation time: 30 to 40 minutes to cook and approximately 1 hour to set

Serves 4 to 6

Ingredients

- 2 cups amasake
- 1 cup organic apple juice or cider
- 1 cup water
- 1 to 2 tablespoons barley malt
- 7 teaspoons agar-agar flakes (also known as kanten flakes)
- ½ cup toasted almonds, finely chopped or crushed

Preparation

- Pour all the liquid ingredients in a saucepan and begin to heat over a medium flame.
- As the liquid begins to warm, add the kanten flakes, then bring to a gentle boil.
- Lower the flame and continue to simmer until the agar dissolves completely.
- Add the barley malt and mix well.
- Ladle the liquid into individual serving dishes or into a flat Pyrex pan.
- Allow the liquid to cool for a few minutes, then top with the almonds.
- The kanten will begin to set as it cools. You may also allow it to cool in the refrigerator.

PUMPKIN CUSTARD

Preparation time: 1 to 2 hours
Serves 6

Ingredients

- 3¾ cups precooked pumpkin (two 15-ounce cans)
- 1½ cups water
- 1 to 1¼ cups brown rice syrup
- 1 teaspoon maple syrup
- 9 to 10 teaspoons agar-agar (kanten flakes)
- Optional: cinnamon and nutmeg to taste and/or my Grandmother's secret ingredient, a splash of good whiskey!

Preparation

- Mix the cooked pumpkin and water together and place in a pot.
- Begin to gently heat the mixture over a low flame.
- Add the kanten flakes and gently cook until the flakes are completely dissolved.
- Add rice syrup and stir to blend thoroughly with the pumpkin.

Serving ideas

- Garnish with chopped and toasted pecans and/or almond crème. Pumpkin custard also makes a great topping for couscous or teff cake, or a filling for pumpkin pie.

BAKED APPLES

Preparation time: 1½ hours
Serves 6 to 8

Ingredients

- 4 apples, washed and cored
- ¼ cup barley malt
- ½ cup rice syrup
- ¼ cup maple syrup
- ¼ teaspoon umeboshi vinegar
- ¼ teaspoon vanilla extract
- 1 cup chopped walnuts
- ½ to 1 cup raisins
- 1 teaspoon extra virgin olive oil
- 1 teaspoon walnut oil
- ⅓ cup apple juice

Cookware

- Deep baking dish
- 2 prep bowls

Preparation

- Preheat oven to 375 degrees.
- Measure the dry ingredients into a bowl and mix well.
- Measure the wet ingredients and pour into a separate bowl and mix well.
- Make a well in the middle of the dry ingredients, then pour the wet ingredients into the well and mix.
- Pour a tablespoon of olive oil and walnut oil into a dish and mix the oils.
- Dip your hands into the oil, then rub each apple with oil.
- Use the remaining oil to oil the baking pan.
- Pour the apple juice into the bottom of the pan and place the apples in the pan, stem side facing up.

- Fill each core with the sweet nut mixture.
- Bake uncovered for 1 hour or until soft.
- Serve in individual dessert dishes.

◦◈◦

STRAWBERRY-BLUEBERRY FRUIT CRUMBLE

This recipe uses strawberries and blueberries, but you can substitute 9 cups of other berries or fruits of your choice.

Preparation time: 1½ hours
Serves 12 to 14

Ingredients

For the fruit filling:
- 4½ cups fresh blueberries, washed and stems removed
- 4½ cups fresh strawberries, washed, stems removed, and quartered
- 6 tablespoons unbleached white flour
- ⅛ to ¼ cup apple juice
- 2 tablespoons rice syrup

For the topping:
- 1 cup whole-wheat pastry flour
- 1 cup cornmeal flour
- 1 cup rolled oats
- ½ cup oat bran flour (or rolled oats whizzed in the blender or food processor)
- ½ cup white flour
- ½ teaspoon sea salt
- ¼ cup barley malt

- ½ cup rice syrup
- ¼ cup maple syrup
- ⅓ cup walnut oil
- ⅓ cup extra virgin olive oil (if possible, choose an olive oil with a buttery finish)
- 1 teaspoon vanilla extract

Preparation

- Preheat oven to 375 degrees.
- Place washed and cut berries in a prep bowl and set aside.
- Use a dry measuring cup to measure the dry topping ingredients into a large prep bowl, and use a pastry blender or two forks to combine well.
- Place the dry topping bowl in the refrigerator while you are preparing the wet ingredients. Measure the wet ingredients into a prep bowl and blend with a spatula.
- Sprinkle the 6 tablespoons of unbleached white flour over the top of the berries. Blend the apple juice and rice syrup together, pour over the fruit, and mix to coat the fruit evenly.
- Oil the baking dish with about 1 teaspoon of olive oil or walnut oil, and add the berry mixture to the dish.
- Take the dry ingredients out of the refrigerator.
- Make a well in the middle of the dry ingredients and add the wet ingredients.
- Blend the wet and dry ingredients together with a pastry blender or two forks. The mixture should form a thick batter.
- Use a spatula to spread the mixture evenly on top of the fruit. Try not to touch the batter with your hands, as the heat and moisture in your hands will affect the texture of the crumble topping.
- Bake uncovered for 30 to 35 minutes.
- Serve in individual dessert dishes.

PIE CRUST

Preparation time: 20 to 30 minutes
Makes a 9-inch pie crust

Ingredients
- 1½ cups pastry flour
- 3 tablespoons olive oil, chilled for 2 hours to make a thicker consistency
- ½ teaspoon sea salt
- ⅓ to ½ cup chilled water. This may vary according to the type of flour you use and your environment.

Preparation
- Pour the olive oil into a flexible container and place in the freezer.
- Let chill until the color changes and it congeals but is still somewhat soft in consistency.
- In a prep bowl use a fork to mix the flour together with a pinch of sea salt.
- Remove the olive oil from the freezer and add it to the flour.
- Use 2 forks to mix together, forming small flaky crumbs.
- Place the crumbs in the refrigerator or freezer for about an hour.
- You can make pie crumbs in advance. Crumbs will keep in the freezer for several months.
- When you are ready to make your crust remove the crumbs from the freezer.
- Dissolve ¹⁄₁₆ teaspoon sea salt in cold water.
- Begin adding the water a little at a time. Use a fork to mix.
- Keep adding the water until the ingredients begin to hold together and you are able to form a ball. At this point use your hands to gently form the dough. Do not over-handle the dough as it interferes with the flakiness of the crust.

- Place the dough ball on a lightly floured pastry cloth and begin rolling out the dough.
- Again, the less you touch it the better.
- Place the dough in a lightly oiled pie pan.
- Use with your favorite pie filling.
- If you just want to make a crust bake at 350 degrees for 10 to 15 minutes or until it is golden brown.

⊸◇⊶

ALTERNATE PIE CRUST USING UNBLEACHED WHITE FLOUR

Preparation time: 20 minutes
Makes one 8-inch pie crust

Ingredients
- ¾ cup pastry four
- ¾ cup unbleached white flour
- ¼ cup olive or walnut oil
- ¼ to ½ teaspoon sea salt
- ¼ to ⅓ cup cold water

Preparation
- Prepare using the same method above. For a variation you can try using walnut oil in place of olive oil.

APPLE PIE

Recipe by my mother, Barbara Schwalm

Preparation time: 50 to 60 minutes
Makes one 9-inch pie

Ingredients
- 8 cups apples, washed and peeled, cut in halves, and then into 1½-inch-thick wedges
- 2 tablespoons pastry flour
- ¹⁄₁₆ to ⅛ teaspoon sea salt
- 1 teaspoon cinnamon
- ¹⁄₁₆ teaspoon nutmeg
- ¼ cup apple juice
- 2 tablespoons brown rice syrup (Suzanne's, Sweet Cloud, or Clearspring)
- 1 tablespoon olive oil

Preparation
- Preheat oven to 400 degrees.
- Begin to prepare the pie dough crumbs and place in the freezer while you prep the apples.
- Wash, peel, and cut the apples, then place in a bowl of water with a pinch of sea salt to prevent oxidation.
- At this point prepare your pie crust. Roll out the bottom crust and place in an oiled pie pan then continue to prep the apples.
- In a separate bowl, mix 2 tablespoons flour with the cinnamon and nutmeg.
- Remove the cut apples from the water. Place in a bowl.
- Add the dry ingredients, then use your hands to mix with the apples.
- Place the apple juice, brown rice syrup, and olive oil in a sauce pan.
- Gently heat for 1 to 2 minutes then pour over the apples.

- Mix well to coat the apples evenly.
- Place the apples in the pie shell.
- Roll out the top crust.
- Place the top crust over the apples, cut off any excess dough.
- Seal and flute the edges.
- Bake at 400 degrees for 30 to 40 minutes.

BLUEBERRY PIE

Recipe by Barbara Schwalm

Preparation time: 45 to 50 minutes
Makes one 9-inch pie

Ingredients
- 4 cups blueberries, washed
- ½ cup rice syrup (Suzanne's, Sweet Cloud, or Clearspring)
- ⅓ cup pastry flour
- 1/16 to ⅛ teaspoon sea salt
- ¼ teaspoon cinnamon
- 1 tablespoon olive oil
- Optional for more sweetness: 1 to 2 tablespoons maple syrup. If using maple syrup, use a little extra flour to coat the berries.

Preparation
- Preheat oven to 425 degrees.
- Wash the blueberries and place in a medium-size prep bowl.
- In a separate bowl mix the flour, sea salt, and cinnamon.
- Sprinkle the dry ingredients over the blueberries and use a spatula to blend.
- In a saucepan gently heat the rice syrup and olive oil.
- Pour over the berries. Use a spatula to coat the berries.

- Allow the berries to sit while you roll out the pie dough.
- Roll out the bottom crust and place in an oiled pie pan.
- Fill the pan with the berries.
- Roll out the top crust and place the top crust over the berries, cut off any excess dough.
- Seal and flute the edges.
- Bake at 425 degrees for 30 to 35 minutes.

⊰◇⊱

MINI APPLE PECAN TART

This is a great way to use up any remaining pie crust, or, if you like, make several smaller pies following the above preparation.

Preparation time: 60 minutes when making crust
Makes one 5-inch tart

Ingredients
- 1 to 1½ cups apples, peeled and sliced
- 1 teaspoon oat flour
- ⅛ teaspoon cinnamon
- ⅟₁₆ teaspoon nutmeg
- ⅟₁₆ teaspoon sea salt
- 2 teaspoons brown rice syrup
- ½ teaspoon olive oil
- ½ teaspoon vanilla
- ¼ cup chopped pecans

Preparation
- Measure the dry ingredients and place in a bowl.
- Use a fork to blend the ingredients.
- In another bowl mix the wet ingredients.
- Wash and peel 2 to 3 apples, then cut into ½-inch-thick slices.

- Pour the dry ingredients over the apples, mix to coat the apples.
- Pour most of the wet ingredients over the apples and mix well.
- Chop the pecans and place them in a prep bowl.
- Pour the remaining wet ingredients over the pecans.
- Roll out the pie dough and place in an oiled pie pan.
- Place the apples in the pie crust.
- Add the pecans evenly over the fruit.
- Bake at 350 degrees for 30 minutes.

BROWN RICE CRISPY TREATS

Although these are more of a kids' snack, everyone seems to love eating these sweet, crunchy treats. This quick snack will keep in a tin or glass container for 1 week.

Preparation time: 15 to 20 minutes
Serves 10

Ingredients
- ½ cup barley malt
- ¾ cup maple syrup
- 1 cup organic currants or raisins
- 1 cup organic peanut butter
- 5 cups organic crispy brown rice cereal

Preparation
- Mix barley malt, maple syrup, and peanut butter in a stainless steel pot. Gently heat on a low flame, then add the fruits and continue to mix. When bubbles appear around the edge of the pot, turn off the flame and add the crispy brown rice cereal. Mix well to blend all the ingredients. Place on an oiled tray to cool a bit, then roll into balls and serve.

Variations

- Substitute almond butter or tahini for the peanut butter. When using tahini, increase the amount of rice cereal by ¼ to ½ cup to maintain a pliable consistency. You can also add grain-sweetened chocolate chips for an extra-special treat.

⊷◈⊶

CHOCOLATE MAPLE WALNUT COOKIES

Preparation time: 25 to 30 minutes
Makes 20 cookies

Ingredients

- 2 cups pastry flour
- ⅛ teaspoon sea salt
- 3 tablespoons organic cocoa
- ½ teaspoon baking powder
- ½ cup chopped walnuts
- ½ teaspoon vanilla
- ½ teaspoon vinegar
- ¼ cup organic olive oil. Use an olive oil that has a buttery taste and no bitter aftertaste.
- 1 cup pure organic maple syrup

Preparation

- Preheat oven to 350 degrees.
- Combine all dry ingredients in a prep bowl.
- Use a fork to blend all dry ingredients.
- Make a hole in the middle of the dry ingredients.
- Add the wet ingredients. Use a spatula to blend all the ingredients.
- Use a large soup spoon to scoop the dough onto parchment-lined cookie sheets.

- Try to keep the spacing uniform, leaving a couple inches between each cookie.
- Bake at 350 degrees for 13 to 15 minutes, rotating the pans halfway through. The baking time depends on how you like your cookies; longer baking equals more crunch.

⊰◈⊱

VANILLA BUTTER PECAN COOKIES

Preparation time: 30 to 35 minutes
Makes 27 cookies

Ingredients
- ½ cup oat flour
- ½ cup corn meal flour
- 1 cup pastry flour
- ½ cup pecan meal or finely chopped pecans
- ¼ teaspoon sea salt
- 1/16 to 1/8 teaspoon nutmeg
- ¼ cup olive oil
- 3 teaspoons or 1 tablespoon vanilla
- 1 teaspoon barley malt
- 2 teaspoons brown rice syrup
- ⅓ cup organic pure maple syrup

Preparation
- Preheat oven to 350 degrees.
- Combine all dry ingredients in a prep bowl.
- Use a fork to blend all dry ingredients.
- Make a hole in the middle of the dry ingredients.
- Add the wet ingredients. Use a spatula to blend the ingredients.

- Use a large soup spoon to scoop the dough onto parchment-lined cookie sheets.
- Try to keep the spacing uniform, leaving a couple inches between each cookie.
- Bake at 350 degrees for 12 to 14 minutes, rotating the pans halfway through. The baking time depends on how you like your cookies, longer baking equals more crunch.

⌖

COOKIE DOUGH PIE CRUST

This is a great crust to use for fruit kanten or custard pies. I have also used it in fruit tarts, following the preparation of apples used in the apple pie recipe. When using this crust for a tart you may have to bake it a little longer.

Preparation time: 40 to 45 minutes
Makes one 10-inch pie crust and a little to spare

Ingredients
- 1 cup pastry flour
- 1 cup oat flour or blended rolled oats
- ½ cup pecans, blended
- ½ cup walnuts, blended
- ¼ teaspoon sea salt
- ½ to ¾ cup rice syrup
- 2 to 4 teaspoons maple syrup. The amount of syrup used may vary slightly depending on the oat flour texture.
- ⅓ cup olive oil
- 1 teaspoon vanilla extract

Preparation
- Preheat oven to 350 degrees.

- Mix dry ingredients together in a bowl.
- Whisk together the wet ingredients in a separate bowl.
- Make a well in the center of the dry ingredients, then add the liquid ingredients.
- Use a spatula to mix thoroughly.
- Press the dough into an oiled pan.
- A thinner metal pan works best for this recipe.
- Bake for 25 to 30 minutes.
- If you are using this crust for a custard, pudding, or kanten filling, allow it to cool before adding the filling.

JUICES

With their light freshness and sweet taste, fresh vegetable and fruit combination juices are perfect for satisfying a sweet craving. They are particularly beneficial to the liver, gallbladder, and pancreas. I like to include juices as a snack or as part of a meal when I create menus for my clients. Juicers: I like using a slow juicer model for vegetables and hard fruits, as they yield more juice than high-speed juicers do. A hand juicer works well for citrus.

All vegetable or vegetable-fruit juices are best when they are made fresh; try to consume them immediately after juicing. Here are some of my favorite combinations.

FRESH CARROT JUICE

Preparation time: 5 to 7 minutes
Serves 1

Ingredients
- 4 to 4½ large carrots, or enough to yield one 8-ounce serving of juice

Preparation
- Wash the carrots and cut into 1-inch pieces.
- Place the carrots in a juicer and juice according to your juicer manufacturer's instructions.
- Pour juice into a glass and enjoy immediately.

CARROT-APPLE JUICE

Preparation time: 10 minutes
Serves 2

Ingredients
- 4 large carrots or 1 cup fresh carrot juice
- 2 apples or 1 cup fresh apple juice
- A squeeze of fresh lemon, optional

Preparation
- Wash the carrots and cut into 1-inch-long pieces.
- Wash and core the apple, then cut into 1-inch pieces. Fill a dish with water and a few grains of sea salt and add the sliced apple to prevent it from oxidizing while preparing the juice.
- Place the carrots in a juicer and juice according to your juicer manufacturer's instructions, then do the same with the apple.
- If you are adding the fresh lemon, squeeze it directly into the juice and blend thoroughly with a wooden utensil.
- Pour juice into two glasses and enjoy immediately.

❖

CARROT-APPLE-ORANGE JUICE WITH A TWIST

Preparation time: 10 to 15 minutes
Serves 2

Ingredients
- 4 large carrots or 1 cup fresh carrot juice

- 1 apple or ½ cup fresh apple juice
- 1 large orange, or ½ cup orange juice
- 2 or 3 lemon wedges, sliced 1-inch thick

Preparation
- Wash the carrots and cut into 1-inch-long pieces.
- Wash and core the apple, then cut into 1-inch pieces. Fill a dish with water and a few grains of sea salt and add the sliced apple to prevent it from oxidizing during the juice preparation.
- Place the carrots in a juicer and juice according to your juicer manufacturer's instructions, then do the same with the apple.
- Peel the orange, cut the wedges in half, and place in the juicer.
- Squeeze the lemon directly into the juice, then use a wooden utensil to stir.
- Mix well, then pour the juice into two glasses and enjoy immediately.

⊶◇⊷

CARROT-CELERY JUICE

Preparation time: 10 minutes
Serves 1

Ingredients
- 3 to 4 large carrots
- 1 to 1½ stalks celery

Preparation
- Wash the carrots and cut into 1-inch-long pieces.
- Wash the celery and cut into ½-inch pieces.
- Place the carrots in a juicer and juice according to your juicer manufacturer's instructions, then do the same with the celery.
- Pour the juice into a glass and enjoy immediately.

LEAFY GREENS JUICES

These juices are mildly sweet and slightly sour. Combining these two flavors relaxes the liver and the gallbladder. These juices are particularly helpful for a spring detox. Of course, you can enjoy them anytime you want a little extra lift.

While these juices might seem tame, they have a very powerful effect on your body. Because of this, we recommend a smaller serving size of these juices. Each juice recipe makes one serving, or half a cup of juice. Since different varieties of leafy greens yield different amounts of juice, I find it helpful to juice directly into a liquid measuring cup, and have specified the ingredients as such. This way you will know exactly how much juice each ingredient yields.

SWEET DREAM OF GREEN (NAPA, GREEN APPLE, CABBAGE)

Preparation time: 10 minutes
Serves 1

Ingredients
- ⅛ cup napa cabbage juice, approximately 2 to 3 leaves napa
- ⅛ cup green head cabbage juice, approximately 1 cup cabbage
- ¼ cup green apple, approximately ½ green apple

Preparation
- Wash and cut the green cabbage into 1-inch pieces.
- Wash and cut the napa cabbage into 1-inch pieces.
- Wash and cut the apple in half. Core one of the halves and cut into 1-inch pieces. Refrigerate the other half in a sealed dish with a little water and a squeeze of fresh lemon juice.

- Place the green head cabbage in a juicer and juice according to your juicer manufacturer's instructions, then do the same with the napa, then the apple.
- Pour the juice in a glass and enjoy immediately.

⟨◈⟩

COOL GREEN CUCUMBER JUICE (NAPA, CUCUMBER, GREEN APPLE)

Preparation time: 10 minutes
Serves 1

Ingredients
- ¼ cup fresh napa cabbage juice, approximately 3 to 4 leaves napa
- ⅛ cup fresh green apple juice, approximately ½ green apple
- ⅛ cup cucumber juice, approximately ¼ to ⅓ cucumber

Preparation
- Wash and cut the leafy greens into 1-inch pieces.
- Wash and cut the cucumber into 1-inch pieces.
- Wash and cut the apple in half. Core and cut into 1-inch pieces. Store the other half in the refrigerator.
- Place the napa in a juicer and juice according to your juicer manufacturer's instructions, then do the same with the green apple and the cucumber.
- Pour the juice in a glass and consume immediately.

GREEN TWIST

Preparation time: 10 minutes
Serves 1

Ingredients

- ⅛ cup green cabbage juice
- ⅛ cup cucumber juice, ¼ to ⅓ of a cucumber
- ¼ cup bok choy juice, approximately 2 to 3 leaves bok choy
- A few sprigs of fresh parsley, approximately ⅛ cup parsley juice
- 1 wedge fresh lemon

Preparation

- Wash and cut the cabbage into 1-inch pieces.
- Wash and cut the bok choy into 1-inch pieces.
- Wash the parsley.
- Wash and cut the cucumber into 1-inch pieces.
- Place the green cabbage in a juicer and juice according to your juicer manufacturer's instructions, then do the same with the bok choy, then the parsley, then the cucumber.
- Squeeze fresh lemon directly into the greens juice and stir.
- Pour the juice into a glass and enjoy immediately.

10-DAY MENU PLANS

Here are two menus for twenty days of macrobiotic eating. If you are new to this way of eating, try one menu plan for just a few days and see how you feel. If you're feeling good, then try the whole ten days. If you love how you feel and want to continue, this menu is designed so that you can go right back to day one. Or you can try the other menu plan. Keep in mind that when making changes to your diet, you might feel a little strange for a few days until your body adjusts to this new way of eating.

ADDING VARIETY

When you repeat this menu plan every ten days, feel free to change the vegetables used in the recipes to include more variety in your diet. For example, bok choy, mustard greens, and collards are all excellent substitutes for kale. Also feel free to explore the other recipes included in this book.

GLUTEN-FREE OPTIONS

I have given some optional grain dishes and substitutions for those who follow a gluten-free diet. If you are gluten-free, substitute gluten-free tamari for any shoyu seasoning, and use brown rice miso instead of aged barley miso.

DAY 1

Breakfast
- Millet with Sweet Vegetables: onion and cauliflower
- Quick Steamed Greens with Fresh-Squeezed Lemon

Lunch
- Brown Rice with Pearled Barley or Brown Rice with Hato Mugi Barley (GF)
- Miso Soup: aged barley miso, wakame sea vegetable, dried shiitake mushrooms, daikon radishes, napa cabbage, finely chopped scallion garnish
- Sweet Vegetable Kinpira: carrots, onions, parsnips
- Blanched Vegetable Salad: bok choy, broccoli, red radishes, served with a few drops of brown rice vinegar

Mid-Afternoon Snack
- Fresh carrot juice or carrot-combination juice

Dinner
- Farro with White Beans and Kale or Peruvian Quinoa Salad with Black Beans (GF)
- Steamed Sweet Potatoes
- Fresh Arugula Salad with Tofu Cheese
- Poached Pear in Balsamic Barley Malt Reduction

DAY 2

Breakfast
- Soft Rice: use leftover rice from yesterday's lunch and season with umeboshi plum, garnish with a half sheet of toasted nori if desired
- Blanched Vegetable Salad: napa cabbage, broccoli, carrots

Lunch

- Leftover Farro or Quinoa
- Miso Soup: sweet-tasting brown rice miso, wakame sea vegetable, onions, turnips, turnip greens or other leafy greens, scallion garnish
- Leftover Kinpira from Day 1
- Quick Steamed Leafy Greens with Fresh Lemon

Mid-Afternoon Snack

- Leftover steamed sweet potato or leafy greens juice

Dinner

- Pan-fried Millet Croquettes: use the leftover millet from Day 1 breakfast, add a little cornmeal to thicken, form into patties and pan-fry on medium-low heat until cooked through.
- Vegan Tartar Sauce: mix together two tablespoons tahini, 2 tablespoons freshly-grated daikon radish, ¼ teaspoon shoyu, ½ teaspoon green nori flakes
- Savory French Lentils with Onions, Leeks, and Fresh Herbs
- Asian-Style Leafy Greens
- Quick Umeboshi Vinegar Pickles: use red cabbage
- Fresh Fruit Kanten

DAY 3

Breakfast

- Steel-Cut Oats with Maple Syrup
- Blanched Vegetable Salad: green cabbage, collards, carrots

Lunch

- Brown Rice with Sweet Brown Rice: garnish with lightly toasted chopped walnuts
- Miso Soup: aged barley miso, wakame sea vegetable, dried maitake mushroom, lotus root, onions, and watercress

- Leftover lentils from Day 2
- Quick Sautéed Vegetables: red onions, bok choy, and carrots

Mid-Afternoon Snack
- Fresh Carrot Juice or Carrot Combination Juice

Dinner
- Fried Noodles: use wheat or gluten-free noodles
- Nishime Vegetables: use sweet root and round vegetables like sweet potatoes, cabbage, onions
- Fresh Salad: hearts of romaine lettuce, cucumbers, pickled red onions, vinaigrette dressing
- Amasake kanten

DAY 4

Breakfast
- Leftover Steel-Cut Oats: top witha sprinkle of ume shiso powder
- Quick Steamed Greens

Lunch
- Vegetable Sushi: use the leftover brown rice and sweet rice from Day 3. Fill with fried tempeh special sauce, sauerkraut, blanched carrots, and cucumber; or cucumber, fresh shiso leaves, umeboshi paste.
- Susan's Special Sushi Sauce: mix together 1 part roasted tahini, 1 part umeboshi paste, and 1 part mustard. Add a small amount of wasabi powder if desired and thin to desired consistency with water.
- Cream of Broccoli Leek Soup: garnish with fresh herbs
- Leftover Nishime
- Quick Sautéed Leafy Greens: bok choy, baby bok choy, olive oil

Mid-Afternoon Snack
- Warm Apple Cider with Fresh Lemon

Dinner

- Couscous with Sautéed Vegetables or Quinoa with Sautéed Vegetables (GF)
- White Beans with Cabbage and Caraway
- Mediterranean-Style Cauliflower
- Fresh Arugula Salad with Tofu Cheese
- Red Grape Fresh Fruit Kanten

DAY 5

Breakfast

- Steamed Sourdough Bread or Gluten-Free Bread: with apple butter or other spread
- Blanched Vegetable Salad: cabbage, kale, and red radishes

Lunch

- Leftover Couscous or Quinoa
- Leftover White Beans and Cabbage
- Quick Steamed Greens: collard greens with fresh lemon
- Quick Umeboshi Vinegar Pickles

Mid-Afternoon Snack

- Fresh Carrot Juice or Carrot Combination Juice

Dinner

- Brown Rice with Wild Rice: top with toasted sunflower or sesame seeds
- Leftover Creamy Soup: with fresh herb garnish
- Sautéed Watercress with Asian seasoning
- Fresh Salad: hearts of romaine, iceberg lettuce, cucumber, radicchio, tofu cheese
- Leftover Grape Kanten

DAY 6

Breakfast

- Soft corn grits: make extra grits, pour into a Pyrex dish, and use on Day 7
- Blanched Vegetable Salad: cauliflower, collards, red radishes or daikon radishes

Lunch

- Fried Rice: use leftover rice
- Miso Soup: aged barley miso, wakame sea vegetable, turnips, turnip greens, chopped scallion garnish
- Arame with Onions, Carrots, Fresh Tofu
- Quick Steamed Greens with Fresh Lemon

Mid-Afternoon Snack

- Warm amasake, slightly diluted with water

Dinner

- Penne Pasta: sautéed broccoli rabe and sun-dried tomatoes
- White Beans with Sautéed Escarole
- Fresh Salad: arugula, pickled red radishes, steamed beets, toasted pine nuts
- Fresh Berries with Almond Crème

DAY 7

Breakfast

- Soft Rice
- Water-Sautéed Watercress

Lunch

- Pan-Fried what you made at breakfast yesterday
- Leftover White Beans

- Blanched Vegetable Salad: napa cabbage, string beans, summer squash, and carrots
- Quick Umeboshi Vinegar Pickles

Mid-Afternoon Snack
- Fresh Leafy Greens Juice

Dinner
- Brown Rice with Lentils and Sautéed Onions
- Miso Soup: aged barley miso, wakame sea vegetable, dried shiitake mushrooms, daikon radishes, and leafy greens
- Leftover Arame
- Quick Steamed Greens: with fresh lemon
- Baked Apple: with toasted walnuts and currents

DAY 8

Breakfast
- Rolled Oats with Umeboshi Plum
- Quick Steamed Greens

Lunch
- Fried Tempeh Wrap: spread an organic steamed wrap with tahini and top with sautéed onions and mushrooms, fried tempeh, and lettuce
- Red Bean Soup with Fresh Herb Garnish
- Sautéed Cauliflower
- Quick Umeboshi Vinegar Pickles: red cabbage

Mid-Afternoon Snack
- Fresh Carrot Juice or Carrot Combination Juice

Dinner
- Leftover Brown Rice with Lentils

- Miso Soup: sweet-tasting brown rice miso, wakame sea vegetable, onions, turnips, tofu cubes, leafy greens, scallion garnish
- Candied Sweet Potatoes
- Arugula Salad with Sautéed Mushrooms
- Leftover Baked Apple

DAY 9

Breakfast

- Sweet Couscous
- Blanched Vegetable Salad: green cabbage, kale, carrots

Lunch

- Brown Rice with Quinoa
- Leftover Candied Sweet Potatoes
- Quick Sautéed Leafy Greens

Mid-Afternoon Snack

- Fresh Leafy Greens Juice

Dinner

- Italian-Style Pasta with Cauliflower Sauce
- Red Bean Soup
- Quick Steamed Greens with Fresh Lemon
- Panna Cotta

DAY 10

Breakfast
- Soft Millet with Sweet Vegetables
- Water-Sautéed Watercress

Lunch
- Fried Udon Noodles
- Miso Soup: aged barley miso, wakame sea vegetable, onions, lotus root, celery greens, scallion garnish
- Roots and Greens
- Blanched Vegetable Salad: napa, broccoli, red radishes served with brown rice vinegar

Mid-Afternoon Snack
- warm diluted apple juice or cider with fresh lemon

Dinner
- Leftover Brown Rice with Quinoa
- Steamed Corn Tortillas, with sautéed onions and mushrooms
- Refried Beans
- Fried Parsnip Chips
- Vegan Caesar Salad with Avocado
- Fresh Seasonal Fruits or Steamed Fruit

Fun Family Menu Plan for Home or Away

Breakfast
- Sweet couscous
- Quick steamed leafy greens with fresh lemon squeezed on individual servings

Lunch
- Tofu Banh Mi
- Steamed sweet potatoes
- Sautéed leafy greens

Mid-Afternoon Snack
- Carrot-apple-orange juice or warm apple cider (or juice)

Dinner
- Brown rice with rye
- Condiment: ½ sheet of toasted nori and walnuts
- Miso soup with wakame, dried shiitake, turnip slices, and leafy greens; scallion garnish
- Stove-top baked beans
- Blanched vegetable salad with cabbage, baby bok choy, and carrots, emphasize the bok choy
- Make enough for the next morning or for lunches.
- Steamed pears

DAY 2

Breakfast
- Rolled or steel-cut oats
- Suggested sweet condiment; maple syrup and walnuts
- Suggested savory condiment: shiso powder or umeboshi plum
- Water sautéed leafy greens

Lunch
- Hummus sandwiches
- Mediterranean-style sautéed cauliflower
- Leftover blanched salad from the previous dinner.

Mid-Afternoon Snack
- Fresh orange slices

Dinner
- Vegetable fried rice using your leftover rice
- Spicy clear soup. Make enough for two days.
- Boiled daikon with sweet miso tahini sauce
- Bibb leaf salad
- Amasake lemon kanten

DAY 3

Breakfast
- Soft rice and leftover oatmeal with umeboshi plum
- Quick steamed leafy greens

Lunch
- Somen noodles served in the leftover clear soup
- Steamed sweet potatoes
- Sautéed leafy greens with tofu and ginger juice
- Fresh grapes

Mid-Afternoon Snack

- Warm soy milk and a nice bowl of nuts

Dinner

- Bulgur with red onions and green peas
- Chickpea stew
- Arugula, beet, and pear salad
- Leftover kanten

DAY 4

Breakfast

- Steamed bread with nut or seed butter topped with sauerkraut or kimchi
- For children who prefer something sweet, fruit jam
- Blanched salad: napa cabbage, broccoli, and red radishes

Lunch

- Leftover bulgur
- Leftover chickpeas
- Leftover sweet potatoes
- Quick steamed leafy greens with fresh lemon

Mid-Afternoon Snack

- Fresh carrot, apple, and orange juice

Dinner

- Brown rice with pearled barley
- Puréed sweet vegetable soup: pick one that suits the season. For variety, use a different vegetable combination the next time you make this soup.
- Sweet and sour red cabbage
- Fresh salad with lettuce, cucumber, red onions, and avocado
- Amasake kanten

DAY 5

Breakfast
- Millet with sweet vegetables
- Quick steamed leafy greens

Lunch
- Leftover brown rice and barley, ½ sheet of toasted nori, and ½ an umeboshi plum
- Leftover puréed sweet vegetable soup
- Leftover sweet and sour red cabbage
- Blanched vegetable salad: cauliflower, collards, and carrots
- Sauerkraut or kimchi

Mid-Afternoon Snack
- Steamed bread with nut or seed butter and fruit jam or a nice bowl of mixed nuts

Dinner
- Pasta with romanesco and fresh tomato
- White beans with leafy greens like escarole or baby kale
- Mushroom fennel and arugula salad
- Fresh grapes or steamed apples

DAY 6

Breakfast
- Leftover soft millet
- Quick steamed bok choy or baby bok choy

Lunch
- Steamed sourdough bread topped with leftover white beans and greens
- Minestrone miso soup (vegetable version)
- Blanched vegetable salad: cabbage, bok choy, and daikon
- Red cabbage or red beet pickles

Mid-Afternoon Snack

- Fresh leafy greens and green apple juice

Dinner

- Porcini farro risotto
- Sautéed broccoli rabe
- Fresh salad with hearts of romaine, cucumber, red onions, and tofu cheese
- Fresh grape kanten

DAY 7

Breakfast

- Rolled oats with maple syrup and pecans
- Blanched salad: napa cabbage, green cabbage, and red radishes

Lunch

- Leftover farro risotto
- Leftover minestrone soup
- Quick steamed leafy greens

Mid-Afternoon Snack

- Warm soy milk

Dinner

- Brown rice with quinoa, ½ sheet toasted nori, and ½ an umeboshi plum
- Cauliflower au gratin
- Mixed arugula and bitter leaf greens salad
- Leftover grape kanten

DAY 8

Breakfast
- Steamed sourdough bread with tahini and sauerkraut or fruit jam
- Blanched vegetable salad: broccoli, baby bok choy, and daikon

Lunch
- Leftover brown rice and quinoa
- Clear soup with enoki mushrooms and watercress
- Leftover cauliflower au gratin
- Quick steamed leafy greens with fresh lemon

Mid-Afternoon Snack
- Fresh carrot, apple, and orange juice

Dinner
- Pasta with zucchini, carrot, and onion sauce
- Green beans with kidney beans
- Mixed lettuce salad with sautéed red onions and sun-dried tomatoes
- Steamed apples

DAY 9

Breakfast
- Soft Polenta
- Condiment: shiso powder
- Quick steamed leafy greens

Lunch
- Brown rice with bulgur wheat and walnuts
- Leftover green beans and kidney beans
- Blanched vegetable salad: broccoli, napa cabbage, and carrots

Mid-Afternoon Snack

- Fresh leafy greens juice

Dinner

- Fried soba noodles
- Cool cucumber soup
- Plain boiled daikon
- Fresh salad with cucumber, red radish, red onion, and tofu cheese
- Fresh orange slices

DAY 10

Breakfast

- Oatmeal with maple syrup and mixed nuts
- Leftover blanched vegetable salad from lunch, or make a fresh one

Lunch

- Leftover brown rice with bulgur
- Condiment: umeboshi plum and ½ sheet toasted nori
- Leftover cucumber soup
- Leftover daikon

Mid-Afternoon Snack

- Fresh carrot and leafy greens juice

Dinner

- Burritos
- Fried polenta with shiso powder
- Steamed sweet potatoes
- Cabbage slaw
- Fresh berries and almond crème

FOOD GLOSSARY

The goal was to keep these recipes simple. Wherever possible, we have used familiar ingredients. We understand that any change in diet requires a rethinking of old food habits; having to learn about new food products presents an additional challenge. You will find, however, that many of the recipes do include unfamiliar ingredients, products that have such strong health benefits and are so delicious that it is helpful to become familiar with them and use them on a regular basis. The following is a list of some of those items:

Farro: Farro is an Italian wheat eaten by Roman soldiers for its strengthening and energizing qualities. It has a pleasant chewy and nutty taste and can be cooked with brown rice or in stews.

Millet: Millet is a small yellow cereal grain traditionally used in Asia, Africa, and Eastern Europe. It is usually cooked with sweet-tasting vegetables as a breakfast porridge, in soups, or as a dinner grain. It strengthens digestion, immunity, and vitality.

Mochi: Mochi refers to a Japanese rice cake made from pounded sweet or glutenous brown rice. It is pan-fried or simmered in soups and is used to strengthen vitality. It may also be shredded and melted on dishes like cheese.

Udon Noodles: These are Japanese wheat noodles. They have a nice light flavor and are free of chemical preservatives. Udon is usually served in a mild shoyu broth but may also be sautéed with vegetables.

Soba Noodles: These are Japanese buckwheat noodles usually made from wheat flour and about 40 percent buckwheat flour. They have a stronger flavor than udon and used to strengthen the intestines and vitality. Udon and soba are usually served in a mild shoyu broth but may also be sautéed with vegetables.

Amasake: This is a mildly sweet beverage made from fermented brown rice. It is energizing and strengthening and is often warmed before drinking. It is also used as a sweetener in desserts.

Un-yeasted Sourdough Bread: This is traditional style European bread made without baker's yeast. It is naturally leavened using a starter made from flour and water that gathers naturally occurring lactobacillus and yeast from the environment. It usually has a mild sour taste. The best quality sourdough breads are made from stone ground organic flours. We recommend steaming it in a steaming basket until it smells like fresh-baked bread and cooling before eating.

Miso: Miso is a remarkable food and is most beneficial when used as a seasoning for soup. Once you get into the habit of using it, you will wonder how you ever managed to cook without it. Miso is a paste made of fermented soybeans, grains, water, and sea salt. Miso is a valuable source of proteins, B vitamins, and minerals. Miso also contains enzymes that aid digestion and strengthen blood quality. Miso soup acts as an antidote to stress by relaxing the nervous system. There are many different types of miso from which to choose. The best kind for daily use is barley miso, also called mugi miso. The other is brown rice miso. Sweet white miso is lighter in taste and will add variety to your meals. Many more types of miso are available and it is fine to use other varieties occasionally; however, for optimum health use barley or brown rice miso on a regular basis. It is important to use only miso that is natural (traditionally made) and that has been aged for two years. Make sure to buy this product at a health food store.

Shoyu: Everyone has used soy sauce, either at home or at a Chinese restaurant. Shoyu is simply traditionally made, naturally fermented soy sauce. What distinguishes it from regular soy sauce is the fact that it is not chemically processed. It is made from soybeans, wheat, sea salt, and water. Use shoyu with a light touch. Do not drown your food in it! Shoyu should be used only for cooking, not at the table. Keep it in the kitchen. Overuse leads to intense thirst and a strong craving for sweets. A small amount of shoyu goes a long way.

Tofu: Tofu, sometimes called bean curd, is made from coagulating soy milk with nigari (magnesium chloride), and pressed into a cake form. It is best steamed, boiled, or made into tofu cheese by mixing with umeboshi vinegar. We use it often or daily in our cooking and meal preparation. It is important to find organic, non-GMO tofu.

Natto: Natto is a fermented soy product with a sticky texture and unusual odor. It's an acquired taste that makes you strong, brilliant, and beautiful. Natto strengthens digestion and vitality, cleans the skin, and clears the mind. It has unique qualities for strengthening the bones and for cleaning the cardiovascular system. Natto is eaten with rice, noodles, in miso soup or in sauces. It is often prepared by mixing it with chopped scallions, toasted nori, mustard, and shoyu and mixed together until sticky. It also combines well with sauerkraut.

Umeboshi Plums: Umeboshi is a salt-pickled plum that has both a sour and salty flavor. The red color of the plums comes from being pickled with shiso leaves. It aids digestion, strengthens blood quality, and is highly alkalizing. Umeboshi plum has the ability to neutralize the harmful effects caused by both animal foods and sugar. Umeboshi plum, or paste, is used to make sauces and dressings and is delicious on corn on the cob.

Umeboshi Vinegar: This vinegar is extracted from the Japanese ume plum. Sorry, I know we promised to keep it simple, but this vinegar is so delicious and so taste-enhancing that we thought you should become familiar with it. The use of umeboshi vinegar will help lighten your digestion.

Shiso Leaves/Shiso Powder: Another digestive aid, used as a condiment with grains or vegetables.

Brown Rice Vinegar: This is a mild vinegar made from brown rice. It has a mild, gentle taste and is very refreshing in light vegetable dishes and salads.

Sea Salt: Sea salt is evaporated from sea water and washed. We recommend unrefined, white sea salt. High-quality sea salt has a soft, mildly sweet taste before tasting salty. High-quality sea salt is as essential for health as it is for taste.

Sea Vegetables: Sea vegetables are the plants of the sea. Kombu and wakame are cooked in small quantities in soups or with vegetables or beans. Arame is a shredded leafy seaweed that has a mildly sweet taste. Hiziki is a stringy seaweed that has a strong and distinctive taste. Arame and hiziki are usually cooked with onions and carrots and other vegetables or tofu as a vegetable side dish. Toasted nori sheets are used as a garnish in grain dishes and soups and are used to make sushi rolls. Nori is probably the only plant source of vitamin B-12. All sea vegetables are packed with vitamins, minerals, and trace elements. They have shown to be protective against heavy metals, various pollutants, and radioactivity.

Kanten: Also called agar-agar, it's a sea vegetable gelatin that is used as a thickener for fruit and vegetable dishes.

Jinenjo/Yamaimo: Sometimes referred to as "Japanese mountain yam." A strong root vegetable that grows in the mountains, Jinenjo aids digestion and strengthens vitality. Jinenjo is usually grated raw, with toasted nori, chopped scallions, and shoyu. Typically served with a sauce over rice or noodles, or in miso soup, Jinenjo can also be cooked like a potato in soups or stews. Usually available in Asian markets.

Shiitake: Shiitake is a mushroom that grows on fallen oak logs. We recommend using sun-dried shiitake in soups and vegetable dishes. It helps reduce fat and cholesterol and promotes immunity and brain function.

Konyaku: Konyaku is a type of potato starch that is made into a rubbery slab and often mixed with kombu powder. It is cooked in miso or shoyu soup or in vegetable stews. The Japanese believe that it improves digestive health and may help with weight loss.

Kuzu: Kuzu is a root starch processed from the mountain-grown kuzu root in Japan. Wild kuzu is considered best. It is used as a thickener for soups, vegetable dishes, and desserts. It strengthens digestion, vitality, and immunity and is often used as a tonic drink for colds and fatigue.

We hope that you found this section helpful and that you enjoy using these ingredients. Once you become familiar with the ingredients, you will find it easy to improvise and come up with variations of your own. Good health is built on the choices we make daily. Don't forget, every day, at every meal, make sure to have both a grain and a separate vegetable dish. Take one or two small bowls of vegetable soup daily. You will be amazed at how much better you will feel.

Acknowledgments

Thanks to our literary agent and friend Danny Astin of March Brown for his passionate support, creativity, and encouragement to do this book.

This book would not be possible without Janie Armfield, who introduced us to her son Claiborne, our publisher.

To Mona Schwartz, our friend and mentor, who encouraged us to develop macrobiotics in a more broad, embracing, and spiritual direction.

We deeply appreciate the support and acknowledgment from T. Colin Campbell and Neal Barnard. These men are inspirations and giants in Science and Medicine and are dedicated to true and lasting health.

To all of our macrobiotic friends and teaching associates, who are too numerous to mention by name.

To many of the people who have been part of our school, Strengthening Health Institute (SHI), including Phillip Abraham, Deborah Albanese, Elizabeth & Misha Balabayev, Bill Bergman, Lear Blitzstein, Robert & Katherine Burdick, Gina Compello, Sheri Demaris, Lori Eckstein, Lee & Irv Fischer, Doug FitzSimons, Susan Harris, Jeremy & Susan Higa, Ralph Jenkins, Warren Kramer, Carlotta Lala, Hyang-Mi Lee, Faina Markov, Don & Mary Marti, Mary McCabe, Michelle Nemer, Natasha Novoselova, Mike & Marlene Pendley, Stephen Prudente, Patrick Riley, Carole & Jack Schultz, Therese Schultz, Tom Spring, Anna Steinberg, Carol Tamburino, and Richard Epstein & Luanne Thomas.

For this book we are indebted to our assistant at SHI Teron Meyers.
—Denny and Susan Waxman

This book is an account of my journey toward and discovery of the process of creating and maintaining lasting health, vitality, and longevity. In a deep sense everyone I have encountered in my life is part of this journey.

The journey begins with my parents Anna and Herman Waxman and brother Howard. It continues with our children and their spouses Nathan and Lindsay, Joe, Nora, Naomi and James, Alisa, Madeline and Ivan, Amy and Ben, Zoe, Andrew and Kelly, Natasha and Sam.

To our grandchildren who are bright shining lights.

To Jared, Barbara, Julie, and Lauren, who have become an important part of my life and family.

I am also indebted to my many teachers and mentors, too numerous to mention fully, who guided and helped mold me on this journey. I especially thank Rod and Peggy House, George and Lima Ohsawa, Shizuko Yamamoto and Michelle Matsuda, and my spiritual parents Michio and Aveline Kushi and Takashi Yoshikawa.

To my wife Susan, who I have shared my life and this book with. Susan cooks like an angel and I am happy you will be able to experience some of her mastery and amazing food through the recipes and insights she shared in this book.

A special thanks to longtime friends Bill Hebden, who guided and nudged me toward the title of this book, and to Sam De Phillippo for his encouragement and guidance.

The many people whose support, guidance, and editing helped create my earlier books, especially Ruth Ann Dubb and Ellen Brodkey.

To my writing assistants Stephanie Bartusis and especially to Jinsey Cox, whose patience, hard work, and endless juggling and reorganizing of many details made this book possible.

—Denny Waxman

I would like to thank my parents Barbara and Jared Schwalm for giving me life, love, and nurturance to help me grow into the woman I am today. You raised me well, taught me the importance of respect and kindness for others, the value of family, and to always try my best.

To all my family, Julie and Loren, Howard and Janet you are the greatest. Thank you to all our children, their spouses, partners, and our grandchildren. I feel grateful and blessed to have you all in our life.

To our kitties Ichi and Cleo for your purrs and affection. You light up our life and lovingly pest us each day.

To my husband, my partner, and a great teacher Denny, for sharing your life and our common dream. I am glad we met and glad we are together.

We make a great team!

To all my teachers, past, present, and future, thank you for your wisdom, guidance, encouragement, and mostly for believing in me.

A special thank you to Michio Kushi and Takashi Yoshikawa, whose encouragement and fatherly advice reminded me that my life had special meaning. Thank you to Ralph for taking me to my first lecture on macrobiotics and for always being there for me. Thank you to my dear friends and mentors Ellen Brodkey and Mona Schwartz, who have helped me to develop as a teacher and grow as a woman.

To my writing assistant Kirin McElwain and Kateri Likourdis for her beautiful photography.

Thank you to all my friends. I appreciate all the good times together, the laughter and tears, and most of all the dream of a happy, healthy world. A special thanks to those of you who tested my recipes on your families.

—Susan Waxman

Index

About the Authors

Susan Waxman, co-author and creator of the delicious recipes found in *The Complete Macrobiotic Diet*, is world-renowned for her culinary creations, which merge health with taste. Using her teachings and years of cooking experience, she is pleased to present an array of new healthy recipes in this book.

Denny Waxman, co-author of *The Complete Macrobiotic Diet*, is an internationally-renowned teacher, counselor, and writer in the fields of health, natural healing, and macrobiotics. Denny is also the founder of the Essene Natural Food Store. Denny runs The Strengthening Health Institute in Philadelphia with his wife, Susan Waxman.